W9-DCD-459

The CLINICAL
NURSE SPECIALIST
HANDBOOK

Second Edition

Edited by

Patti Rager Zuzelo, EdD, RN, MSN, ACNS-BC

Professor of Nursing and CNS Track Director
School of Nursing and Health Sciences
La Salle University
Philadelphia, Pennsylvania

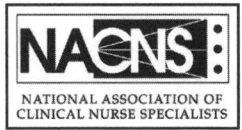

NATIONAL ASSOCIATION OF
CLINICAL NURSE SPECIALISTS

JONES AND BARTLETT PUBLISHERS
Sudbury, Massachusetts
BOSTON   TORONTO   LONDON   SINGAPORE

World Headquarters
Jones and Bartlett Publishers
40 Tall Pine Drive
Sudbury, MA 01776
978-443-5000
info@jbpub.com
www.jbpub.com

Jones and Bartlett Publishers
Canada
6339 Ormindale Way
Mississauga, Ontario L5V 1J2
Canada

Jones and Bartlett Publishers
International
Barb House, Barb Mews
London W6 7PA
United Kingdom

Jones and Bartlett's books and products are available through most bookstores and online booksellers. To contact Jones and Bartlett Publishers directly, call 800-832-0034, fax 978-443-8000, or visit our website, www.jbpub.com.

Substantial discounts on bulk quantities of Jones and Bartlett's publications are available to corporations, professional associations, and other qualified organizations. For details and specific discount information, contact the special sales department at Jones and Bartlett via the above contact information or send an email to specialsales@jbpub.com.

The authors, editor, and publisher have made every effort to provide accurate information. However, they are not responsible for errors, omissions, or for any outcomes related to the use of the contents of this book and take no responsibility for the use of the products and procedures described. Treatments and side effects described in this book may not be applicable to all people; likewise, some people may require a dose or experience a side effect that is not described herein. Drugs and medical devices are discussed that may have limited availability controlled by the Food and Drug Administration (FDA) for use only in a research study or clinical trial. Research, clinical practice, and government regulations often change the accepted standard in this field. When consideration is being given to use of any drug in the clinical setting, the health care provider or reader is responsible for determining FDA status of the drug, reading the package insert, and reviewing prescribing information for the most up-to-date recommendations on dose, precautions, and contraindications, and determining the appropriate usage for the product. This is especially important in the case of drugs that are new or seldom used.

Production Credits

Publisher: Kevin Sullivan
Acquisitions Editor: Emily Ekle
Acquisitions Editor: Amy Sibley
Associate Editor: Patricia Donnelly
Editorial Assistant: Rachel Shuster
Senior Production Editor: Carolyn F. Rogers
Marketing Manager: Rebecca Wasley
V.P., Manufacturing and Inventory Control: Therese Connell
Composition: Auburn Associates, Inc.
Cover Design: Scott Moden
Cover Image: © Jonathan Ross/Dreamstime.com
Printing and Binding: Malloy, Inc.
Cover Printing: Malloy, Inc.

Library of Congress Cataloging-in-Publication Data

The clinical nurse specialist handbook / [edited by] Patti Rager Zuzelo. — 2nd ed.
    p. ; cm.
  Includes bibliographical references and index.
  ISBN-13: 978-0-7637-6114-1 (pbk.)
  ISBN-10: 0-7637-6114-1 (pbk.)
  1. Nurse practitioners—Handbooks, manuals, etc. 2. Nursing—Handbooks, manuals, etc. I. Zuzelo, Patti Rager.
  [DNLM: 1. Nurse Clinicians. 2. Nurse's Role. 3. Nursing Care. WY 128 C64015 2010]
  RT82.8.C5554 2010
  610.7306′92—dc22
                                                                    2009016097
6048
Printed in the United States of America
13 12 11 10 09   10 9 8 7 6 5 4 3 2 1

Contents

Chapter 8:   **Influencing Outcomes:**
Improving Quality at the Point of Care   241

Patti Rager Zuzelo, EdD, RN, MSN, ACNS-BC

Chapter 9:   **Patient Safety: Preventing Unintended Consequences and**
Reducing Errors   291

Patti Rager Zuzelo, EdD, RN, MSN, ACNS-BC

Chapter 10:   **The Basics of Nursing Business   333**

Patti Rager Zuzelo, EdD, MSN, RN, ACNS-BC
Mary Beth Kingston, RN, MSN, NEA-BC

Preface

This second edition of *The Clinical Nurse Specialist Handbook* has been written during a period of time markedly different from that of the first edition. It is rather extraordinary to reflect on the changes that have occurred within the past three years. A new president of the United States has been elected and inaugurated. With this change in leadership comes potential opportunities for dramatic, broad, sweeping revisions in the healthcare system. These changes will certainly affect advanced practice registered nurses (APRNs), including clinical nurse specialists, and will perhaps pave the way for CNSs to influence care processes and outcomes in new ways that are easily recognized, highly visible, and very valued.

Other significant events include finalization of the Consensus Model for APRN Regulation: Licensure, Accreditation, Certification & Education (LACE). The National Association of Clinical Nurse Specialists (NACNS) has endorsed this model after much review. In August 2008, the National Council of State Boards of Nursing (NCSBN) adopted the APRN Model Act/Rules and Regulations. Each state board will make decisions about how to respond to the Joint Dialogue recommendations and APRN regulations; however, potential implications are significant to practice and to education. It is certainly noteworthy that the Consensus Model supports the CNS as an APRN role.

The introduction of clinical nurse leader (CNL) as a master's-prepared generalist, not an APRN, has contributed possibilities and added confusion to healthcare organization dynamics. Administrators are uncertain as to the difference between a CNL with many years of specialty experience and a CNS. It is clear that the CNS is a recognized *advanced* practice role and the CNL role is not; however, articulating differences in real-world practice is challenging. The doctorate in nursing practice (DNP) degree or, the less common, doctorate in research and nursing practice (DRNP) degree, as possible requirements for APRN entry have led to optimism, confusion, and frustration within and between national nursing organizations, organized medicine, universities, healthcare systems, and other stakeholders. There is DNP push-back in the published literature and, as of this point in time, there is no formal commitment by major nursing organizations to DNP as the required level-of-entry degree for advanced practice nursing by the American Association of Colleges of Nursing (AACN) proposed 2015 deadline. Only time will reveal how this degree will alter the nursing practice landscape.

Changes in the Centers for Medicare and Medicaid Services (CMS) reimbursement criteria, particularly nonreimbursement for select hospital-acquired conditions (HACs) that were not present on admission to the hospital, have created threats and opportunities for CNSs. Given their systems expertise, CNSs are in a good position to influence processes and affect outcomes that include HACs. Simultaneously, the sometimes invisible CNS efforts may be too bundled with routine nursing expenditures creating increased CNS vulnerability during times of harsh economic realities and budget cutbacks. CNSs must share their efforts and take credit for the economic benefits reaped by the healthcare systems that employ them. There are also entrepreneurial possibilities available to CNSs that elect to consult for healthcare enterprises having difficulty with establishing and improving systems of care delivery with high numbers of HCA events.

I continue to fervently believe in the work of the National Association of Clinical Nurse Specialists (NACNS). The NACNS conceptualization of CNS practice (NACNS, 2004) has honed CNS practice conceptualization and has led to improved descriptions of exactly what CNSs do to improve processes and outcomes specific to nurses, patients, and systems (Figure P-1).

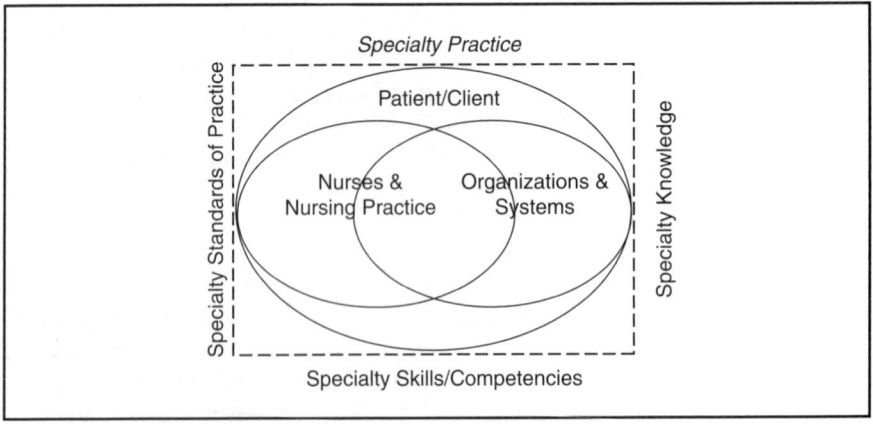

Figure P-1   CNS practice conceptualized as core competencies in three interacting spheres actualized in specialty practice, and guided by specialty knowledge and specialty standards.

Source: © 2004 National Association of Clinical Nurse Specialists. Reprinted with permission.

Threats and opportunities to CNS practice appear limitless and, at times, contribute to stress and role confusion. It is my sincere hope that this book will provide tools and perspectives that may be useful as CNSs continue in established practices or begin the advanced practice journey. For those of you new to CNS practice: count on an interesting, never boring, never static, career. Use the supports available to you through NACNS, other national nursing organizations, and your nursing specialty organizations. Become involved, active, engaged, and determined. The healthcare system needs many more CNSs! I wish you the very best and am hopeful that our paths will cross as you move along in your CNS career trajectory.

The very best,
Patti Zuzelo

Reference

National Association of Clinical Nurse Specialists. (2004). *Statement on clinical nurse specialist practice and education* (2nd ed.). Harrisburg, PA: Author.

Contributors

Janice M. Beitz, PhD, RN, ACNS-BC, CNOR, CWOCN, CRNP
Professor
Director of Nursing Certificate and Distributive Learning Programs
WOCNEP Co-Director
School of Nursing and Health Sciences
La Salle University
Philadelphia, Pennsylvania

Mary Beth Kingston, MSN, RN, NEA-BC
Chief Nurse Executive
Albert Einstein Healthcare Network
Philadelphia, Pennsylvania

Zane Robinson Wolf, PhD, RN, FAAN
Dean and Professor
School of Nursing and Health Sciences
La Salle University
Philadelphia, Pennsylvania

Exemplar Contributors

Geralyn Altmiller, EdD, MSN, APRN
Assistant Professor
School of Nursing and Health Sciences
La Salle University
Philadelphia, Pennsylvania

Carolyn Jacobson, MSN, RN, CCRN
Staff Nurse, Surgical/Trauma Unit
Albert Einstein Medical Center
Philadelphia, Pennsylvania

Jill Stunkard, MSN, RN, CCRN, CNAA-BC
Clinical Director, Institute for Heart and Vascular Health
Albert Einstein Medical Center
Philadelphia, Pennsylvania

Steven Szablewski, BSN, RN, PCCN
Staff Nurse
Albert Einstein Medical Center
Philadelphia, Pennsylvania

CHAPTER ONE

Strategic Career Planning: Professional and Personal Development

Patti Rager Zuzelo, EdD, MSN, RN, ACNS-BC

Clinical nurse specialists (CNSs) are educationally prepared for a variety of career paths. Diverse opportunities are a large part of the appeal of this advanced practice registered nursing role. These opportunities also contribute to the challenges of the role. Many CNSs indicate that there are "not enough hours in the day" or express concerns that juggling competing demands leaves little time for self-care activities.

This chapter focuses on both professional and personal development. Professional development is considered from two vantage points: clinician expertise and professional or scholarly development. Personal development is approached as a requisite component of professional practice, in other words, a call for CNSs to attend to the self and to role model the health-promoting behaviors that CNSs advocate as important for clients, colleagues, and family members.

Reflection

Prior to beginning the activities of this chapter, it is important to reflect on individual accomplishments, learning needs, challenges, expectations, talents, and experiences. Honest appraisal requires self-knowledge. For example, if a CNS is searching for an advanced practice nursing position, it is important to consider the flexibility inherent in the CNS role and to evaluate the aspects that are most appealing and least appealing.

If routine is not appealing and working on diverse projects, taking risks, and addressing systems issues that require rapid change sounds intriguing, a CNS role with a focus on short-term projects, data-driven systems changes, or Six Sigma organizations may be an ideal match. On the other hand, if careful attention to detail, consistency, and an interest in patient education, staff development, and continuous quality improvement activities are of interest, a position as a unit or program-based CNS with shared responsibilities for outcomes management or staff education may be very suitable. For the CNS who feels accomplishment when "watching things grow" and appreciates opportunities to tend to the needs of developing nurses when facilitating professional growth, a position that includes teaching, evidence-based practice, or shared governance activities might be ideal.

Reflecting on the personal self is also a valuable activity and may be useful to do in partnership with professional reflection activities. Professional nurses, including CNSs, frequently advise patients, families, and colleagues to take time out for self-care. CNSs recognize that there is value in leisure, exercise, and physical fitness and that these behaviors are critical for long-term physical and mental health. Yet, many nurses have poor diets with resulting overweight or obesity (Miller, Alpert, & Cross, 2008), smoke, do not exercise, and internalize stress. It is concerning to note that nurses smoke at a rate of approximately 18% in the United States and do experience smoking-related guilt (Bialous, Sarna, Wewers, Froelicher, & Danao, 2004). This statistic is particularly sobering given nurses' role in guiding the public in health promotion and disease prevention strategies.

In addition, nurses recognize that healthy relationships require effort and engagement. However, CNSs may neglect to set aside deliberate time for nurturing relationships that are important to them. Despite advising others to attend to these needs, many times nurses are neglectful of their own personal priorities.

For example, it is not uncommon for CNSs to become involved in local, regional, and, in some cases, national organizations. These activities are rewarding but time consuming. The needs can be great, and nurses are accustomed to taking obligations very seriously. As a result, CNSs may experience personal burnout as they juggle family, clinical work, scholarship, and organizational activities.

It is imperative for CNSs to carefully determine the time that is available for professional work within the context of the priorities of particular periods in life while consciously deciding to recognize and celebrate the events of life. "Living each moment" or "Live life to the fullest" are phrases that may be rather overdone, but they are important to keep in mind during CNS practice.

Reflective Practice

Reflective practice is advocated in the United Kingdom (UK) as a learning process that encourages self-evaluation with subsequent professional development planning. UK practitioners are expected to meet a continuing professional development (CPD) standard, and reflection is a strategy that facilitates meeting this standard for reregistration (Driscoll & Teh, 2001). Much of the work describing reflective practice as a strategy for facilitating continued, lifelong learning and promoting professional competence has been published in UK journals.

In the United States, the term *reflective practice* is increasingly visible in the nursing literature, particularly in education-focused publications. Reflective activities are popular in baccalaureate and graduate nursing programs because the activities are valued as self-discerning. Students learn to question their practice and analyze situations to consider alternative behaviors and develop a plan for future action. Journal-keeping is one particular learning strategy that encourages self-reflection and promotes critical analysis. This useful tool is now available as a feature on many popular distance or Web-based teaching platforms.

Reflection is a useful strategy for CNSs. It is important to differentiate between thinking about daily work versus reflecting on an experience, which requires intentionality and skill (Driscoll & Teh, 2001). Reflective practice demands the ability to analyze situations and make judgments specific to the effectiveness of situational interventions and the quality of outcomes.

Typically, nurses are inclined to keep care practices the same, as there is comfort in routine. Long-established rituals provide security. Reflection encourages CNSs to reveal and consider behaviors, feelings, and ideas that would not ordinarily be examined. For this reason, reflection facilitates professional development. It is also a time-consuming activity that cannot be forced.

Benefits to reflective practice include helping practitioners make sense of challenging and complicated practice, reminding practitioners that there is no end to learning, enhancing traditional forms of knowledge required for nursing practice, and supporting nurses by offering formal opportunities to converse with peers about practice (Driscoll & Teh, 2001). Driscoll and Teh also identified downsides to reflective practice, noting that finding the time, being less satisfied with the status quo, being labeled as a troublemaker, and having more questions than answers are a few of the challenges associated with the deliberate examination of practice.

The Clinical Placement Support Unit (CPSU) of the Health and Community Care (HCC) division of the University of Central England (UCE) offers Web-based information summarizing a variety of models of reflection (CPSU, 2005). The models include Gibbs's model of reflection, Johns's model of reflection, Kolb's Learning Cycle, and Atkins (1995) and Murphy's model of reflection.

In general, the models encourage practitioners to consider a situation in clinical practice. This situation may be positive or negative, but should be important in some sense. After describing the event in writing, practitioners are encouraged to dissect the experience. Practitioners reflect on the emotions, thoughts, and beliefs underlying the experience. They consider the motivation underlying their action choices and think about the consequences of their behaviors. The reflective practitioner is urged to consider alternatives and to challenge assumptions. The final step in the process typically relates to identifying the learning that has occurred and applying this new knowledge in future situations.

Reflective activity is viewed as an opportunity to deliberately think about practice events; evaluate choices, reactions, and behaviors; consider alternatives; develop plans for improvement or identify learning needs; and to follow this action plan in new or similar situations. Johns (2004) warned that stage models of reflection may support the belief that reflection occurs in a sequential fashion moving from step to step. He cautioned that although this approach may be helpful for practitioners new to reflection, in general, reflective practice does not follow a rote stage model.

Johns (2004) offered a model for structured reflection (MSR) that has the potential to guide CNSs to assess the extensiveness of the reflection that is needed for experiential learning (Table 1-1). The reflective cues are logically ordered and are offered as triggers for thought. Each cue is connected to a way of knowing.

Reflective practice is described as holistic practice because it is focused on understanding the significance and meaning of the whole experience (Johns, 2004). Johns recognized layers of reflection that progress from a reflection on experience to mindful practice, which are in juxtaposition with moving from "doing reflection" to "reflection as a way of being" (p. 2).

Reflection is defined as

being mindful of self, either within or after experience, as if [there is] a window through which the practitioner can view and focus self within the context of a particular experience, in order to confront, understand and move toward resolving contradiction between one's vision and actual practice. (Johns, 2004, p. 3)

Reflective practice is increasingly popular in nursing and may provide a means for connecting the art and science of nursing within a caring context. Reflective practice is an active process and supports the development of practical wisdom (Johns, 2004).

CNSs should consider that the tension that exists between vision and current reality are learning opportunities (Johns, 2004). This tension may be uncomfortable, but it offers the opportunity to face and solve the problems creating the anxiety state. Johns suggested that reflection is a learning process that may develop tacit knowledge. One vehicle for reflection is journaling, whereas others include poetry writing, sharing stories, or creating a portfolio.

Professional Portfolio Basics

The act of creating a professional portfolio provides an opportunity to reflect on experiences and establish insights that may inform future decisions specific to practice, education, and professional activities. Portfolio creation compels CNSs to carefully consider a variety of potential items for inclusion and, in doing so, to contemplate the relative worth of each activity and the contribution of the parts related to the "whole" of the individual's practice. CNSs also evaluate the various portfolio components and identify strengths, challenges, and gaps. The professional portfolio provides a context to examine subsets of CNS practice with a focus on self-improvement and self-development. Just as with reflective practice, portfolio development requires self-awareness.

The professional portfolio has become an increasingly popular modality for reflecting on professional development, self-evaluation, creativity, and critical thinking. Portfolios are also useful to track expertise acquisition and to demonstrate competency. McColgan (2008) conducted a literature review to explore current thinking on portfolio building and registered nurses. The literature review revealed four themes: (1) portfolio use as an assessment method for validating competence; (2) portfolio use as a work-based reflective evaluation tool; (3) the relationship between portfolio

Table 1-1   REFLECTIVE CUES—MODEL FOR STRUCTURED REFLECTION

Reflective Cue	Way of Knowing
• Bring the mind home	
• Focus on a description of an experience that seems significant in some way	Aesthetics
• What particular issues seem significant to pay attention to?	Aesthetics
• How were others feeling and what made them feel that way?	Aesthetics
• How was I feeling and what made me feel that way?	Personal
• What was I trying to achieve and did I respond effectively?	Aesthetics
• What were the consequences of my actions on the patient, others, and myself?	Aesthetics
• What factors influenced the way I was feeling, thinking, or responding?	Personal
• What knowledge did or might have informed me?	Empirics
• To what extent did I act for the best and in tune with my values?	Ethics
• How does this situation connect with previous experiences?	Reflexivity
• How might I respond more effectively given this situation again?	Reflexivity
• What would be the consequences of alternative actions for the patient, others, and myself?	Reflexivity
• How do I NOW feel about this experience?	Reflexivity
• Am I more able to support myself and others better as a consequence?	Reflexivity
• Am I more able to realize desirable practice monitored using appropriate frameworks such as framing perspectives, Carper's fundamental ways of knowing, and other maps?	Reflexivity

Source: © Reprinted with permission from Johns, C. (2004). *Becoming a reflective practitioner* (2nd ed.). Oxford: Blackwell Publishing.

building and lifelong learning; and (4) portfolio building as a strategy to motivate and develop nurses.

McColgan (2008) noted that while there is much theoretical discussion concerning the benefits and influences of the portfolio as a vehicle for promoting professional development, there is a lack of empirical evidence supporting these claims. The reflective activities associated with portfolio development intuitively seem connected to self-discovery, self-evaluation, and professional and personal growth; however, evidence-based practice does not prioritize intuition as an effective way of knowing (Duffy, 2007).

Differentiating Portfolios and Profiles

It is important to understand the basic premise of a professional portfolio and to appreciate the differences between a portfolio and a profile. The terms *portfolio* and *profile* are often used interchangeably but they are not the same product. A professional portfolio provides a record of professional development. It is a collection of evidence of products and processes documenting professional development and learning (McMullan et al., 2003). A profile is derived from the personal portfolio. Materials selected for the profile vary according to the audience and the purpose (Jasper, 1995). For example, a CNS applying for advanced practice role recertification might select a photocopy of a published research study, continuing education certificates, and a transcript of a recent pharmacology course from the portfolio to include in a profile that is being submitted with a recertification application.

Portfolios in some form are often encouraged or required in undergraduate or graduate education programs (Alexander, Craft, Baldwin, Beers, & McDaniel, 2002; Joyce, 2005). They also offer opportunities for advanced practice nurses (APNs) seeking credentialing when certification examinations in unique clinical specialty areas are unavailable. The UK requires a professional portfolio to demonstrate continued competency and current professional knowledge. Continued professional development (CPD) is required and is included in the portfolio (Bowers & Jinks, 2004). The portfolio is registered with the UK Central Council and addresses the need for some type of assurance that professional development has continued after basic training is complete.

Professional nurses practicing in Ontario must also meet standards of mandatory portfolio management as part of its quality assurance program (College of Nurses of Ontario, 2008). Recently, the National Council of State Boards of Nursing (NCSBN) considered a proposal for nurses to initiate and maintain a professional profile referred to as the "Continued Competency Accountability Profile (CCAP)" (Meister, Heath, Andrews, & Tingen, 2002). At this point in time, the CCAP is on hold, but NCSBN continues to work on developing methods for ensuring nurse competency to protect the public. Some individual states are testing models for competency that require professional portfolios.

This background information is important for a few reasons. Competency is a hot issue that is likely to increase in its intensity as a focal point of professional practice regulation. Sheets (1998) asserted that meeting basic licensure requirements and subsequently paying a license renewal fee does not warrant public trust in competence.

The variability across states regarding licensure and practice regulations is also concerning and confusing to the public. Some states do not require continuing education, and some do not have CNS title protection with its associated certification requirements and educational mandates. The Pew Report (1998) raised these same concerns related to the state of self-regulation and the need to protect the public.

NCSBN defines competence as "the application of knowledge and the interpersonal, decision-making, and psychomotor skills expected for the nurse's practice role, within the context of public health, welfare, and safety" (2005, p. 1). CNSs must give serious thought to strategies for demonstrating competence, particularly given the breadth and depth of the APN scope of practice. Portfolios may facilitate this process by encouraging reflection, strategizing, and documentation.

Contextualizing the Professional Portfolio

Keep in mind that a portfolio provides a record of growth and change. Think of a portfolio as an evidentiary collection of products and processes (McMullan et al., 2003). The idea of a professional portfolio originated with professionals who were expected to display their work in a portfolio; for example, artists, models, and architects. Portfolios offer the CNS a chance to reflect on achievements, develop goals, and forge new insights. A portfolio is also useful for developing clinical career pathways (Joyce, 2005).

Portfolio contents vary, but most include a résumé or curriculum vitae, selected examples of individual or group projects, letters of recommendation or commendation, awards, transcripts, continuing education certifications, community service activities, publications, and presentation abstracts or handouts. In general, a professional portfolio is an excellent way to organize your best work for personal perusal, but it is also a great vehicle for showcasing your work to future employers or for peer review. Portfolios can also assist in self-evaluation or reflective practice strategies, and they provide a physical structure for organizing materials that support the premise of competency.

Organizing the Portfolio

The physical nature of the portfolio may exist in an expandable file folder, a three-ring binder, or any other type of form that is portable, professional, and visually appealing. The CNS needs to carefully consider the contents of the portfolio. If too much documentation is included, it can become unwieldy and overwhelming. Deciding exactly what to include versus exclude is a reflective process. In general, view the portfolio as a valuable tool for formative assessment rather than summative assessment. Portfolio perusal provides evidence of professional growth over time rather than providing a summary of the CNS's expertise or talents.

Jasper (1995) suggested that the portfolio resembles a scrapbook and noted that Benner's (1984) model of skill acquisition is compatible with the portfolio strategy. Meister, Heath, Andrews, and Tingen (2002) recommended that portfolios include a table of contents, provide section dividers, and use high-quality paper. Bright white paper greater than 90 brilliance with weight greater than 20 pounds will provide a professional look and feel to a hard-copy portfolio.

Binders are available for purchase in a wide range of sizes from 1/2 inch to 6 inches. In general, purchasing a heavy-duty binder is well worth the money. The rings of economy style binders tend to slip open or have gaps when closed, leading to portfolio disarray. Professional portfolios should be contained in a single binder. If there is a lot of documentation, purchase the heavy-duty, 6-inch binders. The CNS should anticipate paying $30 to $40 for this binder style.

When creating the portfolio in paper form, avoid handwritten work. Tables of contents and dividers can be easily created with a word processor. Professional work requires a standard font style. The fifth edition of the *Publication Manual of the American Psychological Association* offers suggestions for professional writing and identifies Times New Roman or Courier, 10- or 12-point font, as appropriate styles. Use black ink and avoid "word art," dramatic shading, or friendly borders. Although such artistry may be appealing in a creative arts project, they are inappropriate for professional work.

Plastic page covers or sheet protectors provide convenient, attractive protection for the portfolio contents. Several styles of sheet protectors are available. A heavyweight, diamond clarity type of protector will allow clear visualization of the covered documents without lifting print. Purchase the acid-free variety for archival quality. Remember that the portfolio is meant to provide formative evaluation data and will be useful for decades.

Electronic Portfolios

Electronic portfolios have many advantages over traditional hard-copy portfolios. There are fewer issues related to storage, costs, handling, and loss (Corbett-Perez & Dorman, 1999). As computers become more accessible and technology skills become more requisite, electronic portfolios become more attractive. The convenience and relatively inexpensive costs associated with compact discs (CDs), digital video discs (DVDs), and flash drives should also encourage CNSs to consider developing an electronic portfolio rather than a paper copy. The electronically produced portfolio also validates the technology skills of the CNS and may suggest that the CNS is current and engaged in using recent technological advances. Certainly such an impression is important given the high-tech nature of many healthcare settings.

Flash drives, which are easily attached to key rings, attaché cases, or handbags, may hold up to eight gigabytes of data and are the size of a stick of chewing gum. Two gigabytes of data is about three times the storage of a standard compact disc (USB Flash Drive Alliance, 2005).

Electronic portfolios allow video, audio, and interactive components to be included in the formative data set. The multimedia presentation maximizes individualism and gives the reviewer a real look at the interactive and presentation skills of the CNS. For example, a hard-copy presentation built in PowerPoint software offers less information than the actual slide show with embedded files and hyperlinks. It is also possible for the CNS to include a video stream of an actual slide show presentation that includes the CNS interacting with the audience.

Web-Based Portfolios

There are an increasing number of Web-based commercial options for maintaining a professional portfolio. In general, the CNS consumer begins by establishing an account for a set fee. Once the account is created, the CNS uploads pertinent documents and enters data into the portfolio system. Data may be retrieved in the form of comprehensive or mini-portfolios, depending upon the situation. Initial data entry may be time consuming; however, once the account is established, portfolio maintenance is simple and very convenient. Web-based portfolio systems are also available for entire departments and institutions. Such a system can be very useful for Magnet certification and recertification processes.

The American Nurses Credentialing Center (ANCC, 2008), Sigma Theta Tau, International, and the National Student Nurses Association use electronic portfolio services offered through Decision Critical, Inc. The Critical Portfolio service costs about $60 annually and provides a vehicle for electronically storing background information, professional development activities, service activities, honors, awards, grants, scholarships, research activities, publications, and any other relevant documentation (Decision Critical, 2009). Profiles may be created in a variety of forms, a useful feature that has the potential to save a lot of time. CNSs may find that the profile development feature is also useful for annual performance evaluation or quarterly productivity documentation.

Portfolio Concerns

Portfolios require reflective practice, a process of self-scrutiny. Ideally, this scrutiny includes peer review. It is very likely that in the process of self-evaluation or peer review, errors or weakness in practice may be identified. When a portfolio is used as a public document to renew professional licensure or regulation, as in Canada or the United Kingdom, it is possible that if an area of practice has been identified as "weak" within a portfolio and a CNS makes an error in this particular area of practice, this may be particularly problematic in lawsuits. At this point in time the concern is unresolved but recognized.

Competing with a Curriculum Vitae

A curriculum vitae (CV) is a comprehensive list of professional accomplishments. The term is derived from the Latin *curriculum* (course of action) and *vitae*, meaning life (Weinstein, 2002). The CNS should view the CV as the "door opener" to opportunity. It should accurately reflect the accomplishments and interests of the CNS to provide the reader with a solid sense of the CNS's professional identity. The CV is a marketing tool as well as a record. The acknowledged "4 Ps" of marketing include *product, promotion, price,* and *position.* Weinstein suggests that the fifth P is *portfolio.*

The CV differs from a résumé (Table 1-2). There are general, customary guidelines for CV structure. Use a standard font and consistent font size. Although bold may be used, avoid designer fonts and elaborate spacing. Customary font styles include Times New Roman, Arial, and Courier in a 12-point size. Do not use a font size less than 10 points. Using spell-check is critical.

CVs should be printed as one-sided documents usually on quality paper. In general, the CNS will not err by selecting bright white paper of 92 or greater brilliance in 24-pound weight. Other paper forms are acceptable, including 100% cotton fiber; however, it is best to avoid pastel or tinted paper unless the color is off-white.

Create a header and include the last name with page number. Although it is acceptable to staple the pages together, there is still a possibility that pages will detach. A header or footer will make it easier to identify missing pages. Also, the CNS may find it necessary to electronically send the CV, and a paginated header or footer will assist the recipient in keeping the CV organized.

The CV is often submitted in response to a query for background information or as an initial step in a job search, particularly in academic environments. The CV is sent electronically or in hard-copy form, depending on the instructions of the request. In both instances, a cover letter is necessary. The cover letter to an electronically attached CV may be submitted as an e-mail message.

If the CV is mailed in paper copy, the cover letter should be consistent with the CV in style and form. The paper or electronic cover letter should include an acknowledgment of why the CV has been forwarded. If there is specific information related to a job opening position number, name of an award, or request, this should be included in the letter. The cover letter should be brief but cordial. Acknowledge the availability of references on request and thank the reviewer for interest in the CV. The CNS should offer to be available for questions or if additional information is required.

One difference between an electronic cover letter and a paper copy cover letter is the addressee. E-mails require an address, but this address is often unrecognizable as an individual's name. Given the succinct, abbreviated nature of e-mail, a salutation of some form may not even be necessary, thereby releasing the CNS from finding out the

Table 1-2   RÉSUMÉ AND CURRICULUM VITAE IN CONTRAST

Résumé	Curriculum Vitae
Overview	Extensive description
One page in length—never more than two	Several pages in length. May be dozens of pages, depending on career length and productivity.
Job application	Multiple uses including professional office, job application, awards, grants, presentations
Employment origins	Academic origins

formal name and title of the intended recipient. If a salutation is preferred, a simple "Dear Employment Specialist" or "Dear Recruiter" may be appropriate.

Paper cover letters require a recipient name and address. The CNS needs to make certain that the addressee's name is spelled correctly and that the job title and credentials are also correct. If there is uncertainty as to any of this information, the CNS should attempt to contact the organization and verify the addressee's information. If contact information is not available and a position title rather than an individual name is provided, the CNS should begin the letter with an appropriate salutation. For example, if a CV is required by an organization for award consideration, the CNS may wish to begin the cover letter with "Dear Awards Committee Representative."

If the cover letter and CV are sent electronically and it is important to ensure that they have been received, use the e-mail system "message options" functions (or use the Help function to search for "read receipt") to request a delivery receipt and a read receipt. The delivery receipt will acknowledge that the electronic message was received by the Internet Protocol address. The read receipt will ask the recipient to acknowledge that the CV was received. These options allow the CNS to verify that the materials were received in a timely fashion.

If a CV is being mailed, particularly if the CV is related to an important professional opportunity, the CNS should consider using certified mail. When certified mail is used, mail travels as first class, and delivery is confirmed. Certified mail is a smart choice for the CNS who may need to substantiate that the CV was mailed. These confirmation and verification suggestions are applicable to any situation in which the CNS is committed to replying to a request for written materials or submitting completed work.

Structuring the CV

Format the pages with the CV's headings flush with the left margins. Consider 1-inch margins or less. In general, begin with name, home address, and home telephone number. Consider including work address and work telephone number. Include electronic mail contact information.

Although some publications recommend including a Social Security number (Hinck, 1997), given the possible distribution of the CV and the increasing threat of identity theft, this may not be a wise decision. Professional license numbers should be included. Do not use pronouns. Use an active voice with appropriate tense and phrases rather than full sentences. For example, avoid, "I developed a research-based protocol for bladder ultrasound in lieu of bladder catheterization with annual savings of $165,000." Instead use, "Designed and implemented bladder ultrasound program with $165,000 annualized savings."

CV formatting varies and is primarily based on personal preference as well as the underlying purpose of the CV. For example, if the CNS is submitting a CV for consideration by a nominating committee of a professional organization for a key leadership position, the CNS may want to consider reformatting the CV to highlight the skills and experiences that are requisite for this type of opportunity. It is generally fairly easy to revise and update CVs now that most documentation is in word-processed form rather than typewritten.

There are many ways to structure a CV (Table 1-3). Most list recent experiences first and move in a reverse chronological order. For example, the highest degree earned is identified followed by the next highest degree. Do not include postsecondary school education prior to college. Include nondegree course work under continuing education or as a separate category.

Professional certifications should be noted on the CV. Certification as an advanced practice nurse is increasingly important for CNS practice, albeit inconsistently mandated at the state level. The CNS should note all types of certifications, including advanced cardiac life support (ACLS), cardiopulmonary resuscitation (CPR), chemotherapy, neonatal advanced life support (NALS), and any other relevant type of certified expertise. It may be useful to include the date of the most recent child abuse clearance and a criminal background check and offer to make these reports available on request. These clearances save time and are increasingly expected, particularly when nurses are working with vulnerable patient or client populations.

All types of publications should be listed. Consider separating publication types: research versus nonresearch, and refereed, nonrefereed, invited, and newsletters. Organize newsletters by professional organization, public organization, institution, department, or unit-based categories. Make certain to include published abstracts, but clearly identify the name of the conference proceedings and whether the abstract was accepted following peer review.

If the CNS does not have many publications, group the publications and order by date. For the CNS without publications, consider this area as a possible area for development. There are beginning opportunities to publish, including book reviews, newsletters, and letters to the editors. These first steps demonstrate an interest in writing and set the CV apart from those without publications in any form. In the meantime, if the CNS does not have publication credit, simply leave this topic off the CV. Do not include the heading and note "not applicable" or "none."

Professional organizations should be included on the CV. Note any leadership positions within an organization. The CNS should critique the depth and breadth of the organizations and contemplate joining a collection of organizations that represent a national nursing interest, clinical area of practice, local or regional organization, scholarly activity or research focus, and an organization that reflects a commitment to relationships, such as an alumni organization. Dues can become burdensome, so it is wise to select carefully. On the other hand, advanced nursing practice demands professionalism. It is difficult to demonstrate professional commitment without any type of national or international nursing organization membership.

Honor society memberships should be included. Sigma Theta Tau, International is the international honor society for nursing, and admission is competitive. Other honor societies should also be listed, including those that are outside nursing; for example, Phi Beta Kappa or Phi Kappa Phi. Honor society memberships outside nurs-

Table 1-3   SUGGESTED CV ORGANIZATION

Curriculum Vitae Organization

Education

Licenses and certifications

Employment history (begin with most recent)

Consultation activities

Professional organizations: Emphasize leadership roles

Presentations

  Papers

    Refereed review

    Nonrefereed review or invited

  Posters

    Refereed review

    Nonrefereed review or invited

Publications

  Refereed

    Research

    Theoretical

  Nonrefereed

  Invited

  Books

Awards

Grants

Continuing education (consider limiting to previous 5 years)

Community service

References: Consider this

Revision and file path

ing are not uncommon, given the increasing numbers of nurses who enter the profession as second-degree students. Social sororities or fraternities may also be included if the CNS is actively involved.

Community activities, including leadership roles, should be documented on the CV. This area of the CV demonstrates citizenship and can be important in a competitive job search. Do not include trivial activities that contribute very little to the overall picture. For example, routinely donating money to a particular charity or tithing to the church are inappropriate to include on a CV. Serving on the church board of directors or volunteering with the Girl Scouts of America are important to include because they require individual sacrifice and benefit a larger societal good in an organized fashion with recognized duties.

Do not include salary information or salary expectations on the CV. If the CV is in response to a potential job opportunity and salary information is requested or required by the employer, this information should be generally addressed in the cover letter.

If the CNS has taught in a formal academic setting, include a brief description of course responsibilities. For the experienced CNS who has been involved in healthcare education, offer specific, factual information about program development and outcomes. If the CNS is a novice, consider including educational activities that were part of the graduate educational program. The CNS should remember that appropriate CV style is terse rather than detailed and narrative.

Résumé

The CNS should keep in mind that résumés are quite different than CVs. A résumé is never more than two pages in length. The résumé is meant to provide an outline of educational background and work experiences with some sharing of professional activities. If more detailed information is needed, a CV may be helpful. Most academic positions require a CV, whereas business settings request résumés.

If the CNS is looking for a position and is considering using a Web-based job search engine, the CNS must keep in mind that electronic résumés will be found only via keywords that have been selected by a potential employer. Some applicant tracking systems search approximately the first 80 words of a document, so be certain to include critical phrases and terms early in the résumé. Avoid graphics, shading, italics, and underlining in electronic résumés; however, this suggestion is reasonable for résumés of any type.

The order of the résumé may be consistent with that of the CV, but the detail will be far less. The résumé may also include a statement of intent or professional interest. This statement is not usually found on the CV.

Résumés may be organized by skill sets or by work and project experiences. The more traditional format is similar to that of the CV but in abbreviated form. In general, continuing education activities are not listed on a résumé; however, the CNS may choose to include a statement about the number of annual hours of completed continuing education.

Many resources are available for creating résumés. CNSs interested in constructing a résumé should use these resources and request guidance from experts. Many resources are Web based and user-friendly.

References

The CNS should give careful thought to references. In general, employers are interested in hearing from individuals who can substantiate the character and abilities of the applicant. Most institutions have a standardized reference form, although reference letters may be acceptable.

New CNSs are often uncertain of whom to ask for a reference. Select an individual who can offer evaluative insight and who has a clear idea of the skill set required of a CNS position. At times, graduate students will request references from professors who worked with the student during beginning graduate courses and who have little to share regarding advanced practice skills or professional attributes. This individual may not be the best referring choice.

Instead, the CNS should consider requesting references from a CNS clinical preceptor, faculty member with responsibility for evaluating end-of-program work, recent employer, or professional organization leader. It is useful to request reference letters before they are needed and include them in the professional portfolio. If references are gathered before the job search process, ask referring individuals if an employer, committee person, or admissions professional has permission to contact them at a later date for validation of the reference. Having written reference letters at the start of a process can save valuable time.

Professional Organizations

Many nursing organizations are experiencing stagnant or declining membership (White & Olson, 2004). This trend is concerning for a number of reasons. Professional organizations provide opportunities for enhancing clinical expertise; keeping apprised of regional, national, and international issues; and developing professional networks. Most groups offer continuing education programs. Some are very involved in political action and have done good work in advancing nursing and societal healthcare agenda items.

There are so many professional organizations that it would be nearly impossible for a CNS to identify an area of clinical or leadership interest that is not represented by an organization. Generally, a Web-based search will identify appropriate professional nursing organizations. It is also useful to visit the American Nurses Association Web site (www.nursingworld.org) or other large nursing organization's Web site and look for organizational links. The links will connect directly to other established, reputable organizations.

Part of the challenge of declining memberships may be that with the proliferation of organizations, nurses feel confusion and pressure specific to selecting the few organizations that are most compatible with their interests and priorities. Another reason for avoiding membership may be that family responsibilities compete for the scarce resources of a nurse's time and money. Given the busy nature of CNS work and the often simultaneous demands of family and other personal commitments, CNSs need to carefully craft a personalized strategy for involvement in professional organizations (Table 1-4). In other words, it may be wise for the CNS to carefully consider the most important aspects of professional organization

---

Table 1-4   PROFESSIONAL ORGANIZATIONS AUDIT: SELECTING AN ORGANIZATION TO JOIN

The CNS should consider each of these criteria:

1. Mission statement
2. Goals and objectives
3. Web-based resources
4. Membership fees
5. Ease of dues payment:
   a. Direct withdrawal from bank account (monthly/annually)
   b. Direct debit from credit card (monthly/annually)
   c. Annual dues by check
6. Continuing education opportunities
7. Journal resources
8. Database access, including evidence-based practice resources
9. Professional activities, including conferences and workshops:
   a. Regional/local activities
   b. National activities
   c. International activities
   d. Relationships to other professional organizations
10. Opportunities to volunteer
11. Opportunities for mentoring
12. Leadership and networking possibilities

---

membership and, having prioritized these concerns, identify the most logical organizations for membership.

Many organizations have broad agendas focused on clinical excellence, research, leadership, and political action. CNSs select these organizations based on a particular clinical focus. A few examples of such organizations include the Oncology Nursing Society (ONS, 2006), American Association of Critical-Care Nurses (AACN, 2006), Association of Rehabilitation Nurses (ARN), American Psychiatric Nurses Association (APNA), and the Association of periOperative Registered Nurses (AORN). It is customary for CNSs to have some type of membership status with their specialized clinical organization.

The National Association of Clinical Nurse Specialists (NACNS) is the only national organization focused on CNS practice regardless of the area of clinical practice. This organization is relatively new, initiated in 1996, and is recognized as an organizational affiliate by the American Nurses Association. Its mission is to enhance and promote the unique, high-value contribution of the clinical nurse specialist to the health and well-being of individuals, families, groups, and communities, and to promote and advance the practice of nursing. Members of NACNS benefit from national, regional, and local efforts of the Association to make the contributions of CNSs more visible. (NACNS, n.d. 1)

NACNS offers a variety of membership benefits and provides opportunities for CNSs to interact with other CNSs. These types of networking opportunities are valuable and allow CNSs to cross disciplines and gain perspectives on the larger issues of advanced practice nursing. Members benefit from a full text online and print subscription to *Clinical Nurse Specialist: The Journal for Advanced Nursing Practice*. Other membership benefits may be reviewed on www.nacns.org.

Stepping Up and Stepping In: Getting Organizationally Involved

New CNSs may be interested in becoming involved within an organization but may be a bit hesitant. This uncertainty is normal and understandable, but it is important to not allow reticence to impede participation. Organizations are eager to have interested, committed, and enthusiastic new members.

Professional organizations face many challenges. Nursing societies are struggling with declining memberships, an aging nursing workforce, increasing expenses, and competition among professional organizations for both members and leaders. Of course, new members should anticipate that involvement usually starts at the local level, if not geographically, then organizationally. Local or regional groups are good places to volunteer as a committee member or to begin participation by attending meetings, offering time to assist at registration tables, or contributing on an as-needed basis.

Many national organizations have committees that are filled by appointments rather than elections. It is not uncommon for organizations to publish requests for participation. Members may be asked to submit a CV and a brief letter indicating interest in the committee work.

As an example, the ONS Web site devotes a section of the membership page to opportunities for involvement in project teams, advisory panels, mentoring programs, or recruitment events. There are also opportunities noted in local chapters or special-interest groups. ONS offers application forms in PDF form on the Web site and is very user-friendly. AACN also offers lots of information on its Web page with a volunteers homepage that describes current needs and provides application forms for download. These opportunities are wonderful networking vehicles for CNSs ranging from novice to expert.

Connecting Professionally in an Electronic World

Listserv Opportunities

There is an increasing number of e-mail lists, discussion boards, and chat opportunities for CNSs. The CNS LISTSERV (CNS-L) allows CNSs to manage, create, and control electronic mailing lists. Registering for the CNS-L is simple and requires only an e-mail address. To subscribe to the CNS-L described on the NACNS Web site, send a blank e-mail to cns-listserv-on@mail-list.com. Send this message from the e-mail address that you will use to read the incoming list materials. At last count, there were approximately 600 CNS colleagues subscribed to this particular listserv (NACNS, n.d. 2). Keep in mind that there is a possibility of receiving a large volume of e-mail.

Upon joining any type of e-mail list, it is a good idea to print instructions for future reference. Instructions for joining always include the instructions for withdrawing from the list. It is interesting to note that LISTSERV is a trademark for a product distributed by L-Soft International. For this reason, LISTSERV is capitalized. The term *listserv* is used in a variety of forms, but those groups using the LISTSERV product refer to it in the aforementioned style.

Generally, there is a moderator or owner of the list. Usually there is a contact person associated with the list to whom questions and concerns may be addressed. LISTSERVs specific to organizations do not typically require membership but do require an e-mail address.

Some groups use the LISTSERV product, for example, the Agency for Healthcare Research and Quality (AHRQ). Others refer to their groups as a "listserv" and use a provider such as Yahoo to organize the group. One such example is the Society of Critical Care Medicine. Regardless of the provider or product, joining the list is easy. The LISTSERV product offers options for organizing and delivering the electronic mail. This feature can be particularly useful when trying to minimize the number of daily e-mails or when working with vacation or part-time schedules. Many LISTSERVs offer the option of a daily summary rather than receiving individual e-mails. This is a particularly important feature when receiving e-mail via portable electronic devices such as cell phones or personal data assistants as the frequent e-mail responses can be quite burdensome.

There are often guidelines for contributing to list discussions (Table 1-5). The CNS must be diligent about remembering the purpose of the list. In other words, each contributed message should relate to the overarching subject of the list. If the CNS is contributing to the CNS LISTSERV, the topic should have some connection to CNS practice. The connection may be weak but must be readily apparent.

CNSs should carefully evaluate the content and wording of postings before clicking the "send" button. Many lists have significant numbers of members. Once the message has been sent, it cannot be retrieved. Other suggestions should be considered and followed prior to participating in a LISTSERV. If each member follows the rules, the communications and connections can be useful and the networking opportunities cannot be beat. CNSs often share policies, procedures, instruments, tools, product evaluations, and sage advice via the LISTSERV.

Discussion Boards and Electronic Forums

Electronic discussion boards and forums are handy and informative. They offer access to a variety of colleagues, sometimes around the world, and can provide important networking when looking for ideas, data, expertise, speakers, and other contacts. Many professional organizations have discussion boards available for members. Registration is free with membership, and participants usually have a self-configured password provided after the registration process is complete.

Numerous electronic forums are also available for nurses that require registration without fees. One forum, www.allnurses.com (2006), boasts over 100,000 members from around the world. Discussion topics vary and are organized by subject. A variety of advertisements are posted on the Web site offering products, including education and employment opportunities, targeted to nurses. NACNS also offers a discussion board, "CNS Exchange." Registration is free and instructions are available at www.nacns.org/bulletin_board.shtml. As mentioned previously, courtesy is required, and discussion board rules are clearly posted for review.

Develop Electronic Expertise

Computer skills are essential. There is simply no way to effectively practice in today's healthcare environment without a basic understanding of commonly used software

Table 1-5   LISTSERV RULES OF ENGAGEMENT

Generic rules for polite LISTSERV participation

1. Absolutely no commercial advertisements of any sort.
2. Remember that LISTSERV participation is open to the world. There are going to be communication challenges related to diversity and language/communication differences. Try to be open-minded. Avoid taking immediate offense, and give the benefit of doubt.
3. Avoid sending messages to the entire subscriber group that are relevant to only a select one or two. Send "thank you" and other pleasantries to the relevant person only.
4. Do not post materials that are under copyright protection.
5. Do not attach files or hyperlinks to LISTSERV comments.
6. No inappropriate or generally offensive language or slang.
7. Do not post personal information to a LISTSERV. Private contact should be handled through e-mail.

products. Technological competence in electronic mail, Excel, PowerPoint, Word, and Internet search strategies are particularly important. Database software familiarity may also be useful; for example, Microsoft Access.

Technological competence is increasingly viewed as a routine expectation of CNSs. Abstracts for professional organization conferences as either poster or paper presentations often require electronic submissions. Many organizations require the use of PowerPoint as the presentation format and expect that presentations will be electronically forwarded to the conference committee to load the presentation for the conference and to develop conference CDs. It is increasingly rare for organizations to use hard-copy forms, and the ease of PowerPoint software makes other presentation media comparatively cumbersome and prohibitively expensive. As an example, 35-millimeter slides and overhead transparencies are not acceptable presentation formats at most national nursing conferences.

There are a variety of ways to develop software expertise. In-house educational programs are ideal. These programs are free to employees and are geared to the software and hardware used within the CNS's place of employment. The challenge lies in arranging the necessary time to attend. Community colleges and university settings offer credit and noncredit courses as do postsecondary technology schools. Online tutorials are available, and there are vendors that sell videotapes designed as user-friendly tools for learners who learn best through visual processes. Microsoft (www.microsoft.com) offers information related to tutorials and software program classes.

Hardware familiarity is also valuable. Blackberry, Palm, and other handheld devices are commonplace and, in some settings, are required as part of the arsenal of workplace tools. CNSs unfamiliar with the capabilities of these devices will be astounded by the features. Drug databases, clinical references, personal scheduling, wireless access, e-mail options, and other resources vary by device. Most are very easy to use and are synchronized through the workplace or home computer making it easy to have consistency across home, work, and pocket.

APRN Certification: A Value-Added Enhancement

CNSs may notice that the terms *advanced practice nurse* (APN) and *advanced practice registered nurse* (APRN) are used interchangeably. APRN is the designated term used by the recent APRN Consensus Work Group and the NCSBN APRN Advisory Committee, otherwise referred to as the APRN Joint Dialogue Group (APRN JDG) report (2008). This group was charged with developing a regulatory model for APRN practice to ensure patient safety and allow for patient access to APRN services. The model has significant implications for CNS practice. The model has been endorsed by many professional organizations and by NCSBN. State boards of nursing have not yet adopted this model into nurse practice acts; however, this model includes elements pertaining to licensure, accreditation, certification, and education (LACE) (APRN JDG, 2008). CNSs should carefully review the JDG report and consider how they need to position themselves specific to professional development, education, and certification within the context of their anticipated career trajectory.

The federal government defines a CNS as a master's degree-prepared nurse educated in a clinical nurse specialist program with certification as an advanced practice registered nurse from an accredited credentialing organization (Zuzelo et al., 2004). To obtain Medicare provider status, the CNS must meet these criteria. The JDG report defines an APRN as a nurse who has met educational criteria for one of the four APRN roles within at least one of the six population foci. Specialization provides depth, but the model specifies that the APRN cannot be licensed solely within a specialty area. This proposal is quite a change and requires careful deliberation as CNSs plan for their professional futures. For example, CNSs may identify themselves as a "critical care" or "oncology" CNS without regard to a population. The APRN Consensus Model would require CNSs to be educated in one of the four roles and at least one of the six population foci: family/individual across the life span, adult-gerontology, pediatrics, neonatal, women's health/gender-related, or psych/mental health (APRN JDG, 2008).

The Certification Quandary

There are challenges associated with the proposed regulatory model as well as with existing APRN definitions. Particularly concerning is the scarcity of specialty certification examinations for CNSs. Additionally, at the state level, CNS title protection is not consistent, and requirements for use of the title "CNS" vary. States that offer CNS title recognition typically require some type of advanced practice certification in a specialty area. States that do not afford the public CNS title recognition do not require certification and may not require a master's degree.

Inconsistencies among states or between the federal government and some state governments have led to confusion and inappropriate titling. The terms *clinical specialist* or *clinical nurse specialist* may be used by nurses and/or employers to represent nurses who are not prepared at the master's level. In fact, there may be nurses using these titles who have not yet completed baccalaureate degrees in nursing. Graduate nursing programs recognize these dilemmas and, as a result, may feel less pressure to reinforce the need for CNS certification than for nurse practitioner or nurse anesthetist students.

When this situation is viewed within the context of a lack of specialty certification examinations, it is readily apparent that certification as a CNS is not a consistent requirement nor an easily acquired status within many specialty areas. Many CNSs use the master's in science of nursing (MSN) degree in posted credentials but have specialization certification at the basic level only. For example, an MSN-prepared CNS may have certification in medical–surgical nursing and may list the credentials as "MSN, RN, C." The certification examination for the "C" credential requires a baccalaureate nursing degree rather than a graduate degree and does not represent an advanced practice credential. CNSs specializing in women's health or wound, ostomy, continence nursing are confronted by similar challenges as there are not CNS certification examinations available within these particular specialty areas. As a result, some CNSs prepare for adult health CNS certification and develop the specialization focus as best as they are able through practice, scholarship, formal educational programs, and continuing education.

It is important for CNSs to appreciate the difference between basic certified clinical specialization and advanced practice certified clinical specialization. Many CNSs practice oncology nursing, and this specialty offers an opportunity for an additional example that is not unique. An oncology nurse with at least 12 months registered nurse (RN) experience within 36 months of examination application and 1000 hours of oncology experience within the 30 months prior to application who satisfies continuing education mandates is eligible to take the certification examination that will award the oncology certified nurse (OCN) credential. A baccalaureate degree in nursing is not required (Oncology Nursing Certification Corporation [ONCC], 2008a). The advanced practice CNS certification is advanced oncology clinical nurse specialist (AOCNS). This examination requires a master's degree or higher in nursing and 500 hours of supervised clinical experience in oncology nursing practice either during or subsequent to the graduate education experience (ONCC, 2008b).

This example illustrates that there are significant differences in requirements within and between clinical specialties for basic certification versus advanced practice certification. It is important for the CNS to consider the meaning of certification and its relationship to demonstrating clinical competence and protecting the public trust.

APRN Certification Opportunities

The American Nurses Credentialing Center (2006) is the certifying arm of the American Nurses Association. It offers nine advanced practice CNS examinations. CNS examinations are also offered by the certification corporations associated with AACN, Orthopaedic Nurses Certification Board, and Oncology Nursing Certification Corporation (Table 1-6). Fourteen CNS examinations are not enough to cover the plethora of CNS specializations. This testing opportunity deficit has made it difficult for CNSs interested in acquiring a certification that truly represents practice expertise.

Certification examination development is expensive. Psychometric testing, examination administration, and test bank development necessitate a high number of users. Tests are not developed for less-popular subject areas. CNSs interested in certification but without access to a specialty examination had few options until the recent development of the CNS core examination.

Prior to the CNS core examination, CNSs often chose to sit for the adult health examination as a "generic" fit. As an example, an MSN-prepared nurse with expertise in wound, ostomy, continence nursing, or women's health, has been unable to certify as a CNS in these practice areas. As a result, since adult health nursing is viewed as the "foundation" to many nursing specialties, a disputable point but a widely held

Table 1-6	CNS CERTIFICATION EXAMINATION OPPORTUNITIES	
Name of Examination	**Sponsoring Organization**	**Web Address**
Advanced Diabetes Management	ANCC (American Nurses Credentialing Center)	http://www.nursecredentialing.org/NurseSpecialties/DiabetesManagementAdvanced.aspx
CNS Core	ANCC	http://www.nursecredentialing.org/NurseSpecialties/CNSCoreExam.aspx
Adult Health	ANCC	http://www.nursecredentialing.org/NurseSpecialties/AdultHealthCNS.aspx
Adult Psychiatric and Mental Health Nursing	ANCC	http://www.nursecredentialing.org/NurseSpecialties/AdultPsychiatricMentalHealthCNS.aspx
Child/Adolescent Psychiatric and Mental Health Nursing	ANCC	http://www.nursecredentialing.org/NurseSpecialties/ChildAdolescentPsychMentalHealth.aspx
Gerontological	ANCC	http://www.nursecredentialing.org/NurseSpecialties/GerontologicalCNS.aspx
Pediatric	ANCC	http://www.nursecredentialing.org/NurseSpecialties/PediatricCNS.aspx
Home Health (only available for recertification)	ANCC	http://www.nursecredentialing.org/NurseSpecialties/HomeHealthCNS.aspx
Public Health	ANCC	http://www.nursecredentialing.org/NurseSpecialties/PublicHealthNurse.aspx
Advanced Oncology CNS	Oncology Nursing Certification Corporation (ONCC)	http://www.oncc.org/getcertified/testinformation/AOCNS/index.shtml
Adult Critical Care Nurse Specialist (CCNS)	American Association of Critical-Care Nurses (AACN)	http://www.aacn.org/WD/Certifications/Content/ccns.pcms?menu=Certification

(continues)

Table 1-6 (continued)		
Name of Examination	**Sponsoring Organization**	**Web Address**
Neonatal CCNS	AACN	http://www.aacn.org/WD/Certifications/Content/ccns.pcms?menu=Certification
Pediatric CCNS	AACN	http://www.aacn.org/WD/Certifications/Content/ccns.pcms?menu=Certification
Orthopaedic CNS	Orthopaedic Nurses Certification Board	http://www.oncb.org/apnexams/apnexameligibility.html

view by some nurses, the graduate degree-prepared nurse may have opted to take this APRN examination and combine it with the basic certification exam available within the specialty.

Of course, adult health nursing is unique, and certification in this clinical area does not presume actual expertise in wound, ostomy, continence care, or women's health. As noted, the option has not been ideal. On the other hand, given that an increasing number of states, as well as federal agencies, require certification, the adult health CNS certification examination was the best option.

A New Certification Opportunity

Recognizing the imperative need to address the lack of CNS certification examinations for all specialties and the practice barrier that such a deficit presents, NACNS and the American Nurses Credentialing Center (ANCC) collaborated to develop a CNS core certification examination. This exam tests the competencies required for the CNS role, regardless of specialty focus, and across the life span (ANCC, 2008). The core exam is intended to provide an opportunity to secure certification as a CNS for practice as an advanced practice nurse within a specialty area that does not have a CNS certification examination. Candidates who successfully pass the core examination may then be required to validate their expertise within a specialty area, depending upon the requirements of the specialty organization or regulatory agency. If and when a specialty organization has enough members to justify the expense of certification examination development and to establish a data set that is valid and reliable, the core examination may not be an option in lieu of the relevant certification examination.

Personal Development and Self-Care

Healthy self-care practices are important for mental well-being, spiritual strength, emotional connectedness, and physical health. Many nurses, including CNSs, attend to their personal needs with far less focus than they attend to the needs of others. It is not uncommon for nurses to smoke, with smoking rates of approximately 28% in the United Kingdom (McKenna et al., 2001) and 18% in the United States (Bialous et al., 2004). Like smokers in the general population, nurses are concerned about the health risks of smoking and are interested in smoking cessation programs. Nurses also experience guilt related to their continued smoking (Bialous et al.).

In addition to the damaging effects of smoking on nurses' health, research findings suggest that nurses who smoke are less inclined to address smoking cessation with patients (McKenna et al., 2001). Nurses need cessation supports similar to smokers in the general population and also need unique supports that address the guilt and shame that they may experience in relation to their persona as a nurse, a person who "knows better than to smoke."

Nurses, including CNSs, are challenged by other conditions that thwart healthy well-being. Many nurses are overweight due to job stress, snacking, inadequate exercise, and a work environment that encourages junk food, end-of-shift desserts, pizza, and pastries (Jackson, Smith, Adams, Frank, & Mateo, 1999). Obese people are generally stigmatized in society (Zuzelo & Seminara, 2006), and these negative attitudes may be particularly pronounced in the healthcare setting. Nurses tend to inconsistently address body mass index measurement with patients and avoid dietary counseling. They worry about hurting patients' feelings. As a result, many nurses avoid difficult conversations with patients about the need to diet, exercise, and lose weight (Zuzelo & Seminara).

Nutritional concerns and the need for self-care may be conversation topics that are even awkward with nurse colleagues. Jackson et al. (1999) call for nurses to engage in and promote healthy lifestyles and confront the mixed message that patients receive when interacting with obese healthcare professionals. These concerns may be more significant when it is the CNS who is overweight with poor physical stamina.

Physical activity is a key determinant of health condition. Midlife women are particularly at risk for inactivity. Nurse demographics reveal that most nurses are in their fifth decade and female. Midlife women tend to experience physiological and psychological transitions that decrease the amount of personal time available for physical activity (Dearden & Sheahan, 2002). Lack of physical activity contributes to weight gain, heart disease, and colon cancer, whereas exercise benefits physical health and mood while reducing distressing signs and symptoms of menopause (Dearden & Sheahan, 2002).

CNSs must evaluate their personal health profiles (Table 1-7). They should think about exercise, smoking cessation, sleep patterns, stress management, habits of health promotion, and weight. The CNS role is incredibly challenging. Nurses commonly place role demands ahead of self-care activities. It is easy to justify a lack of exercise when the physical work of nursing is so demanding; however, a long day at work is not equal to a 20-minute brisk walk or aerobic exercise with weights. Jackson et al. suggest that nurses must begin "walking the walk of a healthy life style" (1999, p. 1), and this directive certainly includes CNSs. The recent attention paid to the historically low rates of influenza vaccination among healthcare providers, particularly nurses and physicians, is an excellent example of the need for CNSs to act on the primary health interventions not only to protect patients but also to protect themselves and their

Table 1-7 PERSONAL HEALTH INVENTORY	
Self-Care Behavior	**Personal Assessment**
1. Do I typically sleep 7 to 8 hours each night?	
a. If I do not sleep enough, how will I increase the amount of sleep time?	
2. Do I smoke?	
a. If I do smoke, when will I stop, and what steps can I take to support my success?	
3. What is my actual body weight?	
a. What is my ideal body weight?	
b. What steps can I take to maintain my current weight or to reduce my current weight?	
4. Do I exercise on a regular basis?	
a. What is my target exercise goal, and how can I reach this target?	
5. Do I have quiet, reflective time for rejuvenating?	
a. If not, how might I increase my opportunity for calm and solace?	
6. What health promotion/disease prevention assessments do I need to schedule?	
a. Blood pressure check	
b. Blood sugar check	
c. Colonoscopy	
d. Mammography	
e. Cholesterol screening	
f. Dental examination	
g. Eye examination	
h. Sex-specific exam: gynecologic or prostate	
7. What age-specific evidence-based health interventions should I consider based upon AHRQ recommendations?	

loved ones while serving as role models to colleagues and the public (Pearson, Bridges, & Harper, 2006) (Figure 1-1).

CNSs who are smokers need to explore options for smoking cessation. Resources are available for nurses who smoke. Tobacco Free Nurses (2008) provides many free resources including a library with reference categories that specifically address nurses, nursing activities, and smoking. These references may be very helpful to CNSs interested in developing and nurturing smoking cessation activities for nurses in the workplace. An electronic support group, QuitNet (Healthways QuitNet, 2008) provides opportunities for networking, support, and tobacco cessation strategies.

It may be difficult for CNSs to attend to personal health needs. Many organizations are more inclined to reward the sacrificing, busy, tired CNS rather than the CNS who insists on time for exercise, healthy lunches, bathroom breaks, and adequate hydration. However, it is empowering and necessary to promote self-health. Leading staff toward positive health practices may improve the quality of health-promotion activities in which nurses engage with patients.

Most CNSs recognize the importance of teaching patients about health promotion and disease prevention. They may be neglectful of promoting these behaviors among nurse colleagues and within their CNS peer group. Self-care is a worthwhile endeavor, but it must be a deliberately planned activity, or it will be unaddressed. Callaghan (1999) claimed that nurses often adopt fewer positive, health-promoting practices

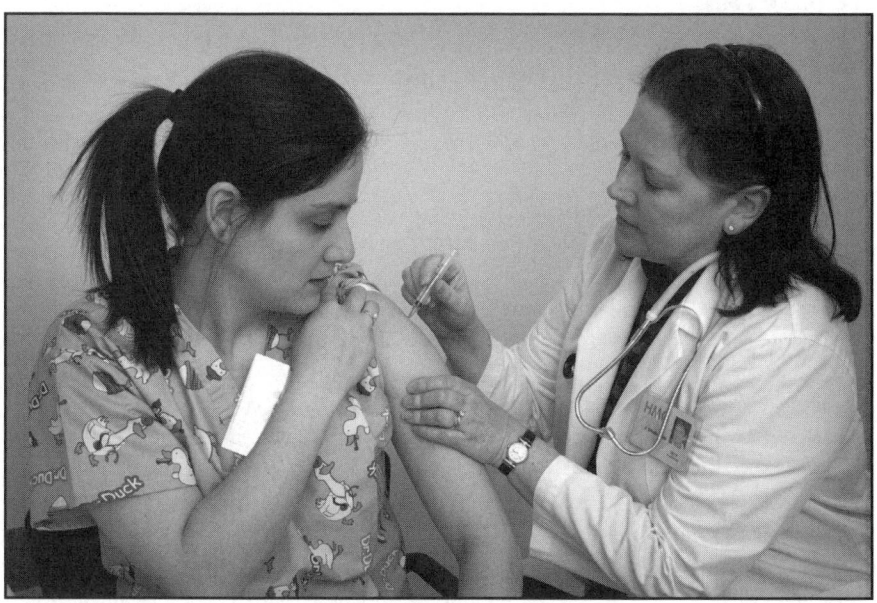

Figure 1-1   Nurse receiving an influenza immunization.
Source: James Gathany, Centers for Disease Control and Prevention.

than laypeople. It is imperative for CNSs to take the lead and promote smoking cessation, regular exercise, normal weight maintenance, snacking avoidance, routine healthy breakfast intake, regular sleep patterns with 7 to 8 hours nightly, and moderate alcohol intake.

Conclusion

CNSs must be strategic as they plan their professional and personal lives. They must proactively address both of these areas, never one at the consistent expense of the other. Professional success is enhanced by a state of personal well-being, and certainly longevity is improved when positive health practices become a routine way of life.

CNSs influence through example. CNSs involved and engaged in professional organizations tend to have more opportunities to share with interested staff. They have an increased ability to mentor because their repertoire of activities and experiences is greater than that of CNSs who are less engaged. This premise applies to self-care practices as well. CNSs cannot be haphazard in their approach to professional practice and must be equally disciplined in their approach to self-care. CNSs who manage their time and activities to benefit their health also benefit their families, colleagues, patients, and the organization.

References

Alexander, J. G., Craft, S. W., Baldwin, M. S., Beers, G. W., & McDaniel, G. S. (2002). The nursing portfolio: A reflection of a professional. *Journal of Continuing Education in Nursing, 33*(2), 55–59.

Allnurses.com. (2006). *Welcome to allnurses.com.* Retrieved July 23, 2006, from http://www.allnurses.com

American Association of Critical-Care Nurses (AACN). (2006). *Volunteer opportunities.* Retrieved July 23, 2006, from http://www.aacn.org/aacn/voluntee.nsf/vwdoc/mainvolunteer

American Nurses Credentialing Center (ANCC). (2006). *ANCC certification. Opening a world of opportunities.* Retrieved July 23, 2006, from http://www.nursingworld.org/ancc/cert/index.html

American Nurses Credentialing Center (ANCC). (2008). *Clinical nurse specialist core exam.* Retrieved December 3, 2008, from http://www.nursecredentialing.org/NurseSpecialties/CNSCoreExam.aspx

American Psychological Association (APA). (2005). *Publication manual of the American Psychological Association* (5th ed.). Washington, DC: Author.

APRN Consensus Work Group and the National Council of State Boards of Nursing APRN Advisory Committee (APRN Joint Dialogue Group). (2008). *Consensus model for APRN regulation: Licensure, accreditation, certification & education.* Retrieved December 3, 2008, from https://www.ncsbn.org/7_23_08_Consensue_APRN_Final.pdf

Atkins, S. (1995). Reflective practice. *Nursing Standard, 9*(45), 31–37.

Benner, P. (1984). *From novice to expert: Excellence and power in clinical nursing practice.* Menlo Park, CA: Addison-Wesley.

Bialous, S. A., Sarna, L., Wewers, M. E., Froelicher, E. S., & Danao, L. (2004). Nurses' perspectives of smoking initiation, addiction, and cessation. *Nursing Research, 53*(6), 387–395.

Bowers, S. J., & Jinks, A. M. (2004). Issues surrounding professional portfolio development for nurses. *British Journal of Nursing, 13*(3), 155–159.

Callaghan, P. (1999). Health beliefs and their influence on United Kingdom nurses' health-related behaviours. *Journal of Advanced Nursing, 29*(1), 28–35.

Cardillo, D. (2000). *Beyond the resume.* Retrieved February 12, 2006, from http://www.dcardillo.com/articles/beyondresume.html

Clinical Placement Support Unit (CPSU). (2005). *Using a model of reflection.* Retrieved December 1, 2008, from http://www.health.uce.ac.uk/dpl/nursing/Placement%20Support/Model%20of%20Reflection.htm

College of Nurses of Ontario. (2008). *Fact sheet. Quality assurance. Reflective practice.* Retrieved December 1, 2008, from http://www.cno.org/docs/qa/44008_fsRefprac.pdf

Corbett-Perez, S., & Dorman, S. (1999). Electronic portfolios enhance health instruction. *Journal of School Health, 69,* 247–249.

Dearden, J. S., & Sheahan, S. L. (2002). Clinical practice: Counseling middle-aged women about physical activity using the stages of change. *Journal of the American Academy of Nurse Practitioners, 14*(11), CINAHL Database of Nursing and Allied Health Literature, 492–497.

DecisionCritical.com. (2009). *Homepage.* Retrieved June 4, 2009, from http://www.decisioncritical.com

Driscoll, J., & Teh, B. (2001). The potential of reflective practice to develop individual orthopaedic nurse practitioners and their practice. *Journal of Orthopaedic Nursing, 5,* 95–103.

Duffy, A. (2007). A concept analysis of reflective practice: Determining its value to nurses. *British Journal of Nursing, 16*(22), 1400–1407.

Healthways QuitNet. (2008). *QuitNet: Quit all together.* Retrieved December 3, 2008, from http://www.quitnet.com

Hinck, S. (1997) A curriculum vitae that gives you a competitive edge. *Clinical Nurse Specialist, 11*(4), 174–177.

Jackson, B. S., Smith, S. P., Adams, R., Frank, B., & Mateo, M. A. (1999). Health life styles are a challenge for nurses. *Image—the Journal of Nursing Scholarship, 31*(2), 196. Retrieved July 23, 2006, from OVID http://dbproxy.lasalle.edu:2249/gw2/ovidweb.cgi

Jasper, M. A. (1995). The potential of the professional portfolio for nursing. *Journal of Clinical Nursing, 4*(4), 249–255.

Johns, C. (2004). *Becoming a reflective practitioner* (2nd ed.). Malden, MA: Blackwell.

Joyce, P. (2005). A framework for portfolio development in postgraduate nursing practice. *Journal of Clinical Nursing, 14,* 456–463.

McColgan, K. (2008). The value of portfolio building and the registered nurse: A review of the literature. *Journal of Perioperative Practice, 18*(2), 64–69.

McKenna, H., Slater, P., McCance, T., Bunting, B., Spiers, A., & McElwee, G. (2001). Qualified nurses' smoking prevalence: Their reasons for smoking and desire to quit. *Journal of Advanced Nursing, 35*(5), 769–775.

McMullan, M., Endacott, R., Gray, M. A., Jasper, M., Miller, C. M., Scholes, J., et al. (2003). Portfolios and assessment of competence. A review of the literature. *Journal of Advanced Nursing, 41*(3), 283–294.

Meister, L., Heath, J., Andrews, J., & Tingen, M. S. (2002). Professional nursing portfolios: A global perspective. *MEDSURG Nursing, 11*(4), 177–182.

Miller, S. K., Alpert, P. T. , & Cross, C. L. (2008). Overweight and obesity in nurses, advanced practice nurses, and nurse educators. *Journal of the American Academy of Nurse Practitioners, 20*, 259-265.

National Association of Clinical Nurse Specialists (NACNS). (n.d. 1). *NACNS mission statement.* Retrieved July 23, 2006, from http://www.nacns.org/mission.shtml

National Association of Clinical Nurse Specialists (NACNS). (n.d. 2). *Subscribe to the CNS listserv.* Retrieved July 23, 2006, from http://www.nacns.org/listserv%20subscribe%20 thankyou.shtml

National Council of State Boards of Nursing (NCSBN). (2005). *Meeting the ongoing challenge of continued competence.* Retrieved February 11, 2006, from http://www.ncsbn.org/ pdfs/07_25_05_continued_comprtencyt_faq.pdf

Oncology Nursing Certification Corporation (ONCC). (2008a). *Get certified: AOCNS eligibility criteria.* Retrieved December 3, 2008, from http://www.oncc.org/getcertified/ TestInformation/ocn/index.shtml

Oncology Nursing Certification Corporation (ONCC). (2008b). *Get certified: AOCNS eligibility criteria.* Retrieved December 3, 2008, from http://www.oncc.org/getcertified/ testinformation/AOCNS/eligibility.shtml

Oncology Nursing Society (ONS). (2006). *Participate in ONS.* Retrieved July 23, 2006, from http://www.ons.org/membership/participate.shtml

Pearson, M., Bridges, C., & Harper, S. (2006). Influenza vaccine of health-care personnel. *Morbidity and Mortality Weekly Report, 55*(RR02), 1-16. Retrieved December 3, 2008, from http://www.cdc.gov/mmwr/preview/mmwrhtml/rr5502a1.htm

Pew Health Professions Commission. (1998). *Strengthening consumer protection: Priorities for health care workforce regulation.* San Francisco: University of California, San Francisco Center for the Health Professions.

Sheets, V. R. (1998). *Supporting careers of competence: A regulatory challenge.* Retrieved March 2, 2006, from www.abms.org/Downloads/Conferences/Sheets%20paper.doc

Tobacco Free Nurses. (2008). *Tobacco free nurses.* Retrieved December 3, 2008, from http://www.tobaccofreenurses.org

USB Flash Drive Alliance. (2005). *USB flashdrive overview.* Retrieved December 2, 2005, from http://www.usbflashdrive.org/usbfd_overview.html

Weinstein, S. M. (2002). A nursing portfolio: Documenting your professional journey. *Journal of Infusion Nursing, 25*(6), 357–364.

White, M. J., & Olson, R. S. (2004). Factors affecting membership in specialty nursing organizations. *Rehabilitation Nursing, 29*(4), 131–137.

Zuzelo, P., Fallon, R., Lang, P., Lang, C., McGovern, K., Mount, L., et al. (2004). Clinical nurse specialists' knowledge specific to Medicare structures and processes. *Clinical Nurse Specialist, 18*, 207–217.

Zuzelo, P., & Seminara, P. (2006). Influence of registered nurses' attitudes toward bariatric patients on educational programming effectiveness. *Journal of Continuing Education in Nursing, 37*(2), 65–73.

Communication Strategies and Tips: Avoiding Problems; Achieving Desired Results

Patti Rager Zuzelo, EdD, MSN, RN, ACNS-BC

Clinical nurse specialists (CNSs) must be effective communicators. The outcomes of CNS practice are dependent on a CNS's ability to wield influence to effect change within and between systems. The ability to influence is essential for effective CNS practice (NACNS, 2004) and positively affects the spheres of influence associated with CNS practice: patients and clients, nurses and nursing practice, and organizations and systems (AACN, 2002; NACNS, 2004). All of this requires exemplary communication skills.

Most CNSs are not in positions of direct authority. They exercise influence using a variety of communication strategies within organizational relationships with indirect or informal reporting mechanisms. CNSs need a repertoire of communication strategies that is effective, powerful, and positive. This chapter provides an overview of the more frequently used methods and modes of communication in healthcare settings. These communication vehicles include electronic mail (e-mail), meetings, presentations, and print.

CNSs interact with a variety of people thereby requiring an appreciation for communicating with diverse personality types. Communication may take place on an individual basis during coaching, consulting, or interviewing. It may also occur in group venues during meetings and presentations. CNSs should critique their communication style, develop their arsenal of communication techniques, and continuously improve their communication skills.

Netiquette

Netiquette is a term used to refer to etiquette practices or manners specific to Web-based or electronic communication. These recommendations apply to a variety of forms including electronic mail (e-mail), discussion boards, Usenet, and listservs. Netiquette resources abound on the Web, and a simple search using the popular search engine *Google* reveals 9,970,000 results. CNSs interested in avoiding a netiquette faux pas will find Web-based resources that offer many valuable suggestions (Tschabitscher, 2008).

E-Mail
Maximizing Impact and Avoiding Pitfalls

E-mail is a popular communication vehicle in work settings and for good reasons. It is much more efficient than voice mail and provides an electronic record of interactions. E-mail is more environmentally friendly than hard print memos and allows for a rapid exchange of information between individuals or within large groups.

The advantages of e-mail contribute to its disadvantages. E-mail is easy and speedy. As a result, there is a tendency for people to respond to e-mails in a reflexive fashion, hitting the "send" button before taking the time to thoughtfully consider the response. A habit of delaying immediate replies to awkward or challenging inbox messages avoids aggravation. Nonverbal and auditory signals are lost with e-mail. The communication process is instant and potentially fraught with the danger of misunderstanding. The problems associated with the rapidity of e-mail are worsened by the enormous volume of messages and the lack of human interaction during message exchange (Brinkman & Kirschner, 2002).

The lack of personal interaction encourages impulsivity and discourages social inhibitions. Firing off a caustic e-mail message or replying to a message using sarcasm and unkind comments may be likened to road rage. The sense of isolation and anonymity in a vehicle encourages people to believe that they have been victimized and provides individuals with poor impulse control an opportunity to retaliate in ways that they might not use during face-to-face encounters.

CNSs should think about the perils and advantages of e-mail and establish personal guidelines for its use (Table 2-1). In general, CNSs need to remember that workplace e-mail is owned and controlled by the employer. As a result, employers have a vested interest in making certain that employees are using e-mail appropriately and within the confines of the law.

Copyright, defamation, discrimination, and harassment regulations that apply to written communication also apply to e-mail. A majority of employers monitor their employees owing to concerns over potential lawsuits. A 2005 survey by the American Management Association found that 75% of employers monitor employees' Web-site visits, and over half review and retain e-mail messages (Privacy Rights Clearinghouse [PRC], 2006).

In general, the best way to approach e-mail is to never send anything that is not appropriate for general viewing by the larger workforce group. There are no guarantees that e-mail messages will not be forwarded. It is also wise to remember to log off e-mail accounts when leaving computer terminals to avoid situations in which other

Table 2-1	E-MAIL GUIDELINES

1. Verify your e-mail settings. Make certain that settings promote efficiency while protecting e-mail retrieval and verification.
2. Establish electronic file folders. Click and drag important messages into appropriate folders.
3. Develop a habit of reading messages and immediately deleting, electronically filing, printing, or forwarding them.
4. Use subject lines.
5. Forward and reply to messages selectively. Follow a need-to-know process to avoid cluttering colleagues' mailboxes.
6. Delete chain mail. Do not forward.
7. Generate a paper copy of important, irreplaceable messages that are sent or received.
8. Do not leave an e-mail account open and accessible when your computer is unattended.
9. Read, review, and reread messages for tone and clarity.
10. Never send an angry e-mail.
11. Use delivery receipts and read receipts selectively.
12. Select high-priority designation infrequently.
13. Clear your inbox of attached files, including pictures, video, and presentations, as soon as possible.
14. Make certain that attached files are not too large for the corporate system to handle before sending them (avoid system crashes).
15. Separate paragraphs with double spaces and keep text succinct.

people send out messages under your account name. Keep in mind that deleted messages may be retained on the workplace server.

Composing E-Mail Messages

Many people use software to filter spam—unsolicited junk mail—from their inboxes. At times, spam filters block legitimate e-mail messages. Blocking is more likely when the subject line entry is not meaningful or is left blank. The sheer volume of e-mail also encourages the use of spam filters as a way to reduce the volume of unimportant inbox messages. CNSs should craft subject-line entries to accurately reflect the nature of the e-mail message. Subject lines should be short and succinct.

Avoid forwarding chain letters through e-mail. It is also helpful to send messages only to people who really need to be in the communication loop. Sending replies to "all recipients" when it is not necessary for the entire group to read the response is impolite. It wastes server space and increases the volume of unnecessary inbox messages.

It is a good rule of thumb to keep e-mail messages as brief and tightly written as possible. If a CNS has a lot of information to convey, it may be best to craft a brief e-mail message and attach a document that can be saved or printed. Make certain to ask permission before sending large electronic attachments or alert the recipient to the size of the attachment within the body of the e-mail. Attachments allow mail recipients to quickly get through the message and return to the information-dense memo at a later time.

CNSs should avoid any sort of sarcastic or threatening messages. The challenge lies in accurately determining whether the recipient will interpret the message as threatening. Without the opportunities of visual and auditory cues, misinterpretation is likely and should be expected.

Emoticons may be used to convey the feeling associated with a message (Table 2-2), but avoid using complex, uncommon symbols that may not be understood by the recipient. Emoticons are increasingly sophisticated and should not be used in any sort of formal e-mail to a supervisor, given the likelihood of confusion. Reserve their use for casual correspondence or to strike a friendly tone :-).

In general, it is best for the CNS to keep e-mail messages and replies brief. Some common abbreviations are used in personal, and occasionally professional, e-mail that may be incorporated into workplace correspondence (Table 2-3). As with emoticons, it is important to make certain that selected abbreviations are easily recognizable. A simple Web-based search using any common search engine provides many examples of frequently used abbreviations. Exclamation points may be useful to demonstrate emphasis or enthusiasm, but make certain to use only one as multiple exclamation points are unnecessary and, at times, may be perceived as irritating.

A few final e-mail caveats deserve emphasis. It is tempting to fire off a response to an incendiary e-mail to immediately set straight the e-mail recipient. As difficult as it may be, the CNS must practice restraint. It is very important to take a time-out before responding.

Table 2-2 EMOTICON EXEMPLARS	
Symbol	**Meaning**
:-) or :)	Smile
;-) or ;)	Wink
:-O or :o	Surprised
:-(or :(	Sad
:-| or :|	Disappointed

Source: Microsoft Corporation, 2006.

Table 2-3	SELECT ELECTRONIC ABBREVIATIONS
Abbreviation	**Meaning**
BFN	Bye for now
IMO	In my opinion
BTW	By the way
LOL	Laughing out loud
HTH	Hope this helps
NRN	No reply necessary
TIA	Thanks in advance

Writing an immediate response may serve as a catharsis for initial emotion; however, once written, the message should not be sent. Most e-mail software gives the user the opportunity to save replies as drafts. Take advantage of the option and save the response. Come back to the original message at a later time, read it again in a calm state, and try to determine whether the initial reaction was appropriate. Then, after reflection, review the drafted response.

Make certain that the written reply is a reasonable, rational, and fair retort. Remember that the response may be circulated to a broader audience or may precipitate an escalated "flame" response. Consider obtaining a second opinion or asking a few clarifying questions.

Quote the original message and backtrack as appropriate. Backtracking involves the use of the caret right (>) sign in front of the words someone else wrote to symbolize quotations (Brinkman & Kirschner, 2002). The CNS must always keep in mind that it takes less time to clarify an issue than it takes to undo the damage associated with an inappropriate, rude, or angry electronic retort (see Exemplar 2-1).

Exemplar 2-1

Taking the Electronic High Road

Richard is a CNS in cardiovascular (CV) care. He has been charged with responsibility for establishing clinical guidelines for managing patients with congestive heart failure (CHF). His multidisciplinary group, comprised of nurses, a CV nurse practitioner, cardiologist, pharmacist, and other nonclinical professionals, has developed evidence-based guidelines that they believe are well suited to the patient population served by this particular acute care setting. The committee has worked for several months and has periodically communicated with various clinicians to solicit input. In preparation for rolling out the guideline, Richard sends a brief, explanatory e-mail with an attached guideline draft to the medical staff. Within an hour, Richard receives an e-mail response from a well-established cardiologist who has been practicing at the hospital for over 30 years. The physician, Dr. Smith, is livid with Richard and the committee and is incensed over the proposed guidelines. The e-mail notes, "The practice of medicine cannot be reduced to a set of guidelines. I refuse to be dictated to by a nurse—go to school, become a doctor, and then try to tell me what to do. My patients trust me and I provide high-quality, individualized care. This guideline is yet another attempt to save money at the expense of our patients! I've already made an appointment to speak with the chairman of the board and will be offering your guideline as yet another example of how patient care is compromised at Get Well Hospital by supposed experts."

Richard's initial response is outrage. He quickly writes a scathing response pointing out the many opportunities for feedback during the guideline development process. Richard notes the importance of evidence-based guidelines and suggests that Dr. Smith would be aware of the importance if he was current in his practice. The e-mail concludes with a hastily constructed, "Go ahead and talk with the chairman. I was assigned this committee job and if my work is not up to par, someone else can do it!"

At this point, it may be wise to consider two possible conclusions.

The First Vignette

Richard hits the "send" button. For a few minutes, Richard feels satisfied in setting straight Dr. Smith. After calming down, Richard becomes increasingly anxious. Dr. Smith is an older physician with long-standing relationships and influence. Dr. Smith is usually rational, and although he can be cantankerous over patient care issues, he is genuinely concerned about his patients. Dr. Smith is considered a nursing champion and is recognized as such by most advanced practice nurses. In fact, Richard usually has an amicable, rather benign relationship with this physician. Richard pulls up his sent response and rereads it. He reads it several times and realizes that although the initial e-mail from Dr. Smith was inappropriate and hostile, Richard has increased the stakes and the hostility by replying in kind. He begins to think about the ramifications of insulting Dr. Smith and writing a flippant comment regarding the chairman. Richard begins to plan a back-out strategy for undoing the predicament in which he now finds himself.

The Second Vignette

Richard rereads his message slowly and looks at his computer screen. Written on a Post-It note is a simple reminder: "Vent it but don't send it." (Brinkman & Kirschner, 2002). Richard saves his response as a draft and leaves his office to get a cup of coffee. He tries to step back from the tone of Dr. Smith's e-mail and consider the variables that may have led to such initial hostility. Richard decides to speak with a cardiologist colleague and get a second opinion.

A few hours later, Richard speaks with his colleague about the guidelines draft and the e-mail response from Dr. Smith. Richard discovers that Dr. Smith is struggling to get insurance company approval for a medical therapy labeled as "experimental" for a middle-aged patient with end-stage congestive heart failure. The patient is doing poorly, and the pressure on Dr. Smith is great. One challenge confronting Dr. Smith is his inability to speak with a physician; rather, the insurance company has him working with a nonphysician representative. The colleague recommends that Richard wait a few days and then approach Dr. Smith personally regarding the proposed guidelines and the angry e-mail response.

Richard returns to his computer, reads his unsent reply, and hits "delete." He has vented his frustration using the computer as a sounding board and now feels calmer. Richard realizes that there was value in writing the response but that sending it would intensify a bad situation and create more work stress for him. Richard's decision does not mean that Dr. Smith is unaccountable for his response. Rather, Richard recognizes that perpetuating electronic hostility is a nonproductive use of his energies and may be counterproductive to the larger goal, approval of the CHF guideline. Richard contacts the cardiology receptionist and schedules a meeting with Dr. Smith.

Tricks for Sending E-Mail

There are times when CNSs need to send a relatively important e-mail that is deserving of immediate review. Similar to making a decision as to whether to send paper mail via first class or priority mail, CNSs need to think about whether an e-mail should be sent with a priority notation. Avoid overusing this function. There are times when individuals use priority designations so frequently that the red font and exclamation mark associated with priority status lose their impact.

Other convenient functions associated with sent messages are the delivery receipt and read receipt. A delivery receipt informs the sender that the electronic message has been received by the designated e-mail address. The read receipt notifies the sender that the message has been read by the recipient.

A word of caution is needed, as most read receipt functions inform the recipient that a read receipt has been requested and ask for permission to notify the sender that the message has been read. If the recipient declines the notification opportunity, the sender will not know that the message has been read. This is why it may be a good idea to consistently send a delivery receipt notification request with a read receipt.

These options are available through most e-mail software, although the function button locations vary. CNSs may also find it useful to access the help function if they are unable to locate the mail priority, delivery receipt, or read receipt functions.

Organizing E-Mail

It is surprising how many CNSs do not use the helpful organizing functions available in most popular e-mail software. The underutilization of filing options and the overuse of server memory can pose significant problems. CNSs should become familiar with the many varied options of the workplace e-mail system to maximize efficiency.

Most e-mail software allows users to select inbox and sent message functions. For example, some systems have an established default that saves copies of all sent messages. The sender is able to modify this default to individually select sent messages requiring a saved copy. This function reduces the number of individually saved messages. By reducing the number of saved message copies, the CNS will also reduce server memory use.

Server memory is an important consideration for the entire e-mail community of the organization. Attachments containing pictures, documents, and PowerPoint presentations can be very large files. CNSs can review their inbox and check the size of each message file. Make certain to clear particularly large files as soon as possible using the Save As function and migrating the files to more appropriate locations. Then delete the e-mail with the attachment.

Inbox messages can usually be read without deciding whether to delete or save the message. It may be tempting for the CNS to quickly read messages without deleting or filing. This e-mail practice can lead to cluttered inboxes making it difficult to retrieve important messages when needed at a later date.

CNSs should consider developing a pattern of inbox message scrutiny that relies on immediate decisions regarding deleting or filing. E-mail software provides options for creating a file directory. CNSs can create files with short clear names that allow inbox mail to be categorized in a meaningful way.

Similar to the filing system popular in Microsoft Windows Explorer, most e-mail platforms allow CNSs to create a file folder, point and click on an e-mail message, and drag the message to an appropriate folder. The individual message or folder can be reviewed and saved or deleted at a later date. Some e-mail messages do not warrant filing and should be immediately deleted after review.

There are times when servers crash, files become corrupted, and systems fail. With these scenarios in mind, CNSs should selectively print hard copies of vital e-mail correspondence. Hard copies should be scarce or the CNS runs the risk of duplicating digital records without good reason. However, there are certainly isolated e-mails that should be saved and protected beyond ordinary digital filing. A reasonable rule of thumb is for CNSs to view e-mail as similar to hard copy files and, as with paper, discard e-mail that is trivial or insignificant.

E-mail has certainly changed communication practices in all venues—including work and home. The advantages of instant communication outweigh the disadvantages. The skillful CNS will recognize the benefits of e-mail and take full advantage of digital communication while remaining wary of its potential for misuse.

Voice Mail and Computer Usage Tips

CNSs need to remember that telephone records, voice-mail messaging systems, and computer terminal activities are employer owned and are not private. Employers have the right to access telephone usage records and may monitor calls, although some states do require employers to notify employees if calls will be recorded or monitored (PRC, 2006). Voice-mail messages may be backed up on magnetic tape in the event that call retrieval is necessary, making it difficult for an employee to know with certainty that calls have been deleted.

In general, CNSs should assume that workplace communications are not private. There are times when personal calls are necessarily placed during work time; however, CNSs may want to consider using a personal cell phone for these types of calls

(PRC, 2006). Another important consideration to keep in mind is that inappropriate communication is neither acceptable nor wise, particularly during work hours. Voice-mail messages may be forwarded, calls may be tracked, and computer usage may be monitored for both time on computer systems as well as specifics related to Web-site activities.

Organizing Successful Meetings

CNSs are often involved in committees as members or as chairpersons. Successful meetings are chaired by effective people who purposively prepare to achieve deliberately selected goals (Table 2-4). Disorganized, poorly planned meetings with no clear goals reflect poorly on the chair and discourage committee members from active engagement in group processes. Agendas drive meetings, and agenda preparation is important.

Arranging the Meeting

Arranging a meeting time that works for multiple committee members can be a daunting task. If a CNS has an administrative assistant available to handle meeting arrangements, it is certainly easier to coordinate a convenient date and time, but scheduling a meeting is still an arduous task. Most CNSs find themselves relying on

Table 2-4   **MEETING PREPARATION CHECKLIST**
Activity
1. Solicit agenda items from committee members.
2. Create an agenda with clear designations of work and responsibilities in preparation for the meeting.
3. Assign a recording secretary for the meeting and place assignation on the agenda.
4. Arrange for a meeting room and refreshments, if appropriate.
5. Distribute the agenda with a copy of the previous minutes. Note the room and time. Request RSVP, regrets only, from committee members.
6. Provide a template for the minutes.
7. Make certain invited guests or committee members have necessary equipment ordered prior to the meeting; for example, overhead projector equipment.
8. Prepare materials for duplicating. If electronic materials are used, send as e-mail attachments with the agenda and old minutes. Make certain that committee members have at least 1 week to review materials. Two weeks is preferable.

multiple e-mails, personal conversations, or telephone messages in an effort to win-now down tentative dates and times for meetings.

There are Web-based scheduling systems available to CNSs that are convenient and free, providing that only basic services are required. Doodle (http://www.doodle.ch/main.html) is useful for scheduling events or polling e-mail recipients. MeetingWizard is a useful tool when scheduling meetings. It provides the CNS with the opportunity to simultaneously send a list of potential dates and times to multiple committee members. The system does not yet permit recurring meeting dates (Meeting-Wizard, 2008) but is a very convenient way to arrange for single meetings.

In the MeetingWizard system, the CNS begins by entering a variety of potential dates and times. The CNS does not need an account to use the basic services. Committee members' e-mail addresses are then entered. Members receive an e-mail asking them to respond to the various date and time combinations. This information is collated by MeetingWizard, and the CNS is notified of the best date and time for the meeting. The resource is Web-based, so it does not require a particular e-mail system. This characteristic is particularly important when committee members include individuals who are not employees of the organization.

Agendas and Goal Setting

Agenda preparation provides an excellent opportunity for meeting planning. The CNS should reflect on the main objective of the meeting, whether this is an agenda for a standing committee that meets on a regularly scheduled basis or a more impromptu ad hoc meeting. The agenda should be distributed prior to the meeting. Include the date, start time, end time, and meeting location.

If recording responsibilities are shared by committee members, it is helpful to identify the meeting's assigned recording secretary on the agenda. This notification alerts the recorder of the need for a laptop, audiotape recorder, or if this particular individual cannot attend the meeting, it places responsibility for finding a substitute squarely on the assigned recorder. Assigning responsibility for minute taking or cajoling members into taking minutes at the start of a meeting conveys a disorganized tone that may influence the dynamic of the committee group process, particularly in more formal meetings.

Consider the desired outcomes of the committee meeting and the preparation that is required of each committee member to accomplish the objectives. Distribute materials as far in advance of the meeting as possible. Remember, members cannot get their work finished if they receive materials at short notice. Many chairs attach old minutes to the new agenda to draw the committee's attention back to previously discussed items that continue to require resolution or ongoing work.

Agenda building may be formal or informal. In general, customary activities lead to a finalized agenda. First, members should be asked to forward items to the chair for the agenda. Timing is important, so make certain to give the members enough time to think about important items but not so much time that the participant places the need for agenda items at the bottom of a to-do list and forgets to submit.

Second, provide committee members with a deadline for agenda items to avoid last-minute changes. The CNS needs to decide whether it is acceptable to include late agenda items. Make certain to carefully discuss agenda items with the person submitting them to avoid any confusion.

Most agendas follow a standard format (Table 2-5). The meeting begins with a call to order. Attendance is checked, and depending on the type of committee, a quorum is established.

A quorum is the minimum number of committee members required to conduct the business of the group. Usually a quorum is defined as a majority; however, this standard varies by committee. In committees with formal structures and processes, the quorum is usually established in the organizational bylaws. Without a quorum, the status quo cannot be changed. If there is not a quorum, any decisions requiring votes, including motions, need to wait until a quorum is available.

The chair may follow the call to order with a brief review of the measurable objectives set for the particular meeting. This strategy focuses the group on the tasks at hand and facilitates a shared consensus about the intent of the meeting. The call to order and brief introduction is usually followed by old business.

New business items are discussed next, followed by announcements. The meeting concludes with instructions regarding the scheduling of the next committee meeting, if an additional meeting is necessary. The meeting concludes with a formal adjournment by the chairperson.

Documenting the Work of the Committee

Committee minutes are critically important. Similar to the popular premise underlying nursing charting, if it isn't documented, it wasn't done—minutes document the work and accomplishments of the committee. They provide a context for evaluating the progress of the committee. Minutes keep people current with the committee's

Table 2-5   STRUCTURING A MEETING
Organization Name
Committee Name
Date of Meeting
I. Call to Order
II. Old Business
A. Items are drawn from previous meeting's minutes
III. New Business
IV. Announcements
V. Adjournment

work by allowing new members, supervisors, and members who miss an occasional meeting to be apprised of the committee's work.

The recording secretary, or in lieu of an established secretary, the chairperson, is responsible for tracking minutes. Minutes should be documented using a word processor during or immediately following the meeting. An electronic record and paper copy should be saved.

At the conclusion of the committee year, usually the fiscal, calendar, or academic year, the minutes may be saved to a compact disc (CD) for easy retrieval. CDs are also convenient during accreditation visits, as missing minutes can be easily replaced and surveyors can quickly scan minutes using a laptop computer. Eliminating paper copies of minutes beyond 1 year can also substantially reduce file clutter, and CD copies protect server memory capacities. Another suggestion is to maintain hard copies of minutes and supporting materials in a 5-inch binder that may be easily transported to meetings and accessed quickly if computer access is unavailable.

It may be helpful for CNSs to develop a standard format for the minutes. Providing a written or electronic template (Table 2-6) can ensure that minutes are recorded consistently between meetings. If recording responsibilities are shared and rotated among committee members, having a template can be a real time saver and is often

Table 2-6   TEMPLATE FOR MINUTES

Name of Organization
Name of Committee
Date of Meeting

Present:
Excused absences:

Agenda Item	Discussion	Outcome
I. Call to Order		
II. Old Business		
A. Agenda Item		
III. New Business		
A. Agenda Item		
IV. Announcements		
A. Next Meeting Date and Time		
V. Adjournment		

Respectfully submitted,
Recording secretary signature
Recording secretary name

appreciated by the recorder. If the meeting's recorder prefers taking handwritten minutes, a template can make it easier for the secretary to follow when word processing.

Isolating a column specific to outcomes related to each item of business facilitates follow-through and helps to clearly establish who is responsible for what and by when. Both the recorder and the chairperson should make certain that each agenda item has an agreed-on outcome or action plan. The chairperson needs to lead the group, and determining end points and responsibilities for the work of a committee is very important. Too often committee discussions are abstract or broad without resolution or measurable outcomes. Compelling an outcome or action plan for each agenda item ensures that members leave the meeting with a clear sense of their assignments.

Minutes are also used to construct the next meeting's agenda. Old business items for the agenda are taken from the previous sets of minutes. New business items should be new to the work of the committee. Minutes provide the necessary data for subsequent agendas. The cycle perpetuates itself, so organizing minutes is well worth the time and effort.

Controlling the Committee

Asserting control in an economical fashion is crucial to ensuring the best use of people's time and achieving the meeting's aims (Banks, 2002). Establishing an agenda is one control mechanism. Asking open questions to stimulate discussion, closed questions to narrow discussion, and directed questions to encourage participation are communication strategies that enhance control and assist in getting work finished (Banks, 2002).

Applying *Robert's Rules of Order* (Robert, Evans, Honemann, & Balch, 2004) is another control strategy that brings order from potentially chaotic meeting situations. Many CNSs have participated in meetings that strictly or loosely follow *Robert's Rules*. As an aside, the rules were originally developed by Henry Martyn Robert in 1876 (Robert's Rules Association [RRA], 2006) after presiding over a church meeting and realizing that he did not know how to effectively use parliamentary law.

Robert was an engineering officer in the regular Army and lived in a variety of places in the United States. He found that different parts of the country had different interpretations of parliamentary procedure, and so he wrote *Robert's Rules of Order*. These rules are now in their 10th edition and are used by many organizations and governments as parliamentary authority (RRA, 2006).

CNSs may find that most committees perform more efficiently when *Robert's Rules of Order* are followed. These rules are very formal and inalienable and so are probably less appropriate for casual meetings or small groups. Chairs may be well-advised to consistently use select procedural rules to avoid chaos (Table 2-7). One specific example might be to allow committee members to speak only after recognition from the chair. This rule prevents members from interrupting others or boisterously dominating a meeting. It also facilitates difficult conversations by directing members to the chair rather than to a member when disagreements arise.

Table 2-7   BASIC STRATEGIES FOR MAINTAINING ORDER

1. Establish a deadline for submitting items to the chair for agenda consideration.
2. Develop a thoughtful agenda appropriate to the length of available meeting time.
3. Distribute the agenda 5 to 10 business days prior to the meeting, depending on the frequency of meetings.
4. Attach previous meeting minutes to the new agenda.
5. Create a minutes template for the recorder. Include action/outcomes column.
6. Follow select parliamentary rules of order.
7. Summarize action plan and members' responsibilities at meeting's conclusion.
8. Follow-up meeting with electronic reminders of agreed-on action items and upcoming meeting date.

In conclusion, CNSs are involved in many sorts of committees, either as members or as officers. Chairing a committee is rewarding work that has the potential to become frustrating if the CNS does not have the requisite skills. Keeping the group focused, controlled within reason, and ensuring documentation of the committee work are a few functions of committee chairs. Preparation is key and can make the difference between a productive committee and an inefficient committee. In general, CNSs are well suited to committee work given their focus on the influence of individuals, groups, and systems.

Communicating Professionalism

The term *professional presentation* usually conjures a vision of a CNS standing in front of a filled room presenting a topic of interest. Sharing work and promoting scholarly practice are certainly integral to the CNS role. It is also important for CNSs to appreciate that each day and in every encounter they present themselves to individuals and groups in both informal and formal settings. Communicating professionalism is a critical component of an individual's practice as a CNS.

Whether a CNS is presenting to a group or presenting her- or himself to others as a professional, understanding the nature of professional behavior is imperative. The word *professional* is used in all types of venues, just as *unprofessional* is used to connote some type of behavior or characteristic that is less than that desired of a true professional. The underlying assumption is that the professional ideal is a shared concept. In fact, CNSs probably have divergent views on professionalism. CNSs know what professionalism is when they see it but may have a difficult time agreeing on its attributes.

Grove and Hallowell (2002) offered an interesting perspective on professional behavior based on their research. They explored what it means to behave as a professional in the United States and uncovered that behaving professionally is a balancing act between contrasting cultural values.

In addition to the seven balancing acts (Figure 2-1), professional behavior includes presentable appearance, reliability, conscientiousness, and a nonjudgmental disposition (Grove & Hallowell, 2002). This model provides an interesting perspective and helps make sense of the tensions CNSs experience as they try to juggle between the contrasting cultural values. It also helps CNSs better appreciate the challenges experienced by foreign nurses, medical residents, and other healthcare professionals as they attempt to navigate the healthcare system.

For example, most CNSs realize that healthcare professionals are conscious of hierarchy while recognizing that American society is based on egalitarian premises. This

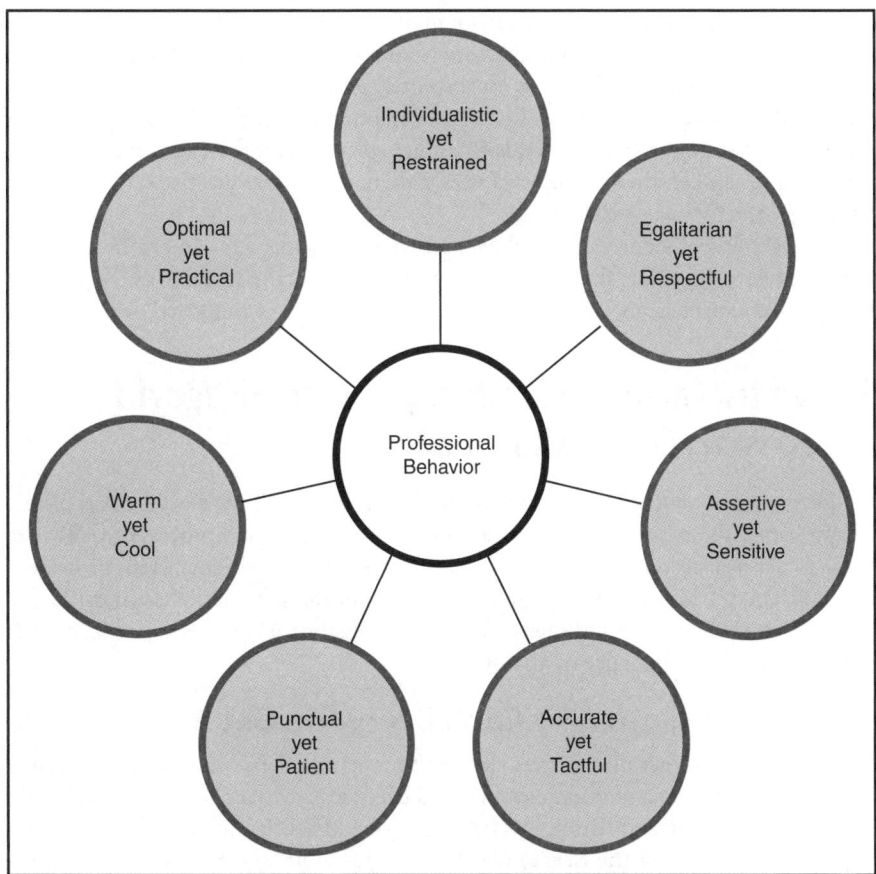

Figure 2-1   Seven balancing acts of professional behavior in the United States.

Source: © Grove, C., & Hallowell, W. (2002). Published by GROVEWELL LLC. Reprinted with permission. Available at: www.grovewell.com/pub-usa-professional.html

idea may explain why CNSs may engage in friendly banter with attending physicians and may interact as colleagues when discussing patient care, yet may refer to attending physicians using the title "Doctor," whereas attending physicians refer to CNSs on a first-name basis without a formal prefix (e.g., "Mrs." or "Mr."). The difference in communication style is anecdotally attributed to social status and traditional female versus male roles; however, the Grove and Hallowell (2002) model suggests that people in the United States are generally conscious of hierarchy, and friendly equality should not be confused with social prestige awarded to and expected by people based on income, education, and history.

CNSs are expected to be warm and friendly while being careful to not become so chummy with staff or other healthcare professionals that they lose the ability to wield influence to improve care or accomplish goals. CNSs are valued as individuals, and being set apart because of a unique attribute can be beneficial, providing the attribute is viewed as individualistic rather than weird or strange. The difficult aspect of these contrasting values is that there are no absolutes. Attempting to describe to the new CNS or the graduate student enrolled in a CNS program the fact that being punctual is good and holding staff accountable for punctuality is appropriate but that this concern with time needs to be tempered with patience begs the questions, "How much patience?" and "When is late too late?"

An awareness of Grove and Hallowell's seven balancing acts can attune CNSs to the necessity of gauging the reactions of colleagues specific to these behaviors and learning the expectations of the culture in which the CNS is employed or practices.

Surviving and Flourishing in a Work World Filled with Difficult People

CNSs are usually effective communicators. They work well with others and have a clear grasp of the basic principles of communication and group processes. CNSs are often asked to intervene in situations that involve difficult patients, staff, or healthcare colleagues based on their prowess as communicators. Nonetheless, most CNSs concur that there are many times in real-world practice when working nicely with others demands the patience of a saint.

The CNS Lament: Why Can't Everyone Get Along?

It is a simple truth that no one gets along with everyone. CNSs may find themselves assigned to committees, working groups, and task forces with colleagues who they do not prefer. Brinkman and Kirschner (2002) described 10 different types of people who are difficult. They offer the *Lens of Understanding* (Figure 2-2) for viewing interpersonal dynamics and understanding the focuses and needs of these 10 types during normal periods and during times of increased demands.

The *Lens of Understanding* is constructed with a normal zone and four primary foci of intents: "get the task done; get the task right; get along with people; and get appre-

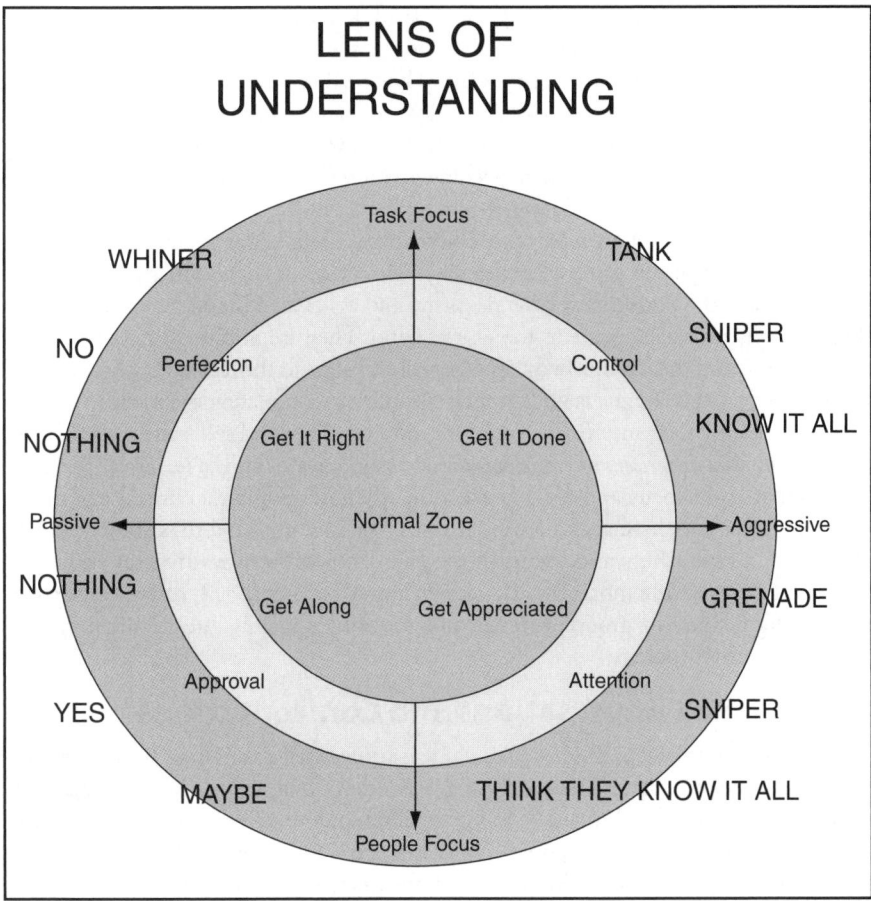

Figure 2-2   Lens of understanding.

Source: © R & R Productions. Published by McGraw-Hill, 1994, 2002. Reprinted with permission.

ciation from people" (Brinkman & Kirschner, 2002, p. 15). As stress is applied to the system, the four basic types of people begin to further differentiate into their more extreme condition. For example, the individual who is motivated to be appreciated by colleagues at work may exhibit attention-seeking behaviors during stressful working group activities. With continued stress, this person snipes at the chairperson or becomes explosive and grenadelike.

The *Lens of Understanding* (Brinkman & Kirschner, 2002) is an excellent resource. Nurses in graduate courses have been encouraged to read this book, and they rave about its helpfulness. The nurses share that they developed a better appreciation for the motivations underlying the behaviors of difficult people. Many times, they have also discovered that *they* are the difficult ones with whom to work.

The four basic intents underlying the difficult behavior categories are general but useful. The CNS may be able to identify colleagues who are primarily focused on getting assigned tasks completed. They want to know what is required and accomplish it as efficiently as possible. These sorts of colleagues can be quite useful on committees, as they tend to take responsibility for completing work and help to keep the group moving. However, once the stakes become greater, these get-it-done colleagues can become aggressive and act as know-it-alls.

Using the *Lens of Understanding*, the CNS may be able to better understand why, when this task-focused person is placed under stress with deadlines or seemingly insurmountable workload, the person may become pushy and aggressive (Brinkman & Kirschner, 2002). Their comments relate to the task at hand. They are not interested in chitchat. Rather, they want the job finished. Whether it is finished to the desired quality standard of the get-it-right colleague is not as much a priority as completing the work.

This typology is an interesting tool for group exercises and self-reflection. It is interesting to apply the *Lens of Understanding* to work groups and to family. If the CNS has a get-it-right focus and seeks perfection when developing a clinical algorithm, there may be interpersonal challenges if this CNS is committed to work with a get-it-done colleague who wants to finish the algorithm without waiting for additional references or reviewing more data. Brinkman and Kirschner (2002) offered many suggestions for facilitating group processes and promoting healthy interpersonal dynamics based on this typology.

High-Stake Conversations and Confrontations

CNSs regularly engage in high-stakes conversations with a variety of healthcare personnel and stakeholders. These exchanges are described as "crucial conversations" (Patterson, Grenny, McMillan, & Switzler, 2002, p. 3) because they are high-stakes discussions involving two or more persons with varied opinions and strong emotions (Patterson et al.). CNSs may find it difficult to effectively handle these dialogues, preferring to avoid them or recognizing that they do not have the necessary skill set to achieve a successful outcome.

There are resources available to assist CNSs with developing and enhancing the communication tools necessary for important conversations (Patterson et al., 2002) and necessary confrontations (Patterson, Grenny, McMillan, & Switzler, 2005). Mastering the ability to transcend habitual, ineffective responses to high-stress conversations is imperative, particularly when working with teams composed of various types of professionals and practitioners. CNSs are recognized as systems experts, and the ability to influence systems of all sorts requires a superb ability to master difficult conversations. High-performing CNSs must know how to confront administrators, physicians, and high-powered colleagues without committing professional suicide (see Exemplar 2-2).

CNSs often work in teams. Some teams work in a parallel fashion, drawing information from each other without developing a common understanding of the issues that could affect the group's work or the problem at hand. Other teams are interprofessional, using inclusive language to share information and collaboratively work to-

Ensuring Accuracy with Tact

Bernie Ward, MSN, RN, ACNS-BC, CDE, is employed by a community hospital to establish community diabetes outreach programs and to assist the nursing staff in their efforts to improve inpatient nursing care related to diabetes management. In particular, Bernie's job is to guide the RN staff to a higher quality of diabetes nursing care. Bernie had 12 years of experience as a certified diabetes educator (CDE) at a local teaching hospital prior to accepting this job at Smithville Hospital. She has been at Smithville Hospital for 7 months. Bernie is smart, conscientious, and reliable. She has a good reputation in general but is warily regarded by the medical–surgical nursing staff, who see Bernie as someone who may report them if diabetes care is amiss.

During a meeting, Bernie is asked to comment on the progress made toward meeting the established inpatient goal of 100% compliance with nursing documentation specific to medical nutrition therapy and self-monitoring of blood glucose for patients admitted with diabetes mellitus as a primary or secondary diagnosis. Bernie shares the lack of progress on one particular nursing unit as compared to two others. She accurately notes that the nurses on the more successful units, 4 West and 6 South, are eager to learn and seem pleased with the opportunity to improve their teaching and documentation, whereas "the nurses on 2 North are pretty disagreeable. It's difficult to get anything done on that unit simply because the nurses are generally disinterested and annoyed by the suggestion that they need to do things differently. The nurses page me for all the patient teaching and seem to be really uncomfortable providing the level of instruction that even nursing students are able to handle."

Bernie was honest in her representation of 2 North staff. However, she was not tactful. The director of nursing (DON) was present at this multidisciplinary meeting and felt that her leadership was reflected poorly by Bernie's comments. This particular unit had experienced administrative turnover several times in the past 2 years and was now managed by an inexperienced nurse manager. The unit's census had been running high due to the closure of an adjoining unit, and the staff was frustrated. These circumstances did not justify the lack of attention paid to meeting the standards for diabetes mellitus nursing care; however, the lack of progress shared by the CNS was perceived as tactless due to the abruptness of the criticism and the lack of explanation related to the context of the perceived inadequacy of nursing care.

Following the meeting, the DON met with Bernie privately to share her assessment of Bernie's unprofessional behavior. Bernie was dismayed, as she believed her brief explanation was accurate and honest, although it may have been less tactful than necessary. The DON reinforced with Bernie that as a result of her indiscreet comments, the new nurse manager and the staff of 2 North were going to feel further alienated from Bernie. The DON reiterated her expectation that Bernie balance honesty with tact and appreciate the impact that accurate but tactless comments could have on the dynamic of the nursing group in which Bernie needed to effect change.

ward a commonly understood end (Sheehan, Robertson, & Ormond, 2007). Learning to discover or invent a mutual purpose (Patterson et al., 2002) may contribute to effective teamwork, particularly for teams striving for a collaborative approach to problem solving.

To successfully build a repertoire of strategies designed to persuade others, avoid anger and hurt feelings, and establish a safe conversational context within which to discuss high-stakes concerns, CNSs must first understand their personal reactions to difficult encounters and learn to monitor their responses to stress (Patterson et al., 2002). CNSs should consider taking stock of their strengths and challenges related to difficult conversations and crucial confrontations by soliciting feedback from valued peers and supervisors. Using self-help resources and attending continuing education programs may also be useful strategies.

The CNS's contribution to effective teamwork must not be limited to the traditional notion of "team." CNSs also need to work toward improving dialogue with practitioners of complementary and alternative medicine (CAM) and integrative medicine. As people increase their demand for CAM, there is an enhanced need for practitioners of all types to better communicate with one another (Benedict, 2007).

The Integrative Medicine Alliance (IMA) fosters communication and collaboration between conventional and CAM practitioners in order to improve the quality of the human experience of health care (IMA, 2008a). This organization provides opportunities for CNSs to connect with CAM practitioners in efforts to improve patients' healthcare experiences. It is a grassroots effort located in Massachusetts and with members from across the country. CNSs interested in learning more about CAM or intrigued by the possibilities of better connecting traditional medication to CAM may be interested in exploring IMA's various educational programs. Select topics include theta healing, medicinal plant walks, Native American spirituality, laughter yoga, and various forms of meditation (IMA, 2008b).

Avoiding Naïveté When Navigating Dangerous Waters

CNSs must be very strategic in their interactions with other health professionals, including physicians. Working strategically requires excellent communication skills, a talent for handling difficult situations without an aggressive or withdrawn stress response, and a keen sense of organizational politics. It is not uncommon for CNSs to have difficulties in the workplace because of an inadequate appreciation for strategic alliances.

"How to Swim with Sharks" (Cousteau, 1987) is a wonderful piece that offers opportunities for personal reflection as well as lively discussion (see Exemplar 2-3). Use this piece as a stimulus for frank group discussion and also to illustrate some of the characteristics inherent in a very political environment. It can be interesting and informative to consider the applicability of the various rules to life in the waters of health care.

Excellent Interviews: Knowing What to Ask and How to Ask It

Conducting a great interview is a skill that can be developed with effort and practical information. It is not uncommon for CNSs to participate in interviewing applicants for positions as advanced practice nurses, administrators, or staff. As shared

Swimming with Sharks: An Interesting Exemplar to Stimulate Discussion

How to Swim with Sharks: A Primer

Voltaire Cousteau

Foreword

Actually, nobody wants to swim with sharks. It is not an acknowledged sport and it is neither enjoyable nor exhilarating. These instructions are written primarily for the benefit of those, who, by virtue of their occupation, find they must swim and find that the water is infested with sharks.

It is of obvious importance to learn that the waters are shark infested before commencing to swim. It is safe to say that this initial determination has already been made. If the waters were infested, the naïve swimmer is by now probably beyond help; at the very least, he has doubtless lost any interest in learning how to swim with sharks.

Finally, swimming with sharks is like any other skill: It cannot be learned from books alone; the novice must practice in order to develop the skill. The following rules simply set forth the fundamental principles which, if followed will make it possible to survive while becoming expert through practice.

Rules

1. **Assume all unidentified fish are sharks.** Not all sharks look like sharks, and some fish that are not sharks sometimes act like sharks. Unless you have witnessed docile behavior in the presence of shed blood on more than one occasion, it is best to assume an unknown species is a shark. Inexperienced swimmers have been badly mangled by assuming that docile behavior in the absence of blood indicates that the fish is not a shark.

2. **Do not bleed.** It is a cardinal principle that if you are injured, either by accident or by intent, you must not bleed. Experience shows that bleeding prompts an even more aggressive attack and will often provoke the participation of sharks that are uninvolved or, as noted previously, are usually docile.

3. Admittedly, it is difficult not to bleed when injured. Indeed, at first this may seem impossible. Diligent practice, however, will permit the experienced swimmer to sustain a serious laceration without bleeding and without even exhibiting any loss of composure. This hemostatic reflex can, in part, be conditioned, but there may be constitutional aspects as well. Those who cannot learn to control their bleeding should not attempt to swim with sharks, for the peril is too great.

   The control of bleeding has a positive protective element for the swimmer. The shark will be confused as to whether or not his attack has injured you and confusion is to the swimmer's advantage. On the other hand, the shark may know he has injured you and be puzzled as to why you do not bleed or show distress. This also has a profound effect on sharks. They begin to question their own potency or, alternatively, believe the swimmer to have supernatural powers.

4. **Counter any aggression promptly.** Sharks rarely attack a swimmer without warning. Usually there is some tentative, exploratory aggressive action. It is important that the swimmer recognize that this behavior is a prelude to an attack and takes prompt and vigorous remedial action. The appropriate countermove is a sharp blow to the nose. Almost invariably this will prevent a full-scale attack, for it makes it clear that you understand the shark's intention and are prepared to use whatever force is necessary to repel aggressive actions.

5. Some swimmers mistakenly believe that an ingratiating attitude will dispel an attack under these circumstances. This is not correct; such a response provokes a shark attack. Those who hold this erroneous view can usually be identified by their missing limb.

6. **Get out of the water if someone is bleeding.** If a swimmer (or shark) has been injured and is bleeding, get out of the water promptly. The presence of blood and the thrashing of water will elicit aggressive behavior even in the most docile of sharks. This latter group, poorly skilled in attacking, often behaves irrationally and may attack uninvolved swimmers and sharks. Some are so inept that, in the confusion, they injure themselves.

7. No useful purpose is served in attempting to rescue the injured swimmer. He either will or will not survive the attack, and your intervention cannot protect him once blood has been shed. Those who survive such an attack rarely venture to swim with sharks again, an attitude which is readily understandable.

   The lack of effective countermeasures to a fully developed shark attack emphasizes the importance of the earlier rules.

8. **Use anticipatory retaliation.** A constant danger to the skilled swimmer is that the shark will forget that he is skilled and may attack in error. Some sharks have notoriously poor memories in this regard. This memory loss can be prevented by a program of anticipatory retaliation. The skilled swimmer should engage in these activities periodically and the periods should be less than the memory span of the shark. Thus, it is not possible to state fixed intervals. The procedure may need to be repeated frequently with forgetful sharks and need be done only once for sharks with total recall.

9. The procedure is essentially the same as described under rule 4: a sharp blow to the nose. Here, however, the blow is unexpected and serves to remind the shark that you are both alert and unafraid. Swimmers should take care not to injure the shark and draw blood during this exercise for two reasons: First, sharks often bleed profusely, and this leads to the chaotic situation described under rule 6. Second, if swimmers act in this fashion, it may not be possible to distinguish swimmers from sharks. Indeed, renegade swimmers are far worse than sharks, for none of the rules or measures described here is effective in controlling their aggressive behavior.

10. **Disorganized and organized attack.** Usually sharks are sufficiently self-centered that they do not act in concert against a swimmer. This lack of organization greatly reduces the risk of swimming among sharks. However, upon occasion the sharks may launch a coordinated attack upon a swimmer or even upon one of their number. While the latter event is of no particular concern to a swimmer, it is essential that one know how to handle an organized shark attack directed against a swimmer.

    The proper strategy is diversion. Sharks can be diverted from their organized attack in one of two ways. First, sharks as a group, are prone to internal dissension. An experienced swimmer can divert an organized attack by introducing something, often minor or trivial, which sets the sharks to fighting among themselves. Usually by the time the internal conflict is settled the sharks cannot even recall what they were setting about to do, much less get organized to do it.

A second mechanism of diversion is to introduce something that so enrages the members of the group that they begin to lash out in all directions, even attacking inanimate objects in their fury.

What should be introduced? Unfortunately, different things prompt internal dissension of blind fury in different groups of sharks. Here one must be experienced in dealing with a given group of sharks, for what enrages one group will pass unnoted by another.

It is scarcely necessary to state that it is unethical for a swimmer under attack by a group of sharks to counter the attack by diverting them to another swimmer. It is, however, common to see this done by novice swimmers and by sharks when under concerted attack.

*Little is known about the author, who died in Paris in 1812. He may have been a descendant of Francois Voltaire and an ancestor of Jacques Cousteau. Apparently this essay was written for sponge divers. Because it may have broader implications, it was translated from the French by Richard J. Johns, an obscure French scholar and Massey Professor and director of the Department of Biomedical Engineering, The Johns Hopkins University and Hospital, 720 Rutland Avenue, Baltimore, Maryland 21203.

Source: Cousteau, V. (1987). How to swim with sharks: A primer. *Perspectives in Biology and Medicine, 30*(4), 486–489. © The Johns Hopkins University Press. Reprinted with permission of The Johns Hopkins University Press.

governance processes become more widespread, staff is also increasingly involved in the interview process and may require the guidance of the CNS. It is important for CNSs to have a basic understanding of interview processes, including the permissibility of certain types of questions. Conducting a successful interview not only leads to the acquisition of useful, accurate information from applicants, it also facilitates relationship building and assists in avoiding litigious situations.

Selecting people with a solid clinical skill set is no longer sufficient to ensuring quality patient care outcomes. Nurses need to be able to work as team members. Communication skills are critical. Nurses must be technically proficient and able to acquire information using the World Wide Web and electronic databases.

Evaluating job candidates for these necessary skills sets is difficult when interviews are unstructured or casual. It may be helpful for CNSs who are involved in preemployment interviews to consider developing an interview query path prior to actually conducting the interview. Soliciting input from staff and colleagues for structured interview guidelines supports consistent interviewing processes within the department. A group interview tool encourages collection of objective data that the group has identified as important (Lindaman, 1997) and also allows for objective comparisons between candidates (Pearce, 2007).

Even with a structured interview format that has been established with group input, there will be differences in interviewers' judgments as to a candidate's desirability. Graves and Karren (1996) suggest that there are four causes of idiosyncratic interview decisions (Table 2-8). These idiosyncrasies may explain how several CNSs interviewing a candidate for a CNS position that is vacant can have very different views of the applicant's suitability for the job.

One possible explanation for the difference in conclusions may be that each CNS has a personal preference for a personality or communication style. Some may be looking for advanced practice registered nursing (APRN) experience, whereas another is more concerned about the type of institutions in which the applicant has previously worked. Some of these issues can be resolved by proactive discussions preceding interviews on what skills, experiences, and attributes are most highly preferred.

Sometimes interviewers' abilities to digest and synthesize information differ, and this difference influences interview decisions. Some interviewees are intent on detail and do a fine job of recalling detail as compared to others who struggle with remembering information.

Graves and Karren (1996) noted that idiosyncratic differences also relate to whether interviewers react intuitively versus analytically to interviewing decisions. They suggest that intuitive judgments may be less accurate and are probably more difficult to defend. CNSs may collaborate with the interview colleagues to develop checklists or data collection forms that would be helpful in the interviewing decision process. These forms would differ depending on the position.

Demographic similarities may also influence interview decisions (Graves & Karren, 1996). When applicants share traits and experiences with the interviewer, they have commonalities and connect on a variety of levels. This connecting experience is different when two people have very little in common.

Table 2-8   CAUSES OF IDIOSYNCRATIC INTERVIEW DECISIONS

1) Interviewers' views of the ideal applicant
   i) Differences in beliefs about the characteristics of the ideal applicant
2) Interviewers' information-processing skills
   i) Differences in the ability to recall information about the applicants and to utilize and combine information about multiple criteria in the decision process
3) Similarity bias
   i) Preferences for applicants who share interviewers' characteristics
4) Interviewers' behaviors
   i) Differences in social competence and general approach to interview

Source: © 1996 by John Wiley & Sons, Inc. Reprinted with permission.

The interviewer's interpersonal skills also affect interview decisions (Graves & Karren, 1996). Personable, engaging interviewers who know how to draw information from applicants elicit more detail from candidates than interviewers with fewer people skills. Inappropriate comments, joking, and personal observations may also influence the interview decision; however, there is variability in what people label as inappropriate behaviors or comments. It is wise to avoid any sort of questionable communications during an interview.

Given the potential for variability in interviewing outcomes based on the interviewer rather than the qualifications of the candidate, it is important for the CNSs involved in interviewing processes to develop some type of guidelines for group and individual interviews. After all, the organization is adversely affected when less noteworthy candidates are hired instead of qualified candidates with potential.

In addition, developing guidelines and developing query paths based on collective input from the CNS group or staff group encourages the professional development of all concerned. Frank discussions help clarify values and compel people to articulate what is important to them.

Graves and Karren (1996) offered five action steps for improving interview decisions (Table 2-9). Increasing the structure of the interview process may result in more

---

Table 2-9   ACTION STEPS FOR IMPROVING INTERVIEW DECISIONS

Step 1—Develop selection criteria.

Determine the knowledge, skills, and abilities required to perform the job, as well as any characteristics needed to function in the broader organizational environment. Determine which of these criteria are most important.

Step 2—Determine how criteria will be assessed.

Determine which of the criteria can be assessed in the interview and which should be measured using other techniques.

Step 3—Develop interview guide.

Develop a semistructured interview guide to assess any criteria identified in Step 1 and determined to be suitable for assessment in the interview in Step 2.

Step 4—Train interviewers.

Train interviewers to use the interview guide and teach them how to have positive interactions with applicants.

Step 5—Monitor the effectiveness of interviews.

Collect data on the job performance, job satisfaction, and retention of new employees. Evaluate and reward managers based on their selection decisions.

Source: © 1996 by John Wiley & Sons, Inc. Reprinted with permission.

uniform decision making. CNSs should consider the usefulness of these action steps for interviews of all types, including interviews for promotions and in-house transfers.

Once an interview structure has been determined and general guidelines have been established, teaching people how to effectively interview is very important. Make certain to begin the interview on time and ensure that the candidate is comfortable. If there are several interviewers, remember to introduce the applicant to each group member and explain the interview process (Pearce, 2007).

Developing questions before the interview helps to avoid inappropriate and potentially litigious situations. However, during the course of a structured interview, it is not uncommon for the interviewer to deviate from the query path and explore areas that have been raised by the candidate. Education programs should address the limits to questions and the rationales for the restrictions.

Falcone (1997) shared 96 effective interview questions that can be used during the preemployment interview. These questions may be modified to meet the needs of the healthcare organization (Table 2-10).

Falcone (1997) recommended asking behavioral questions. These types of questions require quick thinking and self-analysis. Falcone recognized two categories of behavioral questions: self-appraisal and situational. An example of a situational question geared to nursing practice is "Tell me about a time when you took action on a clinically significant problem without getting the nurse manager's or supervisor's prior approval." Falcone offered rationales for each of the suggested questions, red flags that warrant concern or follow-up, and response analyses.

Some questions cannot be asked during an interview (Table 2-11). These restrictions are nonnegotiable. Inappropriate questions include asking about a candidate's age. Asking about college graduation is acceptable because it is not age related; however, queries about high school graduation are not permitted (Falcone, 1997). Other inappropriate question topics include specifics about disabilities, previous arrests, bankruptcy, marriage, child-rearing plans, ethnicity, and religion.

There are ways to obtain the information that is needed for the job interview without violating privacy conditions. For example, the interviewer is permitted to ask whether a candidate will be able to meet the attendance requirements of the job (ED Management, 2008; Falcone, 1997). Avoid unnecessary questions or comments about gender, race, ethnicity, disabilities, or age. Remember that candidates tend to avoid self-blame when considering why a job was not offered. These sorts of gratuitous comments reinforce the possibility that discrimination contributed to the decision to not extend employment to the candidate (ED Management, 2008).

Conclusion

Most CNSs work in demanding clinical settings filled with diverse personalities, multiple agendas, and limited resources. Wielding influence in this type of environment requires excellent communication skills, both verbal and nonverbal, that can be quickly and readily transferred from one type of situation to another. CNSs interact

Table 2-10	SELECT INTERVIEW QUESTIONS TO IDENTIFY HIGH-PERFORMANCE JOB CANDIDATES IN NURSING

Questions

1. Tell me about your greatest strength. What is the greatest asset you will bring to our healthcare organization?

2. What was your favorite nursing position and what role did your manager/CNS/director play in making it a positive experience?

3. What was your least favorite position? What role did your manager/CNS/director play in your career at that point?

4. What makes you stand out among your peers?

5. What has been your most creative achievement at work?

6. What would your current supervisors say makes you most valuable to them?

7. What aspects of your current position do you consider most crucial?

8. What will you do differently in your present position if you do not get this position?

9. What kind of mentoring and teaching style do you have? Do you naturally delegate responsibilities or do you expect staff to come to you for added responsibilities? (Good question for a CNS.)

10. How would you describe the amount of structure, direction, and feedback that you need to excel?

11. How do you approach your work from the standpoint of balancing your nursing career with your personal life?

12. What other types of positions and healthcare organizations are you considering right now?

13. Give me an example of your ability to facilitate progressive change within your nursing unit or department.

14. Tell me about your last performance appraisal. In which area were you most disappointed?

15. In hindsight, how could you have improved your performance at your last position?

Source: © 1997 Paul Falcone, AMACOM. Adapted with permission.

with people possessing varying degrees of social prestige and privilege. They rapidly transition from colleague status to subordinate, supervisor, coach, mentor, leader, practitioner, and friend. CNSs accomplish much with limited position authority.

Without formal power generated by bureaucratic rank, CNSs use influence to affect outcomes, enhance positive work environments, and promote quality care. These

Table 2-11   INTERVIEW QUESTIONS THAT MUST BE AVOIDED
Questions
1. What is your maiden name so that I can check your references and nursing license history?
2. Would your religion prevent you from working weekends?
3. Are you married? Are you planning on having children in the near future?
4. How many days were you sick last year?
5. Have you ever been arrested?

Source: © 1997 Paul Falcone, AMACOM. Adapted with permission.

successes are well established and are directly related to CNS communication savvy. Whether sending e-mails, chairing committees, interviewing applicants, facilitating group processes, or intervening in distressing or awkward group dynamics, the effective CNS demonstrates finesse and aplomb through consistently professional communications. This chapter reviews communication basics with the goal of assisting the CNS with the procedural, structural, and process information necessary to begin building a repertoire of effective communication strategies.

References

American Association of Critical-Care Nurses (AACN). (2002). *Scope of practice and standards of professional performance for the acute and critical care clinical nurse specialist.* Aliso Viejo, CA: Author.

Banks, C. (2002). Taking the hot seat. *Nursing Standard, 16*(47), 96. Retrieved February 5, 2006, CINAHL Database of Nursing and Allied Health Literature.

Benedict, S. (2007). How practitioners do and don't communicate, Part I. *Integrative Medicine: A Clinician's Journal, 6*(6), 52–57.

Brinkman, R., & Kirschner, R. (2002). *Dealing with people you can't stand. How to bring out the best in people at their worst.* New York: McGraw-Hill.

Cousteau, V. (1987). How to swim with sharks: A primer. *Perspectives in Biology and Medicine, 30*(4), 486–489.

ED Management. (2008). Interview questions are dangerous territory. *ED Management, 20*(2), 21–22.

Falcone, P. (1997). *96 great interview questions to ask before you hire.* New York: AMACOM.

Graves, L. M., & Karren, R. J. (1996). The employee selection interview: A fresh look at an old problem. *Human Resource Management, 35*(2), 163–180.

Grove, C., & Hallowell, W. (2002). *The seven balancing acts of professional behavior in the United States. A cultural values perspective.* Retrieved March, 6, 2006, from http://www.grovewell.com/pub-usa-professional.html

Integrative Medicine Alliance (IMA). (2008a). Homepage. Retrieved August 10, 2008, from http://www.integrativemedalliance.org

Integrative Medicine Alliance (IMA). (2008b). Calendar of events. Retrieved August 10, 2008, from http://www.integrativemedalliance.org/ events_calendarofevents.asp

Lindaman, C. (1997). Tools for a successful interview. *Nursing Management, 28*(4), 32B; 32D. Retrieved February 11, 2006, from CINAHL Database of Nursing and Allied Health Literature.

MeetingWizard. (2008). Frequently asked questions. Retrieved July 3, 2008, from http://www.meetingwizard.com/mwiz/home/faq.cfm#faq1

Microsoft Corporation. (2006). *MSN messenger. Emoticons.* Retrieved March 8, 2006, from http://messenger.msn.com/Resource/Emoticons.aspx

National Association of Clinical Nurse Specialists (NACNS). (2004). *Statement on clinical nurse specialist practice and education.* Harrisburg, PA: Author.

Patterson, K., Grenny, J., McMillan, R., & Switzler, C. (2002). *Crucial conversations. Tools for talking when stakes are high.* New York: McGraw-Hill.

Patterson, K., Grenny, J., McMillan, R., & Switzler, C. (2005). *Crucial confrontations.* New York: McGraw-Hill.

Pearce, C. (2007). Ten steps to conducting a selection interview. *Nursing Management, 14*(5), 21.

Privacy Rights Clearinghouse (PRC)/UCAN. (2006). *Employee monitoring. Is there privacy in the workplace?* Retrieved July 1, 2008, from http://www.privacyrights.org/fs/fs7-work.htm

Robert, H. M., Evans, W. J., Honemann, D. H., & Balch, T. J. (2004). *Robert's rules of order, newly revised.* Cambridge, MA: Da Capo Press.

Robert's Rules Association (RRA). (2006). *Short history of Robert's rules.* Retrieved September 10, 2006, from http://www.robertsrules.com/history.html

Sheehan, D., Robertson, L., & Ormond, T. (2007). Comparison of language used and patterns of communication in interprofessional and multidisciplinary teams. *Journal of Interprofessional Care, 21*(1), 17–30.

Tschabitscher, H. (2008). E-mail netiquette tips, tricks and secrets. *About.com.* Retrieved June 10, 2008, from http://email.about.com/od/netiquettetips/Email_Netiquette_Tips_Tricks_and_Secrets.htm

CHAPTER THREE

Influencing Healthcare Quality: Educating Patients, Nurses, and Students

Patti Rager Zuzelo, EdD, MSN, RN, ACNS-BC

Education is a critically important enterprise to the healthcare system and is presumed to directly affect the quality of patient care, systems functions, and institutional efficiency. It can be expensive to develop effective, meaningful education programs, but it is also expensive to educate poorly. High costs associated with a failure to educate include the select liabilities associated with failures in practitioner competency, deteriorating health of patients unable to adequately manage self-care activities due to knowledge deficiencies, and poor publicity or civil suits associated with discriminatory practices or privacy violations in part based on underlying knowledge gaps.

Traditional modes of formal staff education and in-service programming include classroom lecture, continuing education articles with posttests, and unit-based workshops. For the most part, these learning opportunities are packaged in a one-size-fits-all format with little attention paid to experience, age, preferred learning style, culture, or gender. Learning disabilities are rarely, if ever, considered.

Staff is assigned or compelled to attend programs deemed as mandatory. Programs are offered while nurses have colleagues cover their patient assignment, and attendance is often poor. Educators, including CNSs, charged with providing these programs lament the poor participation and the low rate of return on the expensive investment of time while administrators insist on repeated program offerings to increase attendance figures and demonstrate competence to satisfy accrediting and regulatory agencies and to reduce liability exposure.

CNSs also teach patients and families, either directly or indirectly. Patient education concerns differ from those of staff, and yet there are commonalities. Classroom-based instructional programs for patients, families, and community residents are not uncommon. Teaching experiences often follow established routines, including the use of pamphlets, videotapes, and lecture with pretest and posttest evaluation designs. Attendance at postdischarge or preadmission programs is often sporadic, and healthcare professionals decry the perceived disinterest or other barriers to learning. Discharge teaching is offered quickly and supplemented by printed instructions, possibly designed with grade-level readability in mind but perhaps without consideration of overall health literacy concerns.

Nursing students, particularly undergraduates, are taught in clinical settings and are influenced either directly or indirectly by CNSs who facilitate a context of learning within the institution or who teach as adjunct faculty, instructors, or professors of nursing. CNSs may teach as they have been taught using traditional methods of instruction in tried-and-true formats. These teaching strategies may include preconferences, postconferences, or instructor-directed labs and lectures. CNSs are in an ideal position to teach nursing students because their advanced practice role ensures a current knowledge base and the wherewithal to recognize and promote safe clinical decision making. However, many CNSs are unfamiliar with the role of the adjunct faculty member and its associated responsibilities, including processes of student evaluation. They may also be unfamiliar with active teaching strategies, including problem-based learning. CNSs may also be unaware of the cutting-edge topics addressed in nursing education literature.

Relatively new computer technologies are affecting several of these scenarios in positive ways. Web-enhanced learning, intranet opportunities, patient model simulations, and smart classrooms are enhancing the attractiveness of education programs by engaging learners in a variety of instructional modalities that appeal to multiple senses. The need for real-time education is minimized, and nurses can take advantage of learning at a time that suits individual schedules. The World Wide Web has dramatically increased the amount of information available to patients, families, and staff. While patients and providers are satisfied with the easy information access, professionals worry about potential misinformation and overwhelming volumes of data. Many hospitals offer patients, families, and community residents opportunities to access health materials via learning laboratories and public computer stations.

This chapter addresses issues relevant to the education component of CNS practice. Many CNSs are practicing in staff development roles within nursing education departments. CNSs working within a product line or care program practice arrangement also find themselves participating in or orchestrating programs for nursing staff, patients and family, community, multidisciplinary team members, and other individuals operating within the healthcare system. Many CNSs also teach undergraduate or graduate students of nursing. CNSs with doctoral preparation are often employed as professors of nursing, with some having opportunities to practice in joint arrangements with clinical affiliates.

Patient and Community Education

A Description of the Challenge: Literacy in the United States

Nurses are generally aware of the complexities of the English language and recognize that it is a difficult language to master, particularly once people have reached adulthood (Table 3-1). Becoming literate is a more challenging endeavor than the acquisition of conversation skills (Figure 3-1). Health literacy is related to language literacy but is different, both in its components and its usages. Health literacy is an important concern with significant implications for CNS practice.

Many CNSs are involved in patient education programs, either inpatient, outpatient, or through public health initiatives. This involvement requires CNSs to have a clear understanding of health literacy and its influence on patient education. CNSs are often familiar with literacy concerns specific to readability and grade level of written materials but may not have a clear grasp of the enormity of the literacy problem in the United States.

The National Assessment of Adult Literacy (NAAL) was conducted in 2003 to assess English literacy among a nationally representative probability sample of American

Table 3-1   REASONS WHY THE ENGLISH LANGUAGE IS HARD TO LEARN
1. The bandage was wound around the wound.
2. The farm was used to produce produce.
3. The dump was so full that it had to refuse more refuse.
4. We must polish the Polish furniture.
5. He could lead if he would get the lead out.
6. The soldier decided to desert his dessert in the desert.
7. Since there is no time like the present, he thought it was time to present the present.
8. A bass was painted on the head of the bass drum.
9. When shot at, the dove dove into the bushes.
10. I did not object to the object.
11. The insurance was invalid for the invalid.
12. There was a row among the oarsmen about how to row.
13. They were too close to the door to close it.
14. The buck does funny things when the does are present.
15. A seamstress and a sewer fell down into a sewer line.
16. To help with planting, the farmer taught his sow to sow.
17. The wind was too strong to wind the sail.
18. After a number of injections, my jaw got number.
19. Upon seeing the tear in the painting I shed a tear.
20. I had to subject the subject to a series of tests.
21. How can I intimate this to my most intimate friend?

Source: Plain Language Action and Information Network, n.d. 2.

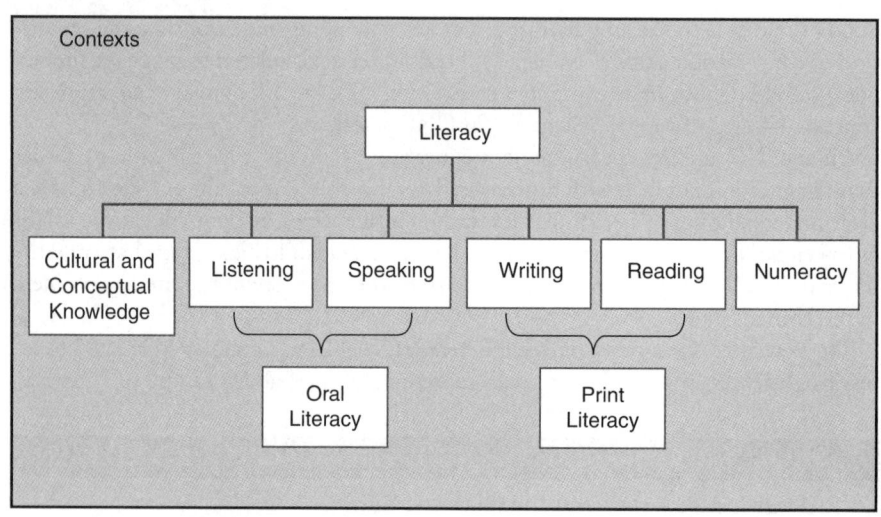

Figure 3-1 Literacy components.

Source: © 2004. Reprinted with permission from *Health Literacy: A Prescription to End Confusion* by the National Academy of Sciences, courtesy of the National Academies Press, Washington, DC.

adults age 16 and older. Data were collected from over 19,000 adults. Subjects were solicited from homes and prisons, both federal and state. NAAL results were compared to the 1992 results of the National Adult Literacy Survey (NALS).

NALS was conducted in three parts and included a national survey of 13,600 people, a 12-state survey of 1000 people per state, and a prison survey of 1100 inmates incarcerated in 80 federal and state prisons. Respondents were scored in three areas: prose, document, and quantitative literacy. The results were ranked into five levels ranging from least to most proficient as designated by level 1 through 5 (National Center for Education Statistics [NCES], n. d.).

A comparison of NAAL to NALS results provides a decade point progress indicator for national adult literacy. CNSs should be aware of these results, as they provide a meaningful description of challenges specific to health literacy and support the need for professionals in the healthcare system to carefully consider the average skill set of the nation that is dependent on it for services. The NAAL has several components that examine the breadth of adult literacy (NAAL, n.d. 1) (Table 3-2).

The NAALS results are concerning, as they demonstrate no significant changes in prose and document literacy when compared to the NALS. There was some improvement in quantitative literacy. Literacy is currently ranked using levels ranging from below basic to basic, intermediate, and proficient (Table 3-3) (NAAL, n.d. 2).

Table 3-2 NAAL COMPONENTS

Component	Description
1. Background Questionnaire	Describes relationships between adult literacy and select respondent characteristics
2. Prison Component	Identifies literacy skills of incarcerated adults
3. State Assessment of Adult Literacy (SAAL)	Statewide literacy estimates for participating states
4. Health Literacy	Ability to use literacy skills in understanding health-related materials and forms
5. Fluency Addition	Measures basic reading skills by examining decoding ability, word recognition, and reading fluency
6. Adult Literacy Supplemental Assessment	Describes the ability of the least-literate adults to identify letters and numbers and to comprehend simple prose and documents

Source: NAAL, n.d. 1.

Findings reveal that 93 million Americans, or approximately 43%, are functioning at below basic or basic levels of literacy (NAAL, n.d. 3) (Figure 3-2). These levels denote an ability to perform tasks at the most basic, uncomplicated level. Tasks include locating information in a short news article or totaling the entry on a bank deposit slip. People with a basic level of literacy have considerable difficulty carrying out tasks requiring them to read and comprehend long texts, and two-step calculations may be beyond their capabilities. A worrisome finding related to the below basic in prose group is that its members are also at greatest risk for compromised health status or societal disenfranchisement (Table 3-4).

Table 3-3 LITERACY LEVELS

Literacy Level	Skill Set
Below Basic	No more than the most simple and concrete literacy skills
Basic	Able to perform simple and everyday literacy activities
Intermediate	Can perform moderately challenging literacy activities
Proficient	Able to perform complex and challenging literacy activities

Source: NAAL, n.d. 2.

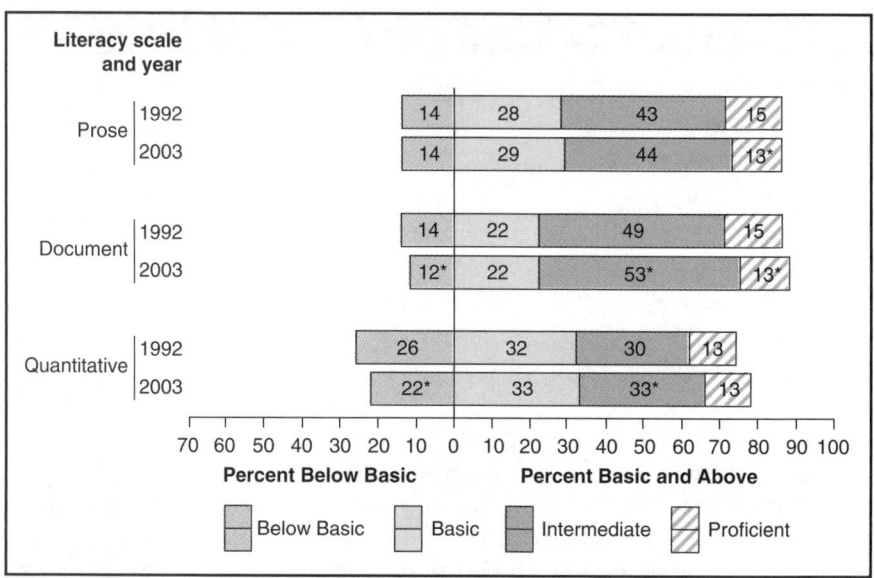

Figure 3-2 Number of adults in each prose literacy level.

* Significantly different from 1992.

Note: Detail may not sum to totals because of rounding. Adults are defined as people 16 years of age and older living in households or prisons. Adults who could not be interviewed due to language spoken or cognitive or mental disabilities (3 percent in 2003 and 4 percent in 1992) are excluded from this figure.

Data from: U.S. Department of Education, Institute of Education Sciences, National Center for Education Statistics, 1992 National Adult Literacy Survey and 2003 National Assessment of Adult Literacy.

Source: U.S. Department of Education, n.d.

Health Literacy: A Challenge within the Context of Literacy

Health literacy is a shared function of social and individual factors (Committee on Health Literacy, 2004) that influence the extent to which individuals are able to obtain, process, and understand basic health information and the services needed to make appropriate health decisions (Office of Disease Prevention and Health Promotion [ODPHP], 2000). Health literacy is not independent of general literacy skills (Rudd, 2007). Health literacy includes the ability to decode instructions, charts, and diagrams; analyze risks to benefits; and make decisions that lead to actions (National Institutes of Health, 2009). Numeracy, or quantitative literacy, is important to the management of daily medications, extracting nutrition information from food product labels, calculating insurance co-payments, or monitoring quantitative data specific to chronic conditions (Wolf, Davis, & Parker, 2007).

The Institute of Medicine (IOM) of the National Academies convened the Committee on Health Literacy to examine the problem of health literacy. The committee report, *Health Literacy: A Prescription to End Confusion*, offers a comprehensive,

TABLE 3-4   CHARACTERISTICS OF ADULTS WITH BELOW BASIC PROSE LITERACY

	Percent in Prose Below Basic Population	Percent in Total NAAL Population
Did not graduate from high school	56	15
No English spoken before starting school	44	13
Hispanic adults	39	12
Black adults	20	12
Age 65+	26	15
Multiple disabilities	21	9

Source: U.S. Department of Education, n.d.

detailed description of health literacy with potential interventions. The report is an excellent resource for CNSs who are interested in examining this problem and developing a better sense of the enormity of the challenge to design effective, targeted patient and family education programs.

The Committee on Health Literacy developed a framework that characterizes health literacy as a synergistic relationship between culture and society, health system, education system, and health outcomes and costs (Figure 3-3). During its work, the committee examined the customary measures of literacy and health literacy and found them lacking.

Responding to these deficiencies, the committee identified three potential points for intervening in the health literacy framework and potentially improving health literacy (Figure 3-4). The committee identified that the health system cannot bear full responsibility for health literacy and that efforts must include both culture and society. The health system and education system were also viewed as important partners in health literacy. This finding needs to influence the ways that CNSs assess and address patient teaching.

Health literacy incorporates a variety of factors, not the least of which includes listening, speaking, writing, reading, cultural influences, conceptualizations, and arithmetic. When CNSs examine patient education materials, they typically use traditional readability measures, such as the SMOG (simple measure of gobbledygook) or the Gunning–Fog indices. These measures are imprecise estimates that do not take into account the broad context of literacy. As a result, materials may seem suitable in terms of word usage and grade-level readability and yet may not affect patients' understanding of the essential truths necessary for health management.

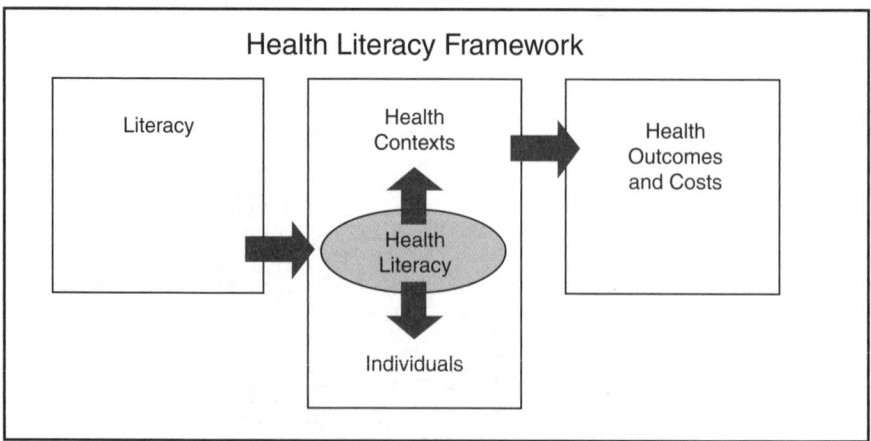

Figure 3-3 Health literacy framework.

Source: © 2004. Reprinted with permission from *Health Literacy: A Prescription to End Confusion* by the National Academy of Sciences, courtesy of the National Academies Press, Washington, DC.

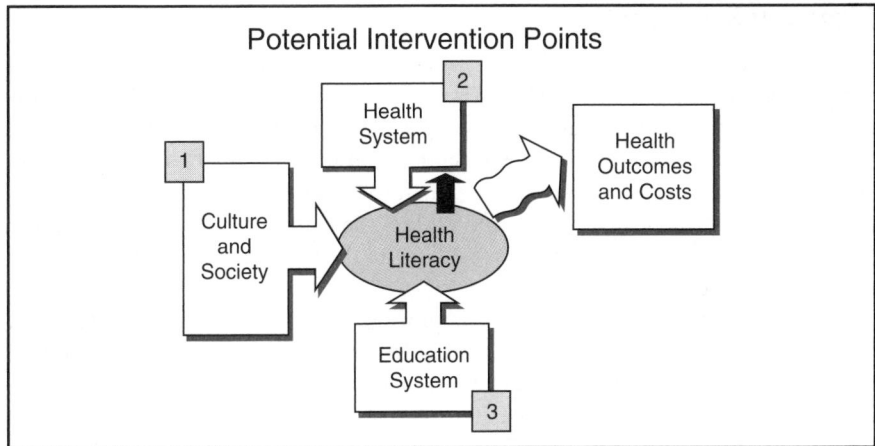

Figure 3-4   Potential points for intervention in the health literacy framework.

Source: © 2004. Reprinted with permission from *Health Literacy: A Prescription to End Confusion* by the National Academy of Sciences, courtesy of the National Academies Press, Washington, DC.

Patients with English as a second language have additional challenges that may be compounded by limited education or age. The committee interpreted available data as suggesting that there is a relationship between health literacy, healthcare use, and healthcare costs. In other words, limited health literacy is expensive fiscally and personally. The Committee on Health Literacy recognized that shame and stigma related to limited literacy skills cause people to refrain from seeking resources to improve health literacy. As a result of limited health literacy, adults have less knowledge of health promotion, disease prevention, and disease management and use preventive services at a comparably lower rate.

The committee asserted that hundreds of studies have demonstrated that health information cannot be understood by most of the people for whom it was intended. The education system does not prepare people for a basic appreciation of anatomy and physiology. Therefore, when a patient experiences pathologies requiring self-management, he or she may not understand even the simple mechanics of functioning that are vital to making decisions about drug dosing, contacting a healthcare professional for follow-up, or returning to the hospital.

For example, a patient with congestive heart failure and coronary artery disease needs to understand the basic premise of coronary artery blood flow, ischemia, anticoagulation, heart rate, and pumping ability. This foundation informs self-management and facilitates recognition of the signs and symptoms that require medical or nursing review. Much of this information is couched in scientific terminologies that are not taught in basic education programs. This knowledge deficit worsens the challenges facing health professionals as they attempt to provide the education needed for self-care efficacy in a time frame that is constrained by inadequate personnel and fiscal resources.

Literacy Resources for CNSs

Health literacy is gaining a lot of attention from both private and public agencies and corporations. As a result, many Web-based resources are available to CNSs at a low cost. These resources may be used to positively affect patient outcomes by influencing the expertise of health professionals within the healthcare system. Resources may also be used to empower patients by helping them to better understand and act on provided health information. CNSs should explore the many Web-based resources and keep in mind that most government sites allow for the free use of materials, providing that they are properly acknowledged.

A number of initiatives are focused on improving health communication and literacy. CNSs should consider exploring the resources available through these programs, as they are typically inexpensive and incorporate best practices using input from a variety of expert sources. A simple Web search using a popular search engine such as Google or Dogpile and the search term *health literacy* reveals a plethora of opportunities.

The Ask Me 3 program was developed by the Partnership for Clear Health Communication to improve communication between providers and patients and to address the relationship between low health literacy and its negative impact on health status (Partnership for Clear Health Communication, n.d.). Ask Me 3 promotes three simple questions for patients to ask their healthcare provider during every encounter:

1. What is my main problem?
2. What do I need to do?
3. Why is it important for me to do this?

The Web site, www.askme3.org, offers a variety of resources for providers, patients, large-scale implementers, and media. The Partnership for Clear Health Communication makes available a variety of posters (Figure 3-5), brochures in both English and Spanish, teaching materials (Table 3-5), presentations, provider recommendations, and the logo at no cost, stipulating that content of the written text cannot be changed, the materials must be appropriately credited, and the logo standards for graphics must be followed (www.askme3.org/PFCHC/download.asp). Funding for the Ask Me 3 program is provided by Pfizer, Inc.

Another helpful Web-based resource is PlainLanguage.gov, a federal government employee initiative designed to facilitate the use of plain language to improve communication. In 1995, a group of federal employees joined together with an agenda to spread the use of plain language. The Plain Language Action and Information Network (PLAIN) created the Web site (www.plainlanguage.gov/index.cfm) to help people learn about and use plain language. There are excellent examples of plain language documents that are in stark contrast to original works (Table 3-6). Wonderful tools are available via this Web site and health literacy is a popular topic. PLAIN offers a document checklist for plain language on the Web (Plain Language Action and Information Network, n. d. 1) (Table 3-7). Each item may be selected using the hyperlink to acquire additional details.

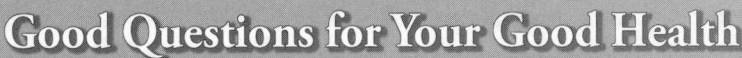

Figure 3-5   Sample "Ask Me 3" poster.
Source: Partnership for Clear Health Communication, n.d.

| Table 3-5 | COMPARISON OF BREAST CANCER PATIENT INFORMATION AFTER REVISION USING PRINCIPLES FOR CLEAR HEALTH COMMUNICATION |

An Extra Step: Mammography

Women in the three high-risk categories —age 50 or more, 40 or more with a family history of breast cancer, age 35 or more with a personal history of breast cancer— may consider an additional routine screening method. This is x-ray mammography. Mammography uses radiation (x-rays) to create an image of the breast on film or paper called a mammogram. It can reveal tumors too small to be felt by palpation. It shows other changes in the structure of the breast, which doctors believe point to very early cancer. A mammographic examination usually consists of two x-rays of each breast, one taken from the top and one from the side. Exposure to x-rays should be carried out to ensure that the lowest possible dose will be absorbed by the body. Radiologists are not yet certain if there is any risk from one mammogram, although most studies indicate that the risk, if it does exist, is small relative to the benefit. Recent equipment modifications and improved techniques are reducing radiation absorption and thus the possible risk.

Original information based on the medical model. U.S. Department of Health and Human Services, National Cancer Institute/National Institutes of Health. Breast Exams: What you should know. 1984. Readability: 12th grade. Retrieved May 28, 2006, from http://www.pfizerhealthliteracy.org/pdfs/Pfizers_Principles_for_Clear_Health_Communication.pdf

What is a mammogram and why should I have one?

A mammogram is an x-ray picture of the breast. It can find breast cancer that is too small for you, your doctor, or nurse to feel. Studies show that if you are in your forties or older, having a mammogram every 1 to 2 years could save your life.

How do I know if I need a mammogram?

Talk with your doctor about your chances of getting breast cancer. Your doctor can help you decide when you should start having mammograms and how often you should have them.

Why do I need one every 1 to 2 years?

As you get older, your chances of getting breast cancer get higher. Cancer can show up at any time—so one mammogram is not enough. Decide on a plan with your doctor and follow it for the rest of your life.

Where can I get a mammogram?

To find out where to get a mammogram:
* Ask your doctor or nurse
* Ask your local health department or clinic
* Call the National Cancer Institute's Concern Information Service at 1-800-4-CANCER

Revised information based on the Health Belief Model. U.S. Department of Health and Human Services, National Cancer Institute/National Institutes of Health. Breast Exams: What you should know. 1997. Readability: 5th grade. Retrieved May 28, 2006, from http://www.pfizerhealthliteracy.org/pdfs/Pfizers_Principles_for_Clear_Health_Communication.pdf

Source: Doak & Doak, 2004.

Table 3-6	BEFORE AND AFTER COMPARISONS: LOSING WEIGHT BROCHURE

Before

The Dietary Guidelines for Americans recommends a half hour or more of moderate physical activity on most days, preferably every day. The activity can include brisk walking, calisthenics, home care, gardening, moderate sports exercise, and dancing.

After

Do at least 30 minutes of exercise, like brisk walking, most days of the week.

Source: Plain Language Action and Information Network, n.d. 3.

Pfizer, Inc., also supports the Clear Health Communication Initiative (Pfizer, 2003) (www.pfizerhealthliteracy.org) and offers a *Patient Education Handbook* (Doak & Doak, 2004) in PDF form and available as a free download. The handbook explores health literacy and offers suggestions, strategies, and examples in an easy-to-read format that exemplifies the simple yet meaningful recommendations it puts forth. This is an excellent resource for CNSs and may be useful to professionals in many disciplines.

The Agency for Healthcare Research and Quality (AHRQ) (Berkman et al., 2004) has developed an evidence report/technology assessment on literacy and health outcomes that is useful and informative. The review addressed two key questions:

- Are literacy skills related to use of healthcare services, health outcomes, costs of health care, or disparities in health outcomes or healthcare service use according to race, ethnicity, culture, or age?
- For individuals with low literacy skills, what are effective interventions to improve use of healthcare services, improve health outcomes, affect the costs of health care, and improve health outcomes and healthcare service use among different racial, ethnic, cultural, or age groups?

Berkman et al. (2004) concluded that low reading skill and poor health are related, thereby legitimizing health literacy and readability as real priorities for CNS practice. The full report is available as a free PDF download.

The Harvard School of Public Health (n.d.) offers a variety of health literacy resources (www.hsph.harvard.edu/healthliteracy/materials.html). The Web site provides information specific to health literacy, health literacy literature, research and policy, innovative materials, print materials resources (Rudd, 2005), health literacy curricula, links, contact information, and updated notifications of talks, presentations, and health literacy studies in the news. The Web site also offers a variety of teaching materials available for downloading, printing, and distributing.

Table 3-7   DOCUMENT CHECKLIST FOR PLAIN LANGUAGE ON THE WEB

1. Written for the average reader

   Know the expertise and interest of your average reader, and write to that person. Don't write to the experts, the lawyers, or your management, unless they are your intended audience.

2. Organized to serve the reader's needs

   Organize your content in the order the reader needs—the two most useful organization principles, which are not mutually exclusive, are to put the most important material first, exceptions last; or to organize material chronologically.

3. Has useful headings

   Headings help the reader find the way through your material. Headings should capture the essence of all the material under the heading—if they don't, you need more headings! You should have one or more headings on each page.

4. Uses "you" and other pronouns to speak to the reader

   Using pronouns pulls the reader into the document and makes it more meaningful to him or her. Use "you" for the reader ("I" when writing question headings from the reader's viewpoint) and "we" for your agency.

5. Uses active voice

   Using active voice clarifies who is doing what; passive obscures it. Active voice is generally shorter, as well as clearer. Changing our writing to prefer active voice is the single most powerful change we can make in government writing. Active sentences are structured with the actor first (as the subject), then the verb, then the object of the action.

6. Uses short sections and sentences

   Using short sentences, paragraphs, and sections helps your reader get through your material. Readers get lost in long dense text with few headings. Chunking your material also inserts white space, opening your document visually and making it more appealing.

7. Uses the simplest tense possible—simple present is best

   The simplest verb tense is the clearest and strongest. Use simple present whenever possible—say, "We issue a report every quarter," not "We will be issuing a report every quarter."

8. Uses base verbs, not nominalizations (hidden verbs)

   Use base verbs, not nominalizations—also called "hidden verbs." Government writing is full of hidden verbs. They make our writing weak and longer than necessary. Say "We manage the program" and "We analyze data" not "We are responsible for management of the program" or "We conduct an analysis of the data."

9. Omits excess words

   Eliminate excess words. Challenge every word—do you need it? Pronouns, active voice, and base verbs help eliminate excess words. So does eliminating unnecessary modifiers—in "HUD and FAA issued a joint report" you don't need "joint." In "This information is really critical" you don't need "really."

10. Uses concrete, familiar words

    You don't impress people by using big words, you just confuse them. Define (and limit!) your abbreviations. Avoid jargon, foreign terms, Latin terms, and legal terms. Avoid noun strings. See our alphabetized list of complex words and simple subjects in the "word suggestions" page on this Web site.

11. Uses "must" to express requirements; avoids the ambiguous word "shall"

    Use "must" not "shall" to impose requirements. "Shall" is ambiguous and rarely occurs in everyday conversation. The legal community is moving to a strong preference for "must" as the clearest way to express a requirement or obligation.

12. Places words carefully (avoids large gaps between the subject, the verb, and the object; puts exceptions last; places modifiers correctly)

    Placing words carefully within a sentence is as important as organizing your document effectively. Keep subject, verb, and object close together. Put exceptions at the end. Place modifiers correctly—"We want only the best" not "We only want the best."

13. Uses lists and tables to simplify complex material

    You can shorten and clarify complex material by using lists and tables. And these features give your document more white space, making it more appealing to the reader.

14. Uses no more than two or three subordinate levels

    Readers get lost when you use more than two or three levels in a document. If you find you need more levels, consider subdividing your top level into more parts.

Source: Plain Language Action and Information Network, n.d. 1.

A few of the Harvard School of Public Health Web-based materials available for download include "Plain Talk About Lupus and Key Words," "Asthma Glossary Key Words in Plain Language," and "Plain Talk About Arthritis and Key Words" (www.hsph.harvard.edu/healthliteracy/innovative.html). A 15-minute video entitled "In Plain Language" is available for viewing as a RealOne Player presentation and addresses health literacy as it relates to medicine and public health. The video link may be an interesting addition to the CNS's health literacy repertoire, particularly when working with nurses and other health professionals interested in improving patient education within a healthcare organization.

EthnoMed (www.ethnomed.org/ethnomed) offers patient education materials tailored to a variety of cultures including Amharic, Cambodian, Chinese, Entrean, Hispanic, Somali, and others (University of Washington, Harborview Medical Center, 2008). The groups represent immigrant groups living in Seattle and other parts of the United States. Cross-cultural links are available. The EthnoMed project began in 1994 with the goal of bridging cultural and language barriers during medical encounters. The project's objective is to make information about culture, language, health, illness, and local resources readily available to healthcare providers working with diverse ethnic groups.

EthnoMed offers CNSs a menu of various cultures. The CNS selects the culture of interest and is presented with options for a cultural profile, clinical topics, or patient education materials. As an example, if a CNS is working with a Vietnamese patient with a cancer diagnosis but the CNS has no experience with this cultural group, the EthnoMed site provides a detailed overview of Vietnamese culture. A list of common Vietnamese symptoms is offered as well as health and illness topics. If the CNS is looking for education materials for this patient, the link to "Patient Education" reveals many resources written in Vietnamese, including a "What Is Cancer?" document available in both Vietnamese and English. The site is an ongoing activity and encourages providers to share information about treatments, resources, and cultural perspectives with the EthnoMed group.

An additional resource is fee-based patient education materials. Some vendors create patient education materials for purchase. Many hospitals and other health organizations choose to purchase patient education materials in the form of text pamphlets with visual aids, Web site development, and specialty program development. These types of products may be useful for streamlining education material resources and protecting the accuracy and consistency of the information provided during healthcare encounters.

Other vendors also provide databases that may be used to develop individualized discharge instructions for a variety of settings, including emergency departments. If this option is interesting, the CNS should request a vendor list from the purchasing expert at the healthcare institution. Vendor information is also available at professional nursing conferences, particularly the larger regional, national, and international conference venues.

A Word About Teach-Back

Teach-back is an easy method that may be used to evaluate patients' understanding of the information taught. This technique is also referred to as the "show me" approach or "closing the loop" (Shillinger, 2004). The method consists of asking patients how they would explain the pertinent procedure, treatment, or other self-care activity to their spouse or family member (AHC Media, 2007). Patients should explain by using their own words. If the patient is incorrect, the nurse should provide clarification using different phrases rather than repeating the previously provided information. To avoid patient feelings of foolishness or defensiveness, nurses should phrase the request for the patient to "teach back" by requesting feedback on the nurse's performance. For example, the CNS teaching the patient how to administer a daily insulin dose might consider saying, "I want to make certain that I did a good job of explaining this insulin dosing to you. Would you please show me how you're going to do this when you get home?"

Although use of the teach-back technique is advocated by health literacy experts, a survey of healthcare professionals attending plenary sessions on health literacy/health communication at 12 different state and national conferences on patient safety and healthcare quality revealed that less than 40% of total respondents ($N = 356$) used the teach-back technique during patient education encounters (Schwartzberg, Cowett, VanGeest, & Wolf, 2007). CNSs should share this simple strategy with nurses and other health providers. As an aside, this may also be a useful method when teaching nursing students and is similar to a bottom-line approach recommended by Zuzelo (1999) to assist students in learning essential information required for success with the National Council of State Boards of Nursing Examination-RN (NCLEX-RN).

Levels of Literacy

Managed care requires people to be increasingly more autonomous in self-care practices. Ownership of self-care responsibilities demands health literacy. Many areas of health management are connected to health literacy (Table 3-8).

Levels of literacy are described by fairly common terms. CNSs should think about these descriptive terms and consider the demographics of the CNS practice within the context of these literacy levels. Low literacy is also referred to as marginally literate or

Table 3-8   HEALTH LITERACY SELF-CARE IMPACT AREAS

1. Patient–healthcare provider communication: health histories, advanced directives, untoward drug reactions, discharge instructions
2. Medication labeling: prescription drug dosing and scheduling, empty stomach instructions, drug interaction precautions
3. Equipment labeling: using durable medical equipment safely and correctly
4. Health information publications and other resources: self-care pamphlets, public health precautions, hazardous materials warnings, household items warnings concerning mixing materials
5. Informed consent
6. Responding to medical and insurance forms
7. Nutrition: food labeling, avoiding allergens, proper food storage, expiration dates, handling instructions

marginally illiterate and designates individuals who are able to read, write, and comprehend information at the fifth- through eighth-grade level of difficulty (Bastable, 2003). Functional illiteracy describes adults with reading, writing, and comprehension skills that are below the fifth-grade level. Literacy categorizations should not be interpreted as akin to intelligence (Bastable, 2006).

Health literacy is one of the health communication objectives in *Healthy People 2010*. Objective 11-2 is to "improve the health literacy of persons with inadequate or marginal literacy skills" (NIH, 2009). To effect change in literacy, *Healthy People 2010* emphasizes the crucial need to develop appropriate written materials for audiences with limited literacy and to improve the reading skills of individuals with limited literacy.

Assessing Patient Education Materials

CNSs should be aware of screening instruments used to determine a patient's literacy and to ascertain the readability and appropriateness of available teaching materials. It is important for CNSs to be comfortable selecting the best-fit instruments and using these tools. Readability is frequently discussed in nursing textbooks, and most nurses are familiar with issues specific to the level of difficulty of materials; however, they may be less familiar with the concept of health literacy. Both measures should be carefully examined when planning patient education.

Readability   CNSs may be familiar with readability tools including the Flesch–Kinkaid Grade Level score and the Flesch Reading Ease score, as these options are available in the readability scores feature of Microsoft Word. Other popular readability measures include the SMOG formula and Fog formula.

The SMOG (simple measure of gobbledygook) index is based on average sentence length and the number of words with three or more syllables in a total of 30 sentences (Potter & Martin, 2006). SMOG is fast and easy to use and has well-established validity. SMOG is based on 100% comprehension of material read, so if the index calculates the readability level to be grade six, it means that 100% of readers able to read at the sixth-grade level should fully comprehend the material. Other formulas rely on 50% to 75% of all persons reading at the sixth-grade level, which explains why SMOG results are often about two grade levels higher than those determined by other indices (Bastable, 2003). The SMOG index follows simple calculation steps (Table 3-9) that may be cumbersome when applied to lengthy documents. Resources are available for passages longer and shorter than 30 sentences that offer conversion tables for ease of use (Bastable, 2003).

The Fog index or the Gunning–Fog index (Bastable, 2006) measures readability of print materials ranging from fourth grade to college level. The formula calculates grade level based on average sentence length and the percentage of multisyllabic words in a 100-word passage. It is an easy formula to use, and the resulting number indicates the number of years of formal education that a person needs to easily understand the text on the first reading (Bastable).

Table 3-9	SMOG INDEX

To calculate the SMOG Index:
1. Count the number of complex words (words containing 3 or more syllables).
2. Multiply the number of complex words by a factor of (30/number of sentences).
3. Take the square root of the resultant number.
4. Add 3 to the resultant number.

The Flesch Reading Ease score rates the text on a 100-point scale, with a high score indicating greater understandability. Microsoft recommends a target score of approximately 60 to 70 for standard documents (Table 3-10). The Flesch–Kincaid Grade Level score rates text on a U.S. grade-school level. A score of 8 indicates that the text can be understood by an individual with the skill set of an eighth grader. For a standard document, the recommended grade level is between seven and eight (Table 3-11). This recommended grade level should be determined by the average reading level of the typical patient with whom the CNS practices.

Readability scores in Microsoft Word are not provided as a default function. To take advantage of this feature, it must be selected. Given its usefulness, CNSs should consider adding the feature to the spelling check function to verify the grade level of written work that directly affects patients, families, or staff. To turn on this function in Word, select Tools from the tool bar. Select Options and then select Spelling and Grammar. There is a box next to Readability Statistics. Check this box and select OK. Readability statistics will now be presented with completed spell-checks. The steps for accessing these statistics vary by software version but may be found in the Help feature of most programs.

Understanding how the reading ease and grade-level scores are calculated will assist the CNS in improving the appropriateness of Word documents by reducing the grade

Table 3-10	FLESCH READING EASE SCORE FORMULA

The formula for the Flesch Reading Ease score is
$$206.835 - (1.015 \times ASL) - (84.6 \times ASW)$$
where:

ASL = average sentence length (the number of words divided by the number of sentences)

ASW = average number of syllables per word (the number of syllables divided by the number of words)

Table 3-11   FLESCH–KINCAID GRADE-LEVEL SCORE FORMULA
The formula for the Flesch–Kincaid Grade-Level score is $$(.39 \times ASL) + (11.8 \times ASW) - 15.59$$ where: ASL = average sentence length (the number of words divided by the number of sentences) ASW = average number of syllables per word (the number of syllables divided by the number of words)

level or enhancing the understandability of the document. In general, a sixth-grade level (rather than an eighth-grade level) may be more appropriate for a large patient audience, depending on the typical demographic profile of the patient group. If needed, consider a fourth-grade level.

The readability tools in software programs may be inaccurate and underestimate the level of text difficulty (Pfizer, 2003). Pfizer recommends using the manual Fry formula because it is not copyrighted, uses a reasonably small sample size of 100 words, has respectability within the reading community, and takes only 15 to 20 minutes to obtain results (Pfizer, 2008). The *Pfizer Principles for Clear Health Communication* (1994) manual offers step-by-step instructions for using the Fry formula and provides the Fry chart for ease of use. The Pfizer Clear Health Communication Initiative Web site offers Fry testing exercises with step-by-step instructions (www.pfizerhealthliteracy.com/pdf/Using-Readability-Formulas.pdf).

There are also online resources that enable the CNS to cut and paste text into text boxes and have the selection evaluated for readability. Wikipedia.com, a free online encyclopedia, provides external links to tools that evaluate the Fog index, Flesch–Kincaid scores, and other readability measures and offers suggestions for enhancing readability (en.wikipedia.org/wiki/Gunning-Fog_Index).

Formatting for Appeal and Impact   In addition to grade level and understandability, CNSs should consider the overall look of printed materials. Graphics can be important visual cues that enhance learning. Elderly patients provided with a leaflet that included graphics were five times more likely to receive a pneumococcal vaccine than were those elders in a control group who received a text-only brochure. They were also more likely to speak with their physicians about receiving the immunization (Jacobson et al., 1999).

CNSs should keep in mind that the average patient is probably a poor reader. Clear headings, bullets rather than full paragraphs, and ample white space are important. Short sentences, active voice, and familiar language with pictures and examples also facilitate engagement and learning (Potter & Martin, 2006). When developing critical materials, it may be useful to consider bringing together a group of intended audi-

ence members and field testing materials to solicit feedback about the effectiveness
and appeal of the written product.

Assessing the Learner

Validated measures for ascertaining health literacy include the Rapid Estimate
of Adult Literacy in Medicine (REALM), REALM-Short Form (SF), and the
Test of Functional Health Literacy in Adults (TOFHLA). REALM measures a
person's ability to recognize and pronounce common health and medical terms
(Potter & Martin, 2006). REALM does not measure understanding but can be used
to assist health professionals in selecting appropriate educational materials and instructions.

REALM comprises 66 items and takes 2 to 3 minutes to administer and score.
Subjects read from a list of 66 medical words arranged in order of complexity as determined by the number of syllables and pronunciation difficulty. Patients read aloud
as many words as they can from the first word and continue until they reach words
that they cannot pronounce correctly. REALM yields a score that estimates a grade
level for reading (Weiss, 2007). A sample kit and pricing information can be obtained
by writing to the developer. REALM has established validity and reliability (Davis et
al., 1991; 1993) and is available only in English. REALM-SF is a revised, shortened
version of REALM (Arozullah et al., 2007).

The TOFHLA is available in both English and Spanish (Weiss, 2007). It measures
the functional literacy of patients using real-to-life healthcare materials. Examples of
these materials include prescription bottle labels, diagnostic test instructions, and patient education information.

The TOFHLA has 67 items and measures numeracy and reading comprehension.
This instrument costs approximately $50 and is available for purchase (Columbia
University School of Nursing, n. d). Scores categorize patients into low, marginal, or
adequate health literacy skill groups. It takes 22 minutes to complete both constructs.
A short form is available, and a shorter form is under development (Weiss, 2007). A
Spanish version is also available for purchase.

Culturally and Linguistically Appropriate Health Care

The Joint Commission views culturally and linguistically appropriate health services
as critical to quality and safety (Joint Commission, 2006a). Many Joint Commission
standards support this requirement, including interpreter and translation services,
food preferences, equal standard of care, informed consent, and many others. Standard R1.2.100 calls for the organization to respect the patient's right to and need for
effective communication (Table 3-12). The rationale for this standard includes concerns with the appropriateness of the selected communication modality as well as the
appropriateness of the language (Joint Commission, 2006a). Interpretation, including translation services, as well as communication aids for patients with vision,
speech, hearing, language, and cognitive impairments create significant challenges
for CNSs.

Table 3-12   JOINT COMMISSION STANDARD RI.2.100
Standard RI.2.100 The organization respects the [patient's/resident's/client's] right to and need for effective communication. **Rationale for RI.2.100** The [patient/resident/client] has the right to receive information in a manner that he or she understands. This includes communication between the organization and the [patient/resident/client], as well as communication between the [patient/resident/client] and others outside the organization. **EP.2** Written information provided is appropriate to the age, understanding, and as appropriate to the population served, the language of the [patient/resident/client]. **EP.3** The organization facilitates the patient in the provision of interpretation (including translation services) as necessary. **EP.4** The organization addresses the needs of those with vision, speech, hearing, language, and cognitive impairments.

Source: © Joint Commission Resources, Inc. *2006 comprehensive accreditation manual for hospitals.* Oakbrook Terrace, IL: Joint Commission, 2006a, p. 3. Reprinted with permission.

Staff Education: Influencing Staff via Educational Programming

Education Programs: Not a Cure-All

CNSs are frequently charged with creating educational programs to correct an identified patient care or indirect care problem. These program requests are often the result of a need to respond to a situation that is viewed as threatening to quality patient care outcomes. Concerns may also be related to institutional liability, patient satisfaction, or safety, among others. Although education may be the correct remedy, it should not always be the only or even the first proposed solution to a concern of interest. Many times practice problems are unrelated to knowledge deficits, but rather are related to competing priorities, workload challenges, or an employee's free will (Exemplar 3-1).

Staff Education: Influencing Staff via Educational Programming

Organizations are responsible for providing opportunities for education so that employees can achieve and maintain the skill set necessary for safe, quality practice. These educational opportunities are opportunities to learn. Employees are obliged to take advantage of these chances to meet their contractual obligation to provide safe care.

Free Will and Missed Opportunities: A Management Consideration

Nurse Robinson, RN, has been employed on South Bay Hospital's telemetry unit for 6 years on 12-hour night shifts. Nurse Robinson is regarded as a competent nurse who works very well under pressure. He is well liked by his coworkers, but supervisors find that he can be a negative influence on the work group when he is dissatisfied with staffing levels or new policies and procedures.

South Bay Hospital has attracted a nationally known bariatric surgeon and intends to develop a bariatric surgery service. Some of the nurses, including Nurse Robinson, are concerned about the impact that this service will have on the telemetry unit. These concerns have been shared and discussed during a variety of unit and department meetings.

In preparation for this new program, the hospital purchased several new patient lifts and bariatric-specific beds. The equipment is not sophisticated but does require staff to learn how to adjust the equipment for emergency procedures and transports. In-services are arranged across all shifts. Educational posters are developed with posttest questions, and access to a Web-based educational module is purchased for a 4-week period. There is also an option of reading a continuing education article and completing the posttest.

Staff is required to select the teaching modality that is most convenient for them. Following this educational session, each nurse must demonstrate correct use of the lift and the specialty bed. The staff has 1 month to complete this educational module and to demonstrate competence with the equipment.

Nurse Robinson fails to complete the education stating, "There is no way I'm coming in on my day off and the other times I've been too busy to leave my patients for an in-service on a bed!" Other nurses agree, resulting in a program completion rate of 60%.

During a meeting with the Director of Nursing Education (DONE), the topic of the bariatric education program is raised. The nurse manager requests that the CNS schedule additional in-services to accommodate the staff who had not elected to attend the previous programs. The bariatric program is progressing quickly, and staff will soon need to use the equipment. The CNS agrees to offer three more sessions. Again, turnout is poor.

Two days following the final education session, an obese woman suffers from respiratory distress. She is in a specialized bariatric bed. The emergency team arrives to intubate the patient but the nurse, Nurse Robinson, is unable to position the bed flat. Other nurses come to the room to assist. After a period of 5 minutes, the patient is successfully intubated. As the team attempts to transport the patient to the intensive care unit, more difficulties arise when they realize that the bed will not fit through the door frame. After a lengthy discussion and several attempts, the nursing team successfully removes the bedrails and transports the patient.

The following morning, the DONE is contacted by the bariatric surgeon regarding the nurses' ineptitude with the bariatric equipment. Although the patient did not suffer harm, the potential for injury was high. He insists that the nursing staff requires education.

The DONE meets with the CNS and nurse manager of the unit. The nurse manager's initial response is, "We'll have to set up more in-services right away. Staff have shared with me that they could not attend the in-services because they were too busy taking care of patients. We'll set up mandatory inservices immediately."

The CNS is asked to respond. After thoughtful consideration, the CNS summarizes the problem:

1. Education programs were offered over a 3-week period on a variety of shifts and a variety of days, including weekends. Attendance was poor.
2. Staff unable to attend the education sessions were encouraged to review the poster information and complete a posttest. Fifty percent of nurses who completed the skills demonstration acquired the necessary information via the poster opportunity.
3. Staff interested in a Web-based learning module were able to access the materials through the vendor's Web site. The posttest used for the poster session was available for these nurses. Forty percent of the nurses who completed the skills demonstration chose this education pathway.
4. Staff were permitted to read a continuing education article, self-study through the instruction booklet, and complete the posttest. Ten percent of staff who completed the skills demonstration acquired the necessary information using this selection.

The CNS identified that the problem was no longer a knowledge deficit but rather was a commitment issue. The CNS worked with the management team to design a strategy. Two nurses, both of whom had completed the education program, were asked for input. The action plan was as follows:

1. Staff who had completed the program and the skills assessment were recognized during a staff meeting.
2. Staff who had not completed the program and the skills assessment were identified as "not yet competent" (Wright, 2005) specific to the bariatric bed and lift. They were not permitted to use this equipment until competency was established. Charge nurses were notified as were the individual nurses.
3. Staff were given 1 week to complete the education program and the skills assessment. The only options for learning were numbers 2–4 noted earlier. No further in-service sessions were available. Self-study time was not paid beyond the shift pay.
4. Evaluative feedback was documented and placed in files to inform upcoming performance evaluations.
5. Staff choosing to not participate in the education opportunities were given the option to meet with the nurse manager to discuss other unit assignments that did not require bariatric equipment skills, given the hospital's decision to prioritize this particular program.
6. Staff discussions during meetings and individual conversations reinforced the new perspective on competency demonstrations. Staff participated in identifying convenient and effective teaching and learning strategies and were encouraged to contribute to competency identification for the upcoming year.

Within the week, each nurse had completed the education program and demonstrated competence with the equipment. Nurse Robinson was reluctant to attend the program; however, alternate assignments within the hospital were unappealing. Nurse Robinson completed the program within the required time frame.

It is reasonable for employees to expect that educational programs will be offered on more than one occasion and in a scheduling pattern that accommodates more than one shift. It also makes sense for educational formats to vary and to include flexible options such as computer-assisted instruction, self-study modules, workshops, poster board formats, or Web-based instruction. These expectations are realistic and may even be obligatory on the part of the employing institution.

Employees have concurrent obligations. They are obligated to make themselves available to educational programs. Nurses are responsible for acquiring and maintaining the skills necessary for the level of practice expected of them by the employing institution and for which they accept compensation. Wright (2005) commented that the organization needs to recognize that employees may not be interested in the direction the organization is moving. If this is the case and the employee is not interested in availing himself or herself of the provided educational opportunities, then the employee should find a different organization in which to practice.

This stance is not threatening; rather, it is an honest appraisal of the situation. As noted by Wright (2005, p. 3), "Employees should periodically reflect on their commitment to their organization's evolution, and if that commitment is not strong, find an organization to work for that is better aligned with his or her personal philosophies and goals."

Nursing administrators may find this position disconcerting. Anecdotal evidence suggests that when systems problems arise, education is often offered as a first-line response. When attendance is poor and nurses' skill sets remain amiss, CNSs or educators are charged with providing more teaching sessions. When low attendance rates persist, nurses are reminded of their responsibility to attend and then cajoled, implored, and threatened.

CNSs may need to consider this loop and more carefully examine the linkages that reinforce the negative behaviors. Could it be that low attendance is the result of two or more influences: an incorrect assumption that education is needed to correct this particular clinical problem, and nurses' realizations that "mandatory" in-services are not truly mandated when there are no clear consequences associated with absences? In fact, employees may have become conditioned to believe that it is the responsibility of organizations to provide carte blanche programming and that this responsibility supersedes the obligation of the nurse to take advantage of the education.

The key point is that a root cause analysis is sometimes needed to identify whether the particular problem is actually related to a knowledge deficit. There are many times when nurses know the correct action or behavior but choose to not act as per policy stipulations or, in the case of equipment, per manufacturer's directions. Understanding the reasons why compromised practice standards or processes occur is important to correctly remedy the situation.

At times, the remedy is education. At other times, the solution relates to management interventions. This sort of analysis may be more time consuming than the typical "let's teach—that will fix the problem" reaction but will save money and needless effort by targeting interventions that will correct the underlying problem. The challenge may lie in changing the culture of nursing to one that views competence as radically different from education program attendance.

The Creating and Recognizing Excellence (CARE) program of Albert Einstein Healthcare Network (AEHN) is a unique strategy for rewarding desirable nurse behaviors and promoting professionalism (Exemplar 3-2). This program offers a good example of an opportunity that was initiated by administrators to specifically reinforce employee behaviors that were important to the organization. Rather than providing monetary incentives for overtime or bonuses, a strategy that perpetuated a work culture motivated by pay incentives for time, CARE financially recognizes nurses who demonstrate professional excellence. The impetus for this program was similar to the challenges currently faced by many CNSs when trying to ensure competence in a work environment that devalues educational programming. There may be lessons learned from AEHN's CARE program exemplar that are applicable to other types of organizational challenges.

Exemplar 3-2

Creating and Recognizing Excellence (CARE) Program

Jill Stunkard, MSN, RN, CCRN, CNAA-BC

The CARE Program, Creating and Recognizing Excellence, was developed at Albert Einstein Healthcare Network (AEHN), Philadelphia, Pennsylvania, as a joint venture between Nursing and Human Resources. AEHN was responding to a regional and national nursing shortage and the additional challenge of attracting nurses to an inner-city location. The intent of the program is to improve patient and employee satisfaction, as well as to promote teamwork and improve quality of care.

Program objectives specifically include:

1) differentiate the organization as an employer of choice,
2) reward behaviors that are most beneficial in helping to achieve the institution's mission and goals,
3) retain and attract talented employees in hard to recruit areas,
4) promote career development, and
5) provide excellent clinical service.

Specific activities of nurses and both individual and team goals that should be rewarded were identified. Rather than continually offering bonuses for working long hours, this program financially recognizes steps nurses take to foster professionalism in their own practice and the organization in which they work. The organization's Chief Executive Officer (CEO) and senior leadership team show commitment to the program by providing financial incentives to frontline employees who achieve measurable results that are aligned with the organizational goals of the institution.

The CARE Program consists of four main components, all of which are aimed at retaining registered nurses and other direct patient care providers. Most offer rewards for achievements. The components are an RN Excellence program, Medical/Surgical Team Incentive, Loan Repayment, and Leadership Incentive, a program rewarding managers.

1) One component offered to RNs throughout the Network is the RN Excellence Incentive Program. Initially developed by the Network Nursing Council, this program most importantly promotes development and personal growth of direct patient care RNs. Financial incentives are awarded for achieving excellence in one or more of three areas: Clinical Practice, Leadership/Citizenship, and/or Education/Professional Growth.

2) The Medical/Surgical Care Team Incentive is an innovative program, which focuses on rewards for multidisciplinary teamwork. In addition to RNs, other members of the team may include LPNs, Patient Care Associates, medical clerks, Environmental Service workers, Food and Nutrition staff, physical therapists, and pharmacists. Team members set targets that are reviewed monthly. Assuming the unit meets their target, the reward is divided among the unit members. The three metrics targeted in the first year of this program included patient satisfaction, turnover of licensed staff, and a quality measure. Many units chose decreasing the patient fall index because it was something on which each team member could have an impact.

3) As a method of enhancing educational benefits to RNs, Loan Repayment is offered for RNs employed in Medical/Surgical areas. These RNs are eligible for up to a $10,000 lifetime benefit to be used for repayment of nursing school loans.

4) The final program is a leadership incentive, which is based on five key areas or indicators. These include quality of care, patient satisfaction, staffing, fiscal performance, and professional development. The financial award varies, depending on an eligible leader's role and success in achieving the mutually agreed upon target goals.

Program requirements for CARE were developed collaboratively among nursing managers, staff nurses, and Human Resources (HR). Through AEHN's nursing shared governance model, staff nurse councils assembled members from each specialty area to assist in development of the program. Members of care teams, administration, and HR met to discuss what aspects should be rewarded. The facility also held focus groups to gauge interest in the program and determine what the staff found motivational.

Metrics required within each category often deliberately overlap, so that managers and staff are working toward a goal collectively. RN Excellence, the Medical/Surgical Care Team incentive, and the leadership incentive are all aligned with the goals of the nursing department and the organization as a whole. The monetary reward notwithstanding, active participation in these programs contributes to individual growth and development that benefits not only the individual, but the organization as a whole. After a year of planning, the program was launched in the summer of 2004.

Initially meetings were held with nursing management and education to provide them with specific information about the CARE Programs. Subsequently in July 2004, there were presentations to staff by nursing leadership via Town Meetings, unit staff meetings, and publishing of the "RN Excellence Resource Kit." Nurse managers, Clinical Nurse Specialists, and educators have proven to be significant resources for RNs aspiring to meet the criteria defined in the RN Excellence program. At first glance many people find the requirements overwhelming and value input from nursing leadership.

In order to qualify a nurse must be employed at AEHN for at least 1 year, have no active disciplinary action, and meet baseline criteria on their annual performance review. The plan is for an interested RN to meet with their manager to determine appropriate projects, which would both fulfill the established criteria and be of benefit to the nursing unit where the RN is employed. Nurses must meet various criteria within a category to fulfill requirements, which may include: being a preceptor, acquiring a determined number of continuing education credits, spearheading a performance improvement activity, or attaining certification (see the figure following this exemplar). All three categories of practice (Clinical Excellence, Education/Professional Growth, and Leadership/Citizenship) are valued the same and have similar intensity of criteria. An applicant may select any or all of the three categories in any order they desire, however a monetary award can be earned only once for each category per fiscal year.

The nurse is responsible for creating a portfolio highlighting his/her achievements thereby demonstrating fulfillment of the criteria selected. Once reviewed by the RN's manager, the portfolio is evaluated by the RN Excellence Review Committee. This group of ten is comprised of staff nurses, a nurse manager, a nursing director, the Nursing Career Specialist, and a Human Resources representative. When a nurse's portfolio is approved in one of the categories, he/she receives a $4,000 bonus. Approval in subsequent areas can earn $2,000 for each category. Individuals whose portfolios are not approved are provided with feedback, which almost all have utilized in revising and resubmitting their work.

In March 2005, the "RN Excellence Resource Toolkit" was placed on AEHN's intranet to provide convenient access. A Portfolio Development Seminar was held in April 2005, at which time mentoring by Review Committee membership and RN Excellence Award recipients was initiated. There has been periodic education regarding the program at nursing management meetings.

Nurses are acknowledged for involvement in a variety of projects including in-services, committees, and research. The program has encouraged nurses to think about ways of improving their workplace and their practice. In the first year of the program, $142,000 was paid to 29 nurses who submitted a total of 43 portfolios. Year-to-date March FY06 there have been 30 portfolio submissions by 26 RNs. The number of certified RNs has increased in the past year, anecdotally attributable to the RN Excellence Program.

The RN Excellence Committee is in the process of attempting to determine measurable indicators of the success of the program. They are also making minor adjustments to make some of the criterion more understandable. Plans are underway to create pins, which will be presented to award recipients at a program where nurses will be asked to present some of their projects to their colleagues. Modifications to the program are being considered to include smaller monetary rewards for individuals who finish a project, but feel overwhelmed at the prospect of completing an entire category.

Clinicians are embarking on endeavors that will undoubtedly have an impact on nursing practice and patient outcomes. Continuing evaluation is needed to determine if rewarding professionalism and professional growth contribute to desired outcomes.

Source: © 2004 Albert Einstein Healthcare Network. Reprinted with permission.

MANDATORY REQUIREMENTS FOR THIS CATEGORY:			
Candidate is required to attain 12 contact hours or one (1) college credit in nursing (or related area) in the 12 months prior to submission of their portfolio. Copies of contact hours or proof of a grade of C or above must be provided. Candidate is required to provide evidence of effective utilization of the nursing process — assessment, planning, intervention, and evaluation. Provide evidence of twelve (12) randomly selected charts/year (3 per quarter) that appropriately document all the above stated components of the nursing process. See attached evaluations completed by 1) nurse manager, 2) peer (selected by nurse manager), and 3) candidate-selected peer, manager, or educator (approved by nurse manager). The RN must also submit documentation of attainment of three (3) other of the following criteria:			
Criteria:	Met	Unmet	Comments
1. National certification in the specialty in which the RN currently practices, as recognized by an accepted organization.			
2. Teach a structured educational offering to staff, patients, family, or community a minimum of twice a year (such as BLS, ACLS, PALS, diabetic class, spinal cord injury class, NRP instructor, "Handle with Care," specialty "core," or unit-based in-service). Copies of course coordinator/nurse manager evaluation and attendance sheet must be provided.			
3. Participate in writing and/or revising patient education materials, documentation tools, protocols, policies, and/or procedures. Must be able to demonstrate an evidence-based approach. Provide written documentation signed by a nurse manager.			
4. Be a primary preceptor/mentor for new hires/less-experienced team members a minimum of twice/year. Meet criteria for goal setting, evaluation of goal attainment, collaboration with management and/or CNS as appropriate, and completion of all required documentation. May include coordination/facilitation of student rotations depending on complexity. Evidence of preceptor workshop or "refresher course" completion required. See attached evaluations completed by 1) manager, 2) CNS/clinical educator, and 3) orientee [must have a total rating of ≥ 39 with no "1" (never) rating].			
5. Poster or oral presentation at a professional conference. Copy of program brochure must be provided.			
6. Completion of a quality improvement or process improvement initiative. (May include oversight of the entire project, writing abstract, presenting at PIC (Process Improvement Council), and/or relaying information to the staff via a report, bulletin board, or poster presentation.) *Please note: identification of a problem and/or data collection alone does not qualify to meet these criteria.*			
7. Active participation in Nursing Shared Governance or other entity network committees or councils. Attendance records and minutes must be provided. Attendance records (showing attendance at 80% of meetings) and minutes must be provided.			
8. Author or coauthor of an article in a nursing-focused media (e.g., professional journal or magazine, chapter in a book). If the publication is a peer-reviewed journal, the date of the letter of acceptance will be utilized (not the date of publication).			

Nurse Manager/Clinical Director and/or Clinical Nurse Specialist must initial Met/Unmet in each category.

Initials: _____ Signature: _____

Initials: _____ Signature: _____

Source: © 2004 Albert Einstein Healthcare Network. Reprinted with permission.

Developing Competence with Competencies

There is confusion surrounding the definition of competence (Tilley, 2008), and there are many problems with its measurement (Watson, Stimpson, Topping, & Porock, 2002). The root of this confusion may relate to the lack of a conceptual definition of nursing competence, making it difficult to establish measurable operational definitions (Waddell, 2001). Cowan, Norman, and Coopamah (2005) suggested that nursing requires complex combinations of knowledge, performance, skills, and attitudes, and this complexity necessitates consensus on a conceptual and operational definition. Tilley (2008) described the attributes of competency as the application of skills in all domains for the practice role, instruction focusing on select outcomes or competencies, allowances for increasing levels of competency, learner accountability, practice-based learning, self-assessment, and individually tailored learning experiences.

Identifying domains of competence may be useful, as domains offer possibilities for practical evaluation strategies. Lyon and Boland (2002) suggested that competence domains may include knowledge, technical, cultural, and communication. del Bueno (2001; del Bueno, Barker, & Christmyer, 1980) offered technical, critical thinking, and interpersonal domains as a model of competence. These domain models are consistent and may be useful to the CNS when developing multifaceted strategies for developing nursing competencies and assessing nurse competence.

The terms *competence* and *competency* also require definition, as they are often used interchangeably and may, in fact, be unique but related entities. Competence is often defined as a capacity to perform based on knowledge, whereas competency is the actual performance (Nolan, 1998; McConnell, 2001).

Distinguishing competence from performance is also challenging, and there is no clearly established link from these two concepts to capability and expertise (Watson et al., 2002). Although the notion of protecting the public by ensuring competent practitioners makes sense, the level of performance that actually demonstrates competence in practice has not been determined. An example of this concern is illustrated by a scenario in which an RN completes a medication administration examination for a critical care unit position. The RN scores a 90%. Does this score reflect medication administration competence, or is competence demonstrated only by a 100% score? If the RN scores an 85%, does this score indicate incompetence? Competence may seem simple, but it is a sophisticated issue.

Many healthcare agencies are investing time and money into systems to assess competency of nursing professionals. One example of such a system is the Performance-Based Development System (PBDS). This particular system uses video simulations, written out-of-context exercises, and visual out-of-context exercises to evaluate critical thinking manifested primarily as clinical judgment (del Bueno, 2005).

Aggregate results for competency assessment of new RNs using PBDS indicates that clinical judgment abilities are lacking. del Bueno (2005) suggested that clinical judgment may be best promoted by asking questions and inquiring as to the evidence available or needed to evaluate the effectiveness of nursing interventions. These strategies more effectively promote judgment building than multiple-choice exams offering a choice of written potential solutions (del Bueno, 2005).

del Bueno's (2005) findings and suggestions should be carefully considered by CNSs as they work with newly graduated RNs and as they coach and educate more experienced staff. Assessing competence must be done using more than multiple-choice tests offered immediately following an educational program. This evaluation strategy may be appropriate in certain situations but does not provide credible evidence that a nurse is competent.

In addition, CNSs must remember that attendance at an educational program does not ensure competence with the particular topic or skill. It is probably also true that demonstrating a performance in a controlled laboratory situation with a single skill in a simple environment as compared to a complex, stressful, real-world environment also does not denote competence. Of course, the more sophisticated and labor intensive the competency assessment, the more the activity costs. This is a legitimate concern that cannot be easily dismissed.

Competence assessment involves some form of evaluation by one person of another (Watson et al., 2002). When human interaction is involved in competence assessment, reliability is a potential concern due to the influence of social processes on the consistency of evaluative scores (McMullan et al., 2003; Watson et al., 2002). Validity is also a problem related to the lack of psychometrically established instruments used to determine competence. Reliability concerns are not often raised when CNSs are planning skills labs assessments. Validity is discussed even less frequently. Both of these topics are critically important to the notion of competent practice (Exemplar 3-3).

Exemplar 3-3

Validity and Reliability as Applied to Competencies

A CNS identifies a need for professional nurses to improve their recognition of acute myocardial infarction (AMI) electrocardiogram (ECG) patterns after a potentially serious clinical event in the telemetry unit during which several nurses failed to recognize AMI ECG changes in a 52-year-old female patient. The CNS designs a program to develop competence in AMI ECG interpretations and creates outcomes measures to ascertain competency. The CNS selects a posttest and case study exercise as strategies for verifying competency. In addition, a mock clinical scenario using a simulation model is developed. This simulation experience will take place 2 weeks after the program and will be scored by one or two CNSs. The experience will consist of acute myocardial infarction electrocardiogram recognition and three associated scenarios: (1) acute destabilization with dysrhythmias, pulmonary edema, and hypotension; (2) preparation for and administration of thrombolytic therapy; and (3) immediate preparation for cardiac interventional therapy.

The CNS conducts a literature search and software search to locate an infarct pattern test. None is located, and the CNS creates an examination. The case study exercises are actual 12-lead ECGs from patients who have had a variety of cardiac events and nonevents, including infarcts and angina episodes. Several staff nurses have agreed to supervise small groups of case study sessions and grade the tools.

Reflection Questions

1. Reliable measures are consistent measures. Where are the potential measurement problems specific to reliability?
2. Valid measures accurately reflect the true nature of what is being measured. A valid measure is a truthful measure. What validity concerns are associated with this competency program?
3. How might the CNS improve the reliability and validity of this competency program?
4. Why do the posttest, case study, and clinical simulation work well together to evaluate competence with AMI ECG interpretation and treatment? What does each single evaluation strategy evaluate?

Skillful Nurses and Competency Assessment

Wright (2005) offers very specific, practical suggestions for competency assessment. She asserted that competency assessment follows a continuum that evolves as the requirements of the nurses' jobs evolve (Figure 3-6). Competency assessment for the new hire should differ from that of the established RN. Wright suggested that competency assessment must be perceived by staff as a valuable process, or it will be perceived as a time waster.

One strategy for competency assessment is to engage staff in identifying the competencies that are required for safe and professional practice. Once the competency is determined, verification strategies should match the competency categories. Nurse leaders need to support and sustain a culture of success by promoting, nurturing, and rewarding positive employee performance related to competency assessment (Figure 3-7).

This suggested model is quite different from the traditional competency assessments used in many healthcare organizations (Figure 3-8). Wright's Competency Assessment Model is outcome focused and holds employees accountable for managing their competency verifications. Competency assessment forms are useful as documentation templates for competency identification, verification methodologies, and action planning (Table 3-13).

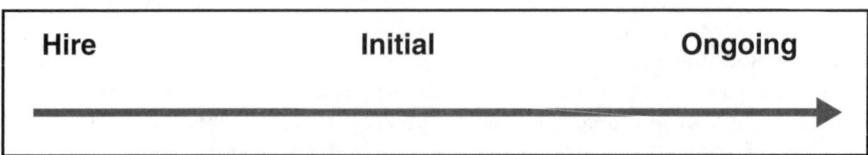

Figure 3-6   Competency continuum.

Source: From *The ultimate guide to competency assessment in health care* (3rd ed.) by Donna Wright. ©2005 Creative Health Care Management. Used with permission.

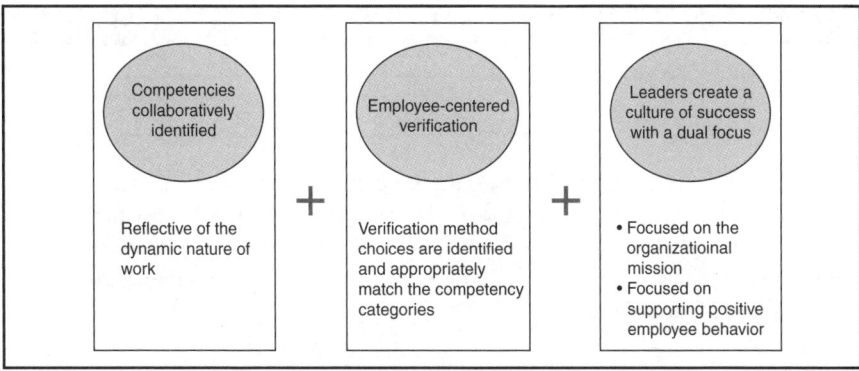

Figure 3-7   Donna Wright's Competency Assessment Model.

Source: From *The ultimate guide to competency assessment in health care* (3rd ed.) by Donna Wright. ©2005 Creative Health Care Management. Used with permission.

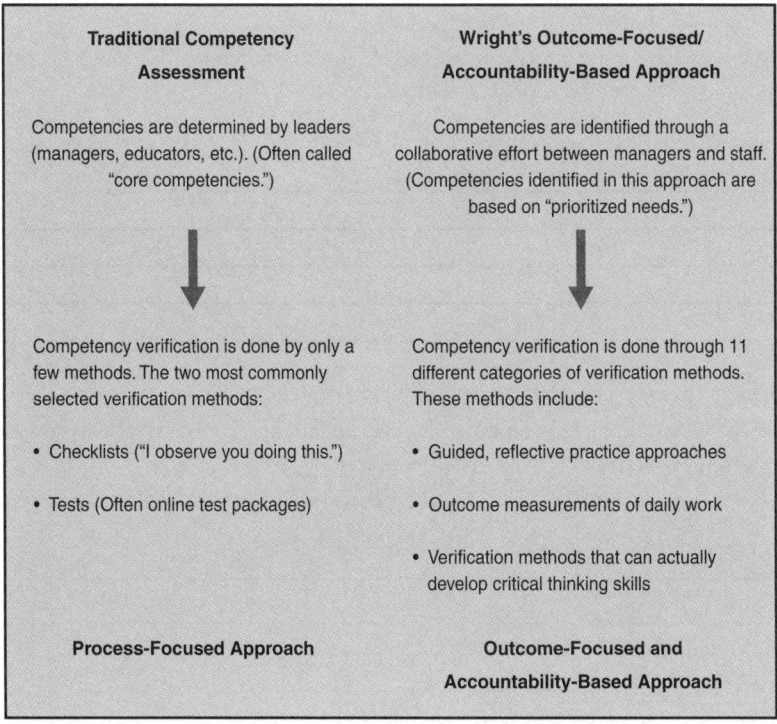

Figure 3-8   Traditional assessment versus Wright's Competency Assessment Model.

Source: From *The ultimate guide to competency assessment in health care* (3rd ed.) by Donna Wright. ©2005 Creative Health Care Management. Used with permission.

Table 3-13   COMPETENCY ASSESSMENT FORM

Competency Assessment Form for ——————— through ———————
                                        (job title)   (competency assessment period)

Name: ——————— Job Class: ——————— Work Area: ———————

This form is to be completed by the employee. For each of the competency statements listed below, the employee may select which method of verification he or she would like to use for validation of his or her skill in that area. See the method of verification for details. When this form is complete, submit it to the area supervisor as indicated.

Competency	Method of Verification	Date Completed

For added effect, this form can be categorized into three domains of skill (technical, critical thinking, and interpersonal).

The following is a list of organizational activities required for this job. Select the method of education/verification that you prefer.

Organizational Education and Other Requirements	Method of Education/ Verification	Date Completed

This section to be completed by the supervisor:

With consideration of the employee's performance and competency assessment, this employee is competent to perform as a/an:

——————— on/in ——————— ❑ YES ❑ NO (Not yet deemed competent)
   (job class)   (work area)

Action Plan:

Employee Signature ——————————— Date ———————

Supervisor Signature ——————————— Date ———————

Source: From *The ultimate guide to competency assessment in health care* (3rd ed.) by Donna Wright. © 2005 Creative Health Care Management. Used with permission.

Regulating Competency Assessment

External agencies such as the Joint Commission provide powerful motivation for competency development and implementation. Wright (2005) observed that many times organizations are cited as deficient on a particular standard by an external agency because of an internal policy. For example, the Joint Commission (2006b) requires that organizations ensure that staff abilities meet the requirements of the job. Management of Human Resources Standard HR.1.20 states: "The organization has a process to ensure that a person's qualifications are consistent with his or her job responsibilities" (p. 8).

The elements of performance specific to this standard are variable and include elements related to nonemployees, students, and employees. One of the Joint Commission (2006b, p. 4) elements is "Staff supervises students when they provide client care, treatment, and services as part of their training." This element is written in a general way that is open for interpretation by the individual organizations.

When the organization is crafting policy that meets this external agency standard, the organization must give careful thought to the best policy for its particular circumstances and design the policy parameters to be reasonable and consistent with its operations and resources. If the organization drafts a policy mandating that each student have an RN assigned for direct supervision and that the assigned RN will be designated on the daily assignment sheet, then this is what the Joint Commission will expect to find. Wright (2005) cautioned that external agencies can cite organizations for noncompliance with the organizations' established internal policies. It is very important for institutions to craft policies and standards that are realistic, reasonable, and effective within its particular practice setting.

Essentials for Educating with Excellence: Academic Teaching and the CNS

Many CNSs are interested in teaching undergraduate nursing students, whereas others find that precepting graduate students is more to their liking. There are many opportunities to participate in nursing education at both the undergraduate and graduate levels. The nursing profession and the healthcare system are challenged by the shortage of professional nurses, including advanced practice nurses. Faculty shortages are contributing to this nursing shortage because baccalaureate program enrollment figures cannot exceed the availability of nurse educators.

The American Association of Colleges of Nursing (AACN) has identified that budget constraints, an aging faculty, and increasing competition from clinical agencies for graduate-degree nurses have contributed to the nursing faculty shortage (AACN, 2005). In 2004, nursing schools in the United States turned away 32,797 qualified applicants from college/university undergraduate and graduate programs because of insufficient resources, including faculty and clinical preceptors. A July 2004 AACN report revealed that 717 faculty vacancies were identified at 395 nursing schools with baccalaureate and/or graduate programs. This lack of faculty contributes to the nursing shortage which, in turn, adversely affects the provision of safe patient care (Allen, 2008).

The shortage of formally prepared nurse educators coupled with the need for clinical experts puts CNSs in an ideal position to consider opportunities in clinical instruction, professorships, and part-time employment as adjunct faculty members. CNSs need to have a clear understanding of the differences between these roles, the expectations of each, a general sense of the right questions to ask, and a handle on the responsibilities and challenges associated with the teaching role.

Undergraduate Clinical Teaching

There are a number of ways for CNSs to become involved in basic nursing education. In general, most nursing programs require a master's of science in nursing (MSN) degree of faculty. Although some individuals using the title "CNS" or "CS" do not have an MSN, specifically in those states that do not recognize the title "CNS," most CNSs do hold an MSN degree, usually from a graduate program providing CNS preparation. Specialty certification is not usually required for clinical teaching, although it may be desirable to demonstrate expertise within a particular specialty area.

Some nurses prefer to work as a CNS on a full-time or part-time basis and to teach as an adjunct faculty member for a university, 4-year college (baccalaureate program), or community college (associate of arts/science degree of nursing [ADN]). This type of teaching position is referred to as "adjunct" because the clinical instructor is a supplemental teaching resource who contributes to the overall education of the students and the quality of the program but does not have the responsibilities of a full-time faculty member.

Other CNSs may elect to teach on a full-time basis while practicing clinically on a part-time basis. This clinical practice may be in the form of agency or per diem work, part-time employment, or in a joint appointment. A joint appointment is a combined position that links academic work to clinical practice. The CNS holding a joint appointment position typically straddles both worlds, academic and service, with varying accountabilities to administrators in each setting. This type of role can be challenging in its duality but is also stimulating. Challenges associated with joint positions include a high workload, lower salaries as compared to clinical practice alone, and role conflicts (Lewallen, 2002).

Adjunct or part-time clinical instructor positions are also available in basic nursing programs at the diploma (hospital-based) level. The more typical terminology is *part-time* clinical instructor rather than *adjunct* faculty and probably relates to the historical differences between the hospital-based and university-based programs. There are also fewer diploma programs in the United States than other types and, therefore, fewer opportunities for CNSs. For the purpose of this chapter, academic opportunities relate to college or university settings.

What Are Creative Teaching Strategies?

The descriptive phrase "creative teaching strategies" is commonly used by nurse educators. Some institutions of higher education use this phrase on evaluation forms as an aspect of teacher evaluations. In general, this phrase is a catchall term for a variety of teaching methods that are designed to engage the student in the process of learning as an active participant rather than as a passive receptacle of information.

Creative teaching or active learning strategies may include concept mapping (Billings & Halstead, 2005; Hsu & Hsieh, 2005), problem-based learning activities (Zuzelo, Inverso, & Linkewich, 2001), case studies, simulation exercises, games, logs, journals, and role playing, as well as others. Billings and Halstead (2005) provide helpful descriptive summaries for multiple teaching strategies. These descriptions, as well as the identified supplemental resources, may be very useful to the novice CNS educator.

Clinical Teaching vs. Clinical Practice: Duality and Harmony

It is common for CNSs to express an interest in teaching nursing students. Many CNSs have an interest in education and a commitment to clinical practice excellence. Clinical expertise is an advantage to nursing students as CNSs' expertise contributes to the overall quality and relevance of the educational experience.

CNSs may find that their expertise is associated with unique challenges. It can be difficult to instruct students in settings that are challenged by a lack of experienced staff or a culture of mediocrity. Staff may approach the CNS for advice, assistance, or troubleshooting. CNSs may feel inclined to participate in decision making and care provision that is not within their purview as nursing instructors but, rather, belongs with the RN employees of the host institution.

CNSs may also find it difficult to teach at a rudimentary level when their usual practice is much more advanced. It can be tempting to launch into a discussion of abnormal physical assessment findings, complex pharmacology, or advanced pathology topics with students who are eager to learn and interested in everything and anything that the CNS may be willing to share! At the same time, these students may not have had a pharmacology course or medical–surgical content or have practiced beyond providing fundamental care to a single patient assignment. Although the instructional conversations may be interesting, CNSs teaching as academic instructors need to stay focused on facilitating progression toward the final course objectives. This duality as educator and clinician can work in harmony if the CNS is clear about the responsibilities and focus of clinical teaching experiences.

Exploring the Possibilities of Teaching

Gathering information about clinical and classroom teaching is a good first step for the CNS interested in nursing education. Lewallen (2002) provides an excellent overview of academic nursing and tailors this discussion to CNSs. Lewallen suggests that there are questions that CNSs should ask when considering an academic position (Table 3-14). These questions are an excellent starting point, but other preparatory questions may also be useful.

The school of nursing's philosophy is an important consideration, as the philosophy should provide a context for educational experiences. The school's philosophy

Table 3-14   **ACADEMIC POSITION CONSIDERATIONS AND QUERIES**
1. What is the school's philosophy?
2. What does the job description say?
3. What about tenure?
4. How are the courses sequenced?
5. How do I begin to prepare for classroom teaching?
6. How do I make the transition from clinical nursing to clinical teaching?
7. What regulatory and accreditation issues will I face?
8. What will my students be like?

Source: Lewallen, 2002.

must be congruent with the philosophy of the larger university or college in which it exists. The university's philosophy and mission relate to the ways in which nursing education is provided.

As an example, a university dedicated in the traditions of the Christian Brothers and a Roman Catholic, private, urban institution may have a different perspective on faculty obligations and student-to-faculty relationships than a large, publicly funded state university located in a rural region. Students may also have differing expectations of their selected program, depending on school type. The school of nursing exists within the confines of the university's mission. CNSs need to consider the university's philosophy and make certain that it is compatible to their personal philosophy of education.

Reviewing the position's job description is important to understand the responsibilities of clinical instructors. Job descriptions may be written in broad terms to address the generic responsibilities associated with any type of nursing course. CNSs need to be aware of the different responsibilities associated with the different teaching roles within the school.

For example, the responsibilities of a clinical instructor, classroom teacher working in a team, and course coordinator or single classroom professor are markedly different. These differences may not be clearly articulated in a job description. CNSs should review the syllabi for their course assignment and discuss the responsibilities of the course specific to clinical faculty or assistant classroom faculty. It is often helpful to construct questions specific to clinical (Table 3-15) and classroom (Table 3-16) teaching responsibilities to assist in developing a very clear understanding of the commitments and expectations of each type of position.

CNSs considering an opportunity to take responsibility for coordinating and teaching a course may find that they have additional obligations including communicating with clinical instructors, arranging student experiences at affiliating agencies, and organizing paperwork, evaluations, and documentation specific to student perfor-

Table 3-15	SAMPLE QUERY PATH FOR FLEDGLING CLINICAL INSTRUCTORS

Questions to Ask:

1. How large is a typical clinical group?
2. How does the instructor become familiar with the clinical setting? Is there an orientation program, and if so, who arranges this orientation?
3. The name, job title, credentials, electronic mail address (e-mail), and telephone number of the clinical agency contact person.
4. How are the students oriented to the agency?
5. What is the appropriate dress, including identification, for clinical faculty?
6. Is there a student handbook that describes policies and procedures for medication administration, charting, student illness, absenteeism and lateness, dress code, and clinical preparation requirements?
7. How long is the clinical day? What is the typical schedule?
8. How are assignments shared with students? Are they posted at the clinical agency, and if so, when should they be posted?
9. What is the required student preparation for clinical, and when should this preparation occur?
10. How should an instructor respond to the poorly prepared student?
11. Secure a copy of the required clinical paperwork. What criteria are used to evaluate the preparatory work? When should the work be returned to the student? How does the clinical instructor respond to inadequately completed paperwork?
12. When are students evaluated? Secure a copy of the evaluation tool.
13. What resources are available to assist the student who is performing poorly or unsafely in the clinical setting?
14. What is the policy for office hours?
15. Is parking available at the clinical agency?
16. Is a preconference session required?
17. Is a postconference session required?
18. Are clinical activities scheduled solely at the clinical agency, or are there required activities that are scheduled for additional, outside sites?
19. How does inclement weather affect the clinical learning experience, and who makes decisions regarding early dismissal or clinical experience cancellations?
20. Are phone chains required? What is the expected mode of communication between the clinical instructor and the students?

(continues)

Table 3-15   (continued)

21. What circumstances should be described and forwarded to the immediate course supervisor?

22. What are the clinical expectations for students specific to numbers of patients, intravenous and medication therapies, discharge planning, teaching, physical assessment, and charting?

23. How will course content and concerns be communicated to the clinical instructors to connect clinical and classroom learning activities?

24. How are instructors addressed in the clinical setting? Are formal titles required, or do instructors work with students on a first-name basis?

mance issues. Differentiating between these roles and asking appropriate questions prior to accepting the position may help the CNS avoid problems or surprises during the semester.

Many CNSs become initially involved in nursing education as part-time clinical instructors. Be aware that the responsibilities of clinical instructors can vary between schools and/or within schools. As an example, some programs require clinical instructors to participate in grading student assignments. CNSs need to seek information specific to the turnaround time for grading assignments as well as any opportunities for asking questions and seeking validation from more experienced colleagues that grades have been correctly assigned.

Difficulties associated with grading tend to relate to the clarity and detail of the assignment flyers. If grading activities rely on the subjective evaluation of the clinical instructor, the CNS may find it helpful to ask that the instructor group meet to share insights and critiques prior to returning grades to students. This activity promotes interrater reliability and prevents the variability in grading that students perceive as unfair. Some programs do not require clinical instructors to grade assignments but may require paperwork evaluations using satisfactory versus unsatisfactory criteria. Again, this is an important area to explore before signing a contract.

Clinical Instruction: Control the Urge to Nurse

New clinical instructors often find it difficult to establish boundaries with the staff on the assigned nursing unit. CNSs are accustomed to serving as the clinical expert and typically enjoy interacting with staff and troubleshooting patient care dilemmas. As a result, the CNS may feel conflicted when a situation develops on the assigned unit that appears to require the expertise of the CNS.

Although it may be tempting to fully participate in the problem-solving activities of staff, the CNS is on the unit in the capacity of a nurse educator. Within this capacity, the instructor must attend to the learning needs of the students rather than the unit activities. CNSs need to remember that each student is relying on the instructor

Table 3-16	QUESTIONS TO ASK WHEN CONSIDERING CLASSROOM TEACHING OPPORTUNITIES

Didactic Instruction

1. How large is a typical classroom group?
2. Is there a general orientation to the university?
3. Is there an orientation to the school?
4. Copy of the academic calendar including withdrawal dates, semester holidays, examination schedules at midsemester and final-semester.
5. What is the policy and procedure for printed materials?
6. What resources are typically used for testing (e.g., test scoring equipment, Scantron sheets, pencils, laptops), and how are arrangements made for secure testing?
7. What is the policy and procedure for missing or making up a class due to attendance at a professional conference or illness?
8. Are guest speakers encouraged, and if so, are they paid? How is this pay generated? Is there a resource list of speakers?
9. What is the process for textbook selection?
10. How are texts secured for faculty?
11. Is there a notification process to alert students when their academic progress is below the required passing mark?
12. What is the policy for office hours?
13. Is there a platform for Web-based/computer-based instruction as a supplement to the course? If so, how does the professor access this resource?
14. How is the instructor addressed by the students? First-name basis or formal titles?
15. Who is responsible for developing and updating the course syllabus? Is it an individualized activity or a group activity with other faculty members?
16. How are final grades entered into the university system? What are the reporting mechanisms associated with all grades? Failing grades?
17. Is there a policy for missed examinations?
18. Is there an honesty code, and if so, how is this policy enforced?
19. Are professors required to tutor, and if so, how are rooms reserved?
20. Explore the availability of office space and secretarial support.
21. Is there a required format for course syllabi? What topics are included on the syllabus? What other additional forms should be generated for a course?

to make certain that learning is occurring and that patients are safe. If the instructor becomes too involved in isolated patient care situations or practice dilemmas, students are left unsupervised, and patients are receiving care from individuals who are not licensed or prepared to practice with autonomy.

Another boundary challenge relates to complex patient care scenarios. There are times when patients' conditions deteriorate. Depending on the academic standing of the nursing student and the responsibilities and activities of the other students in the clinical group cohort, the CNS instructor may be able to engage in prioritizing and intervening in the complex patient care situation with the intent of promoting student learning.

However, the reality of this type of situation is that deteriorating patient circumstances demand time and attention. Acute instability may require medication orders, initiating a rapid response team consult, and, perhaps, verbal orders. These responsibilities are more appropriately met by the employed RN. It may be possible for a student to work closely with the RN and either assist or observe; however, the CNS must step out and focus on the learning experiences of the remaining students.

Lewallen (2002) cautioned that clinical instructors need to realize that they are not on the unit as direct care providers. Instructors are on the unit to teach. There are times when students will be unable to accomplish the tasks of patient care. These activities will need to be turned back to the staff. The CNS clinical instructor cannot perform nursing care outside the purview of teaching students. It is difficult to acknowledge that total care has not been completed and to return these responsibilities to the staff; however, clear communication processes and ongoing updates assist in preventing misunderstandings.

Another potential problem area relates to the relationship between ancillary staff members and students. This relationship is a frequent "hot button" and has been known to create much stress for clinical instructors. It may be helpful to meet with the nurse manager and/or charge nurses before beginning the clinical experience to establish rules and procedures prior to the first day of clinical.

In general, it is important to recognize that neither the students nor the instructor are agency employees. In fact, the clinical learning group is a guest to the institution. Ancillary staff members are paid employees. As such, certain responsibilities and tasks are assigned to them, for which they are paid. The employed RNs are responsible for assigning work to the ancillary staff members and for supervising this work.

Within this context, it is useful to explain to students and reinforce to staff that ancillary staff assigned to patients are required to meet the needs of the patients. If a student is also assigned to the patient, the student is responsible for completing assigned patient care activities as demanded by his or her learning needs. These needs are delineated on the course syllabus.

In other words, students are at the clinical agency to learn, whereas ancillary staff members are at the agency as employees. When a nursing assistant (NA) receives a patient care assignment, the NA is responsible to the employed RN assigned to the particular patient. The NA is not accountable to the student; however, the student is also not accountable to the NA.

Rather, NAs should go about their work as they are paid to do within the confines of the usual practice patterns on the unit. If a nursing student is assigned to the same patient, the NA should not abdicate responsibility for patient care because "the patient has a student today." The student may or may not have responsibility for learning and practicing fundamental skills.

If a student is required to learn discharge teaching and planning, physical assessment, or other aspects of professional nursing care, the morning care routines of beds, baths, and weights may or may not be required of the student. Communication is absolutely critical in these scenarios. The clinical instructor needs to recognize that tact, kindness, and respect for others should be paramount in the interactions with staff members. Otherwise, issues with ancillary staff and professional staff may negatively affect student learning experiences. Instructors should view these interactions as opportunities to role model professional communication processes.

This same rationale explains why students should not be inappropriately used for patient transport, pharmacy pickups, and other routine tasks. When students spend too much time in these activities, they become resentful and frustrated because these activities take time away from critical experiences, thereby undermining the educational value of the day. Of course, in the event of a true patient care emergency, students may need to be flexible and assist as team members. It is important for the clinical instructor to recognize what sorts of situations are emergencies as compared to situations that are predictable and related to short staffing, sick calls, or poor planning.

Typically Atypical Nursing Students

Nurse demographics are changing, and the profession is welcoming, even encouraging, these changes. Society needs an increased number of nurses, and both society and the profession need these nurses to reflect the richly diverse cultural montage of the country. These needs are encouraging professional nursing organizations and foundations to increase recruitment efforts directed toward diverse students, including people from low socioeconomic backgrounds (Zuzelo, 2005).

The aging nursing workforce is also a concern and provides additional incentives for recruiting potential nurses from underrepresented groups. It is anticipated that by 2010, the average age of nurses will be 45.4 years, with approximately 40% of the workforce beyond age 50 (U.S. General Accounting Office [GAO], 2001). These concerns, coupled with the desires of disadvantaged and disenfranchised people to improve their quality of life, are changing the demographics of the nursing classroom. CNSs working in academic nursing need to be prepared for the joys and challenges of a student body that includes people of all ages, even those near retirement age, races, religions, and socioeconomic backgrounds.

Zuzelo (2005) asserted that disadvantaged students present challenges to nurse educators who may be unprepared to identify and respond to the unique needs and characteristics of this group. Disadvantaged students come to higher education programs with different background experiences than do advantaged students. These past experiences may affect the ways that the student engages with classmates and faculty.

When an instructor values a consistent approach to students, there may be a tendency to use a one-size-fits-all teaching style. The problem with this approach is that it discounts the differences in the opportunities to learn. In other words, disadvantaged students may not have the same real-life opportunities to learn as a student who is academically and psychologically ready to learn at the college level. Educators need to keep these differences in mind as they work with clinical groups and classroom sections and strategize appropriately to meet the needs of these students, within reason (Table 3-17). It is important for faculty to be fair and rigorous in expectations while simultaneously assisting students from all types of backgrounds to be as successful as their skills and abilities permit.

Handling the Angry Student

CNSs may also find it important to note that there is an increasing body of published literature suggesting that student incivility is a significant problem in nursing education. Whether described as "attitude" (Zuzelo, 2005, p. 29) or categorized as incivility, aggression (Luparell, 2005), or "maladaptive anger behavior" (Thomas, 2003, p. 17), hostile and aggressive behaviors are increasingly witnessed in nursing education settings. Incivility and threatening behaviors may be viewed as manifestations of a more aggressive society; however, nurse educators need to have a ready repertoire of strategies for dealing with student behaviors that may be unpredictable, uncivil, offensive, or even dangerous (Table 3-18).

Table 3-17   STRATEGIES FOR AFFIRMING DISADVANTAGED STUDENTS
1. Recognize the lack of role models for disadvantaged students and fill the void by personally reaching out.
2. Evaluate reading assignments, class activities, patient care assignments, and speakers to ensure that they reflect pluralism and diversity and are relevant to the experiences of students from a variety of backgrounds, including disadvantaged backgrounds.
3. Recognize that self-confidence, assertiveness, and teamwork are part of the hidden yet important curriculum of nursing education programs.
4. Counter student hostility with calm, quiet, and immediate discussion.
5. Offer additional supports to disadvantaged students, including students who are disadvantaged within the university setting because of minority status.
6. Consider joint projects between instructors and disadvantaged students, remembering that these particular students may be less likely to volunteer or ask for such experiences.

Source: Zuzelo, 2005.

Table 3-18	STRATEGIES FOR RESPONDING TO INCIVILITY, THREATS, OR DANGER

Recommended Strategy

1. Clearly describe behavioral expectations using both verbal and written instructions (Luparell, 2005).

2. Explain the purpose and necessity of constructive criticism (Luparell, 2005).

3. Engage in circumspective self-evaluation and consider personal behaviors and teaching strategies that may be perceived as disrespectful by students (Luparell, 2005).

4. Anticipate the possibility of an uncivil response from students (Luparell, 2005). Keep office doors open without violating student privacy. Meet in common rooms rather than in an isolated office.

5. Prepare for occasions when negative feedback needs to be delivered to a student (Luparell, 2005).

6. Respond promptly to incivilities and disruptive behaviors—mediate the form of the response based on the severity of the behavior (Luparell, 2005).

7. Establish a zero-tolerance policy for violent behavior.

8. Avoid appointments with students in isolated settings during off-business hours.

9. Establish a security or alert system to intervene when student behaviors are threatening.

10. Utilize safety and security services on campus or at clinical affiliates as appropriate.

Source: Zuzelo, 2005.

Although incivility is not a hallmark of nursing students in general, it is a phenomenon that is increasingly worrisome and should be not unexpected. There have been incidents of fatal violence directed at professors from students as well as stalking incidences and assault (Thomas, 2003).

Student anger may be triggered when students feel "different" or isolated from the normative group (Zuzelo, 2005), feel the perceived pressures associated with constructive criticism (Luparell, 2005), or experience one of five common triggers (Thomas, 2003). Thomas noted five common causes of nursing students' anger: (1) perceptions of teacher unfairness, discrimination, or rigidity; (2) unreasonable expectations of faculty; (3) overly critical instructors; (4) reactions to unanticipated changes; and (5) unresolved family issues that influence and inform reactions to situations in the educational setting. CNSs considering educator roles should think about these triggers and contemplate strategies to minimize the likelihood of evoking an unreasonably angry student response to an unreasonable teacher behavior (Table 3-19).

Table 3-19	ANGER TRIGGERS FOR STUDENTS

1. Receiving only negative feedback without recognition of jobs well done.
2. Treating students differently based upon sex. Avoid making gender-based requests such as, "I need one of the male students to assist with a transport."
3. Criticizing students for their opinions or feelings when honesty is requested.
4. Insulting or criticizing students in public forums including nursing stations, patient rooms, or during clinical conferences.
5. Making unexpected changes to clinical schedules, assignments, or locations and providing little to no notice.

Source: Adapted from Thomas, 2003.

Exemplar 3-4

The Unprepared Student

Background:

Suzanne Perkins is a 21-year-old junior nursing student entering her second semester of nursing courses. She has completed the Fundamentals of Nursing course as well as the Health Assessment and Health Promotion course. Suzanne is presently enrolled in a Medical–Surgical Nursing course that focuses on the adult client. Her clinical experience takes place at a local university hospital on a busy medical unit. The clinical instructor is responsible for a total of eight nursing students. The instructor reviewed the clinical objectives with the students during the first week of class. The evaluation tool was carefully reviewed with the students and questions were encouraged. The students were informed that the following week, they needed to be prepared to provide comprehensive nursing care to one patient. This assignment would include medication administration, with the exception of intermittent intravenous medications. Clinical paperwork would be collected at the end of the clinical day. Students who attended preconference without satisfactory evidence of clinical preparation would be sent off the clinical unit for the day. The instructor made certain that the students had her office phone number and e-mail address. Policies for absences and lateness were reviewed.

Week One:

Suzanne presented to preconference on time and adequately discussed her nursing plan of care for the day. She claimed to have had difficulty finding two of her assigned clients' medications and was unaware of the patient's bladder irrigation therapy required for hemorrhagic cystitis (she had not yet had this topic in nursing class). Her care provision for the day was organized, and she was professional and friendly on the unit. When dispensing medications, Suzanne was able to identify Digoxin as a "cardiac glycoside" but was unable to relate the Digoxin to the patient's long history of atrial fibrillation. Additionally, she identified Capoten as an "ACE inhibitor" but was unaware of what this term meant and believed that her patient required such for hypertension, despite the fact that her patient had no such history noted on his record. The instructor reviewed these concerns with Suzanne and related these issues to inadequate clinical preparation. Suzanne's comment to these concerns was, "I spent 4 hours getting ready for clinical! It's unrealistic to expect me to spend more time!" The instructor discussed strategies for clinical preparation with Suzanne and made certain that the student knew how to find information in the chart, how to prioritize multiple diagnoses, and how to fine-tune her medication preparation. The student expressed understanding and appreciation.

Week Two:

Suzanne was assigned two patients; one patient required partial assistance with care, whereas the other required minimal assistance. The first patient was in the hospital with the diagnosis of deep vein thrombosis (DVT) and was receiving concurrent heparin and Coumadin therapy. Suzanne was able to discuss DVT and the nursing care associated with such. She was unable to identify signs and symptoms of pulmonary embolus. Suzanne also was unable to explain why the patient was receiving both heparin and Coumadin. Suzanne did adequately discuss the nursing care associated with anticoagulation therapy in general. After preconference, the instructor approached Suzanne about her inadequate preparation. Suzanne stated, "We haven't had any of this in class yet. You can't expect me to learn all of this the night before clinical. Besides, I think my preparation was as good as anyone else's!" After further discussion, Suzanne reluctantly acknowledged that her preparation was superficial and vowed to be more focused the following week.

Week Three:

Suzanne was assigned one patient with total care needs. The patient was receiving continuous enteral feedings via a PEG tube. The patient had a Stage III decubitus ulcer on her left hip requiring dressing changes twice daily. Additionally, she was receiving intravenous fluid at 80 cc/hour. The patient was alert and oriented to person and place with a diagnosis of hemiplegia secondary to an embolic cerebral vascular accident (CVA). Suzanne satisfactorily discussed the physical care needs of this patient. She was unable to relate the patient's CVA to her atrial fibrillation despite the fact that this information was noted in the chart on several occasions. Additionally, although she was aware of the patient's diarrhea, she was unaware of the patient's diagnosis of Clostridium diffocele and treatment with Flagyl.

Reflection Questions

1. Was this student's clinical preparation satisfactory? How do you determine whether a student has "adequately" prepared for the clinical day?
2. Is information not yet covered in the classroom fair game for clinical?
3. How would you respond to Suzanne's comment, "Besides, I think my preparation was as good as anyone else's"?
4. In what ways could this performance issue with Suzanne affect the rest of the clinical group?
5. What types of documentation should the instructor maintain as she works with Suzanne?
6. What is the role of the course coordinator in this situation?
7. Identify your concerns when you place yourself in this scenario as the instructor.
8. Identify your concerns when you place yourself in this scenario as the student.
9. Develop a possible action plan for Suzanne.

Evaluating Students

Setting the tone for the clinical learning experience is important and should be carefully contemplated before the first day of clinical. The CNS instructor should develop a loose script for the orientation day and make clear the behaviors required for satisfactory performance. The tone of the initial meeting and the clarity of shared information affects students' perceptions of the rigor associated with the clinical experience. Ultimately, these perceptions influence student behaviors and affect student performance evaluations.

A word of caution: Clinical instructors occasionally confuse rigor with meanness. Students should not feel threatened, bullied, or diminished by instructors. High expectations are able to coexist with warmth, friendliness, and genuine concern. Reading the riot act to students as a method of ensuring hard work and discipline is not an effective teaching method. Rather, it may perpetuate itself in practice when nurses "beat up" new colleagues or are intolerant of the needs of colleagues.

Clinical instructors are responsible for evaluating students' performance. This may be one of the more difficult aspects of academic nursing. CNSs may have experience with evaluating the performance of new or established employees; however, evaluating students is somewhat different. The Clinical Instruction Algorithm (Figure 3-9) (Zuzelo, 2005) is a useful pictorial representation of clinical instruction and evaluation processes. Instructor feedback suggests that it is easy to follow and a rapid way to understand the larger context of clinical instruction.

Students should be evaluated on an ongoing basis. The clinical instructor should be making conclusions based on patterns of behavior with the purpose of developing students and assisting them in their efforts to become proficient beginner clinicians. If a student is performing at an unsatisfactory level, inform the student immediately and follow an organized process for supporting the student in attempts to improve and develop competence (Table 3-20). There are strategies and guidelines available to assist the instructor with meeting the needs of the struggling student (Zuzelo, 2000), including probationary processes, remedial supports, or systematized warnings.

Most institutions require a midsemester and end-semester clinical evaluation. A general guideline to consider is that students should not be surprised by the contents of their performance evaluation. Ideally, students should have an ongoing sense of how they are performing as measured against the clinical objectives (Zuzelo, 2000).

The Contractual Obligations of a Syllabus

Students should be evaluated against the clinical objectives of the course, and these objectives should be theoretically consistent with the overall course objectives delineated on the syllabus. This syllabus is a contract that instructors and students are obliged to follow.

CNSs need to appreciate the serious nature of contract obligations and rights established through school and course policies and procedures to avoid misunderstandings related to compromised due process requirements stemming from property rights

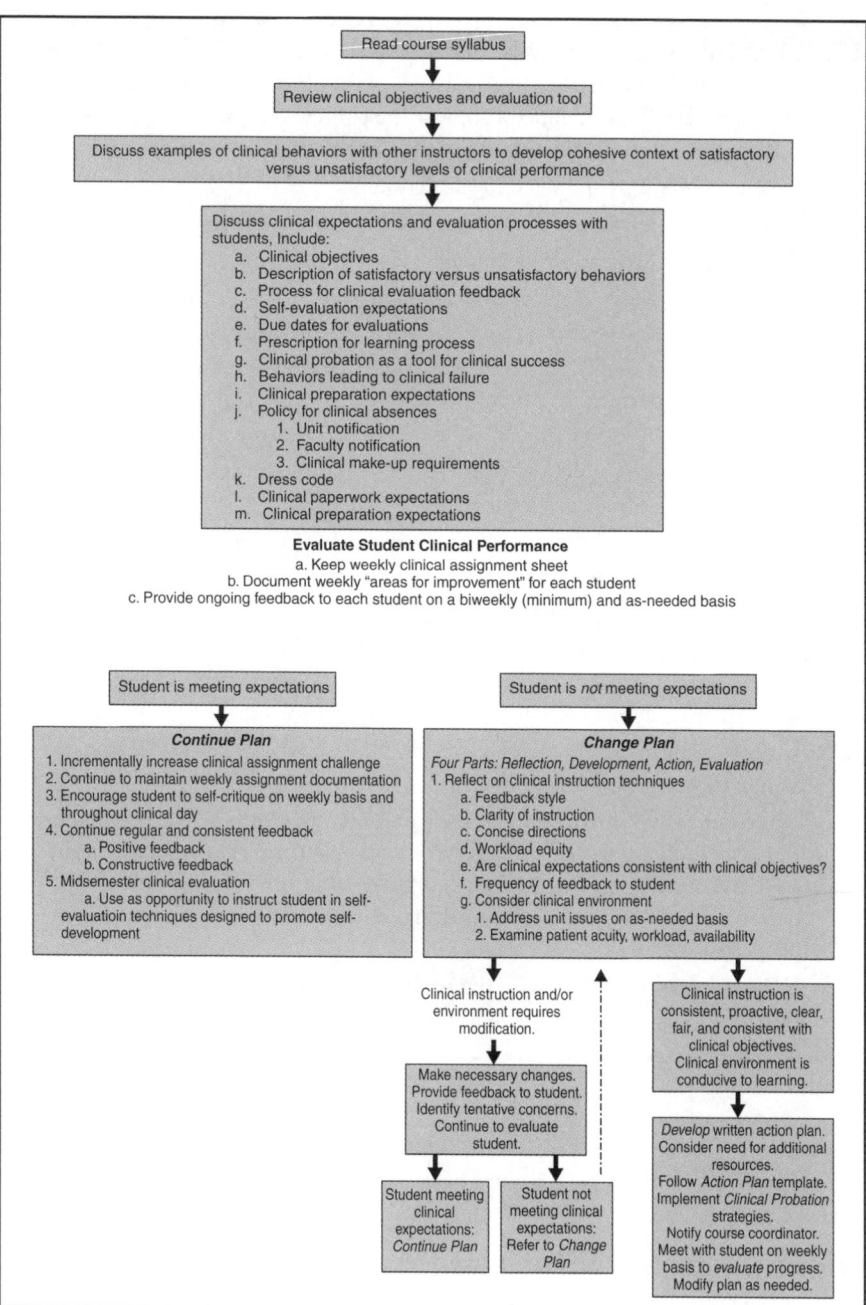

Figure 3-9   Clinical evaluation algorithm.

Source: © 2006 Patti R. Zuzelo. Reprinted with permission.

Table 3-20   CHECKLIST FOR CLINICAL ADVISEMENT

1. Has the student received a written copy of the clinical objectives/ requirements? This includes a copy of the clinical evaluation tool, written criteria from the clinical instructor, and course syllabus criteria.
2. Has the student participated in the action plan?
3. Is the action plan signed and dated by each party with each meeting?
4. Are copies being kept of the student's written work?
5. Do you have copies of the weekly assignments?
6. Keep objective anecdotal records. Are these records available for all students in the clinical group cohort, or is excessive rigor being applied to the poorly performing student?
7. Review school policies and follow.
8. Better to use clinical probation early than late. Remember, student success is the goal; therefore, as early a notice as is realistic is best for the student.
9. Think about support services. What else can be offered to the student, and who else can be involved?
10. If meetings are uncomfortable or angry, bring in a consistent third party.
11. Are other students asking questions? Firmly but kindly assure them that their concerns are understood, but one student's issues cannot be discussed with other students.
12. Is staff curious? Do not share information. Reassure staff that the student is supported in the learning process.
13. Are parents calling? Do not discuss the student with them. Rather, suggest that they come in with their child to discuss the concerns. Remember, the student controls this interaction, and the student needs to speak with his or her parents and arrange the meeting at the mutual convenience of all parties.
14. Was written notice regarding the particular student's performance issues provided to the course coordinator?

(Exemplar 3-5). The clinical instructor is obliged to provide feedback, both positive and negative, to students on a regular basis through informal communication or in brief, written comments.

Communicating with Students

CNSs should give careful thought to the method of shared communication. Some instructors prefer to distribute their personal cell phone numbers or home numbers,

Exemplar 3-5

Critical Thinking Question: CNS as Clinical Instructor

Due process rights emanate from the ideas of a property right or a liberty interest. They are constitutional rights. The Fourteenth Amendment protects citizens from having property denied without due process of law. Public universities must protect these rights. Private universities do not have to protect constitutional rights, but they must fulfill their contractual obligations with students. Of course, the private institution cannot make a mistake by protecting due process rights, so it is always best to keep due process in mind when making student decisions.

Property is defined as "anything that one possesses." A contract is property. Students have a contractual relationship with the college/university. A contract is a promise or a set of promises obligating parties, student and school, to perform or behave in certain ways.

Contracts may be written or oral, expressed or implied. The academic handbook is an example of a written, expressed contract. The course syllabus or clinical guidelines are also examples of written contracts.

When students are admitted to programs of study, certain contractual obligations follow. Private institutions, although not governed by constitutional obligations, are governed by the terms of the contracts.

Reflection Questions

1. What are the implications of contract law and constitutional requirements for the clinical instructor teaching at a public university? How do these obligations differ from those associated with teaching at a private college or university?
2. How should these constitutional and contractual protections inform and influence the clinical instructor who is evaluating the poorly performing student at risk of failing the course and, potentially, needing to leave the nursing program?

Discussion Points

1. Follow the course guidelines and the school guidelines for academic/clinical advisement, support, disciplinary proceedings, and failure.
2. Make certain that the student has been clearly informed of the criteria required for clinical success.
3. Document required outcomes and the ramifications of unsatisfactory performance.
4. Make certain to keep ongoing records documenting exchanges.
5. Be objective. Although it can be difficult, do not perceive the probationary student as an "adversary."
6. The obligations may be daunting, but at stake is patient safety, the reputation of the program, and an obligation to the public and profession that graduates of nursing programs are prepared for entry into practice. Evaluations must be honest, well documented, and fair and follow the established policies and procedures.

Source: Adapted from Hendrickson, 1999.

whereas others prefer e-mail and voice-mail messages in the event of missed experiences. Many professors have experienced problems with students lacking a clear understanding of boundaries and telephoning faculty at inappropriate times of day, calling about minutiae, or to engage in general conversation. Clinical instructors subjected to these demanding telephone conversations need to set immediate limits and expeditiously end the call with a reminder to the student that e-mail may be a more reasonable mode of communication for nonessential concerns.

In addition to inappropriate student calls, clinical instructors may also experience family calls. It is not uncommon for unsatisfactorily performing students to share the instructor's cell phone number with family members, including parents. Not only are these particular calls uncomfortable and surprising, they also place the instructor in an awkward position. Students over the age of 18 are entitled to privacy. Their scholastic performance is considered private information, regardless of who is paying the tuition bills.

Parents are occasionally frustrated by the privacy restriction, but instructors cannot share information about a student's performance with family, friends, or acquaintances unless the student has granted permission. In general, it may be wise to provide students with contact numbers and addresses that are solely work related rather than home phone numbers, addresses, or personal e-mail addresses.

Fitting into the Academic Environment

Many faculty organizations encourage adjunct faculty members to attend meetings and contribute (Lewallen, 2002) through voice but restrict voting to the full-time professoriate. If a CNS is working as an adjunct or part-time instructor, it is important to share the "adjunct point of view" during faculty meetings. Today's educator shortage frequently creates a dichotomy of classroom faculty and clinical faculty. At times, this relationship is cantankerous as educators struggle with resource and workload challenges that are not much different from those experienced in service settings. Full-time faculty members regard highly those clinical instructors who attend meetings, communicate regularly with course faculty, offer well-written and organized evaluation data, and exert positive influences on students. Highly regarded instructors usually enjoy long-term relationships with professor colleagues and have opportunities for participating in academic research, mentoring, and other types of support.

Conclusion

CNSs enjoy teaching and tend to be effective educators. There are many opportunities to teach in nursing, and it is not uncommon to find CNSs participating in educational activities across many venues, including hospitals, universities, and public agencies. First teaching occasions can be nerve-wracking as the CNS attempts to learn the ropes and develop a teaching plan that is appropriate for the particular learner.

Most nursing programs address the basics of teaching and learning at the undergraduate level. As a result, the majority of CNSs are comfortable with creating a teaching plan that is based on learner assessment and framed by measurable objectives and goals that are evaluated using outcome-driven data. CNSs are less likely to understand health literacy. They may not appreciate the wealth of materials that are freely available in electronic form. CNSs may also not appreciate the complexity of student teaching and learning or the practical challenges associated with teaching nursing students.

Teaching can be an exciting enterprise, and excellent educators are needed in so many areas within and outside healthcare organizations that CNSs can have their pick of opportunities. It is rewarding to facilitate growth in others, and the teaching role, when satisfied with excellence, is satisfying personally and professionally. The skills that distinguish the expert CNS are readily transferable to and sorely needed in all types of education venues.

References

Agency for Healthcare Research and Quality (AHRQ). (2004). *New evidence report illustrates links between health literacy and health care use and outcomes.* Agency for Healthcare Research and Quality, Rockville, MD. Retrieved December 17, 2008, from http://www.ahrq.gov/news/press/pr2004/litpr.htm

AHC Media, LLC. (2007). Joint Commission focuses on improving communication in light of literacy issues. *Patient Education Management, 14*(4), 37–48.

Allen, L. (2008). The nursing shortage continues as faculty shortage grows. *Nursing Economics, 26*(1), 35–40.

American Association of Colleges of Nursing (AACN). (2005). *Faculty shortages in baccalaureate and graduate nursing programs: Scope of the problem and strategies for expanding the supply.* Retrieved December 17, 2008, from http://www.aacn.nche.edu/Publications/pdf/05FacShortage.pdf

Arozullah, A. M., Yarnold, P. R., Bennett, C. L., Soltysik, R. C., Wolf, M. S., Ferreira, R. M., et al. (2007). Development and validation of a short-form, rapid estimate of adult literacy in medicine. *Medical Care, 45*(11), 1026–1033.

Bastable, S. B. (2003). *Nurse as educator: Principles of teaching and learning for nursing practice* (2nd ed.). Sudbury, MA: Jones and Bartlett.

Bastable, S. B. (Ed.). (2006). *Essentials of patient education.* Sudbury, MA: Jones and Bartlett.

Berkman, N. D., DeWalt, D. W., Pignone, M. P., Sheridan, S. L., Lohr, K. N., Lux, L., et al. (2004). *Literacy and health outcomes. Summary, evidence report/technology assessment No. 87.* AHRQ Publication No. 04-E007-1. Rockville, MD: Agency for Healthcare Research and Quality. Retrieved December 17, 2008, from http://www.ahrq.gov/downloads/pub/evidence/pdf/literacy/literacy.pdf

Billings, D., & Halstead, J. (2005). *Teaching in nursing: A guide for faculty.* St. Louis, MO: Elsevier Saunders.

Columbia University School of Nursing. (n. d.). *Health literacy assessment tool.* Retrieved December 31, 2008, from http://www.nursing.columbia.edu/informatics/HealthLitRes/assessTool.html

Committee on Health Literacy, Board on Neuroscience and Behavioral Health, Institute of Medicine. (2004). *Health literacy: A prescription to end confusion.* Washington, DC: National Academies Press.

Cowan, D., Norman, I., & Coopamah, V. (2005). Competence in nursing practice: A controversial concept. A focused review of the literature. *Nurse Education Today, 25*, 355–362.

Davis, T. C., Crouch, M. A., Long, S. W., Jackson, R. H., Bates, P., George, R. B., et al. (1991). Rapid assessment of literacy levels of adult primary care patients. *Family Medicine, 23*(6), 433–435.

Davis, T. C., Long, S. W., Jackson, R. H., Mayeaux, E. J., George, R. B., Murphy, P. W., et al. (1993). Rapid estimate of adult literacy in medicine: A shortened screening instrument. *Family Medicine, 25*(6), 391–395.

del Bueno, D. (2001). Buyer beware: The cost of competence. *Nursing Economics, 19*(6), 250–257.

del Bueno, D. (2005). A crisis in critical thinking. *Nursing Education Perspectives, 26*(5), 278–282.

del Bueno, D., Barker, F., & Christmyer, C. (1980). Implementing a competency-based orientation program. *Nurse Educator, 5*(3), 16–20.

Doak, L. G., & Doak, C. C. (Eds.). (2004). *Pfizer principles for clear health communication* (2nd ed.). Retrieved December 31, 2008, from http://www.pfizerhealthliteracy.com/pdf/PfizerPrinciples.pdf

Harvard School of Public Health. (n.d.). Health literacy studies web site. Retrieved November 12, 2008, from http:www.hsph.harvard.edu/healthliteracy

Hendrickson, R. L. (1999). *The colleges, their constituencies, and the courts* (2nd ed.). No. 64 Monograph series. Dayton, OH: Education Law Association.

Hsu, L., & Hsieh, S. (2005). Concept maps as an assessment tool in a nursing course. *Journal of Professional Nursing, 21*(3), 141–149.

Jacobson, T. A., Thomas, D. M., Morton, F. J., Offutt, G., Shevlin, G., & Ray, S. (1999). Use of a low-literacy patient education tool to enhance pneumococcal vaccination rates. A randomized controlled trial. *Journal of the American Medical Association, 282*(7), 646–650.

Joint Commission. (2006a). *2006 comprehensive accreditation manual for hospitals.* Oakbrook Terrace, IL: Author.

Joint Commission. (2006b). *2006 hospital requirements related to the provision of culturally and linguistically appropriate health care.* Retrieved December 31, 2008, from http://www.jointcommission.org/NR/rdonlyres/A2B030A3-7BE3-4981-A064-309865BBA672/0/hl_standards.pdf

Lewallen, L. P. (2002). Using your clinical expertise in nursing education. *Clinical Nurse Specialist, 16*(5), 242–246.

Luparell, S. (2005). Why and how we should address student incivility in nursing programs. In M. H. Oermann & K. T. Heinrich (Eds.), *Annual review of nursing education: Strategies for teaching, assessment, and program planning* (pp. 23–36). New York: Springer.

Lyon, B. L., & Boland, D. L. (2002). Demonstration of continued competence: A complex challenge. *Clinical Nurse Specialist, 16*(3), 155–156.

McConnell, E. (2001). Competence vs. competency. *Nursing Management, 32*(5), 14–15.

McMullan, M., Endacott, R., Gray, M. A., Jasper, M., Miller, C., Scholes, J., et al. (2003). Portfolios and assessment of competence: A review of the literature. *Journal of Advanced Nursing, 41*(3), 283–294.

National Assessment of Adult Literacy (NAAL). (n.d. 1). *What is NAAL?* Retrieved December 17, 2008, from http://nces.ed.gov/NAAL/index.asp?file=AboutNAAL/WhatIsNAAL.asp&PageId=2

National Assessment of Adult Literacy (NAAL). (n.d. 2). *Performance levels. Overview of the literacy levels.* Retrieved January 3, 2009, from http://nces.ed.gov/naal/perf_levels.asp

National Assessment of Adult Literacy (NAAL). (n.d. 3). *National assessment of adult literacy—overall. Demographics.* Retrieved December 31, 2008, from http://nces.ed.gov/naal/kf_demographics.asp

National Center for Education Statistics (NCES). (n.d.). *1992 national adult literacy survey.* Retrieved June 4, 2009, from http://nces.ed.gov/pubsearch/pubsinfo.asp?pubid=199909

National Institutes of Health (NIH). (2009). *Clear communication. An NIH health literacy initiative.* Retrieved December 17, 2008, from http://www.nih.gov/clearcommunication

Nolan, P. (1998). Competencies drive decision making. *Nursing Management, 29*(3), 27–29.

Office of Disease Prevention and Health Promotion (ODPHP). (2000). *Healthy people 2010: Terminology.* Retrieved December 17, 2008, from http://www.healthypeople.gov/document/html/volume1/11healthcom.htm#_Toc490471359

Partnership for Clear Health Communication. (n.d.). *Ask me 3.* Retrieved April 24, 2009, from http://www.npsf.org/askme3

Pfizer, Inc. (2003). *Clear health communication. Improving health literacy.* Retrieved May 18, 2006, from http://www.pfizerhealthliteracy.org/improving.html

Pfizer, Inc. (2008). *Pfizer clear health communication initiative.* Retrieved December 17, 2008, from http://www.pfizerhealthliteracy.org/index.html

Plain Language Action and Information Network (PLAIN). (n.d. 1). *Document checklist for plain language on the web.* Retrieved December 17, 2008, from http://www.plainlanguage.gov/howto/quickreference/checklist.cfm

Plain Language Action and Information Network (PLAIN). (n.d. 2). *Reasons why the English language is hard to learn.* Retrieved April 24, 2009, from http://www.plainlanguage.gov/examples/humor/englishishard.cfm

Plain Language Action and Information Network (PLAIN). (n.d. 3). *Before and after: Losing weight HHS brochure.* Accessed December 17, 2008, from http://www.plainlanguage.gov/examples/before_after/pub_hhs_losewgt.cfm

Potter, L., & Martin, C. (2006). *Health literacy fact sheets 6 & 7.* Center for Health Care Strategies, Inc. Retrieved December 17, 2008, from http://www.chcs.org/publications3960/publications_show.htm?doc_id=291711

Rudd, R. E. (2005). *How to create and assess printed materials.* Harvard School of Public Health: Health Literacy Studies. Retrieved December 17, 2008, from http://www.hsph.harvard.edu/healthliteracy/materials.html#two

Rudd, R. E. (2007). Health literacy skills of U.S. adults. *American Journal of Health Behavior, 31*(Supplement 1), S8–S18.

Schwartzberg, J., Cowett, A., VanGeest, J., & Wolf, M. (2007). Communication techniques for patients with low health literacy: A survey of physicians, nurses, and pharmacists. *American Journal of Health Behavior, 31*(Supplement 1), S96–S104.

Shillinger, D. (2004). *Case & commentary. Lethal cap. Web M & M: Morbidity and mortality rounds on the web.* Retrieved January 4, 2009, from http://www.webmm.ahrq.gov/case.aspx?caseID=53#figure1back

Thomas, S. P. (2003). Handling anger in the teacher–student relationship. *Nursing Education Perspectives, 24*(1), 17.

Tilley, D. (2008). Competency in nursing: A concept analysis. *Journal of Continuing Education in Nursing, 39*(2), 58–64.

U.S. Department of Education. Institute of Education Sciences, National Center for Education Statistics. (n.d.). *Demographics—overall.* Retrieved January 3, 2009, from http://nces.ed.gov/NAAL/kf_demographics.asp

U.S. General Accounting Office (GAO). (2001). *Nursing workforce. Emerging nurse shortages due to multiple factors.* GAO 01-944. Washington, DC: Author. Retrieved December 17, 2008, from http://www.gao.gov/new.items/d01944.pdf

University of Washington, Harborview Medical Center. (2008). *EthnoMed home page.* Retrieved December 17, 2008, from http://ethnomed.org/ethnomed

Waddell, D. (2001). Measurement issues in promoting continued competence. *Journal of Continuing Education in Nursing, 32*(3), 102–106.

Watson, R., Stimpson, A., Topping, A., & Porock, D. (2002). Clinical competence assessment in nursing: A systematic review of the literature. *Journal of Advanced Nursing, 39*(5), 421–431.

Weiss, B. (2007). *Health literacy and patient safety. Help patients understand* (2nd ed.). Retrieved December 17, 2008, from http://www.ama-assn.org/ama1/pub/upload/mm/367/healthlitclinicians.pdf

Wolf, M., Davis, T., & Parker, R. (2007).The emerging field of health literacy research. *American Journal of Health Behavior, 31*(Supplement 1), S3–S5.

Wright, D. (2005). *The ultimate guide to competency assessment in health care* (3rd ed.). Minneapolis, MN: Creative Health Care Management.

Zuzelo, P. (1999). Professional practice and the NCLEX examination. A bottom-line approach. *Nurse Educator, 24*(3), 11–12, 28.

Zuzelo, P. (2000). Clinical probation: A supportive process for the at-risk student. *Nurse Educator, 25*, 216–218.

Zuzelo, P. (2005). Affirming the disadvantaged student. *Nurse Educator, 30*, 27–31.

Zuzelo, P., Inverso, T., & Linkewich, K. (2001). Content validation of the medication error worksheet. *Clinical Nurse Specialist, 15*(6), 253–259.

Supplemental Resources

Stevens, B. (2003). How seniors learn. *Center for Medicare Education, 4*(9), 3. Retrieved December 17, 2008, from http://medicareed.org/PublicationFiles/V4N9.pdf

Mastering Performance Appraisal: Tips for the CNS

Patti Rager Zuzelo, EdD, MSN, RN, ACNS-BC

CNSs are often involved in performance evaluation processes. Most CNSs do not have line authority; in other words, most do not have subordinate employees reporting directly to them. However, CNSs are frequently asked to contribute to formal employee evaluations and may be responsible for participating in action plans designed to improve employee job performance or to substantiate a need for employee dismissal.

CNSs participate in evaluating performance on a day-to-day basis. They provide feedback, recommend nurses for additional responsibilities, address patient care problems related to nursing performance, and frequently give nurses a "thumbs up" related to their care practices. These informal performance appraisals often contribute to formal performance appraisals.

There are important do's and don'ts associated with written or formal evaluation processes. Many people are intimidated by evaluation processes and would prefer to avoid them entirely. CNSs are no exception; however, consider evaluation sessions as opportunities to establish relationships, support motivated colleagues, or redirect disengaged or frustrated nurses. Performance appraisals are here to stay, so it is important to learn how to make them work. This chapter addresses performance appraisals: employee evaluations (satisfactory and unsatisfactory) and peer reviews. Strategies, techniques, and human resource guidelines are offered, and exemplars provide coaching opportunities for self-instruction.

Employee Evaluation

Understanding the Process of Evaluation

There is not a lot of evidence to support the premise that performance appraisals improve performance (Zemke, 1991). Goal setting may be useful in performance improvement processes providing the conditions are right. Goal-setting theory (Locke

& Latham, 2002) was formulated on the idea that conscious goals affect action. CNS input into staff evaluations, including goal setting, may affect whether performance improves, so whether contributing to a manager's employee appraisal or evaluating a new hire, CNS input is critical.

The performance appraisal process has several purposes, including rewarding and recognizing good employees, coaching nurses who are having difficulties, staying in touch with staff, and avoiding legal trouble in the event of employee disciplinary actions, up to and including termination. Work performance appraisals have utility when making personnel decisions related to promotions or transfers (Chandra, 2006). Performance appraisals are also useful when evaluating new hires for purposes of determining whether the employee meets the required standards set for the end of the probationary period. Unit-based CNSs are often very involved in orientees' evaluations and are wise to keep evaluative responsibilities in mind when working with new employees during the probationary period. CNSs usually have good rapport and close working relationships with the staff, enabling them to contribute personalized and accurate assessment data to performance evaluations.

Performance appraisal may be viewed as one component of performance management. Shaneberger (2008) suggests that performance management consists of eight elements:

1. An accurate, well-written job description
2. Initial competencies that describe the knowledge and skills required of the nurse
3. Appropriate orientation to the role and its expectations
4. Goal setting and performance planning
5. Annual competency assessment
6. Coaching, mentoring, and recognition
7. Performance evaluation conducted by the employee and by a peer
8. A performance enhancement plan

Preparing for the Evaluation

CNSs need to think about staff performance appraisals before they happen. A proactive stance will provide the data necessary for a fair evaluation. In some ways, employee performance appraisal is similar to the nursing process (Figure 4-1).

Spend time gathering employee assessment data. Diagnose strengths, challenges, at-risk behaviors, and unacceptable behaviors. Share this feedback with the employee and develop goals. Evaluate progress within at least 1 year, earlier if appropriate, but make certain to follow established polices. Remediate or reward and reevaluate. Thinking about employee appraisal in this systems fashion makes the evaluation process less overwhelming.

Collecting well-balanced appraisal data is critical to a fair evaluation process. Employees have both strengths and weaknesses. Recognizing both types of performance goes a long way toward demonstrating to the employee that you acted fairly. In the rare event of employee-initiated grievances or lawsuits related to the outcomes of an

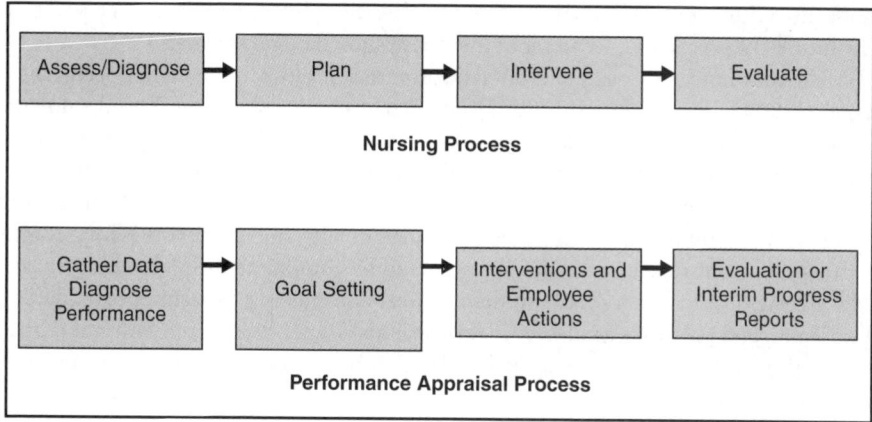

Figure 4-1   Parallel processes.

evaluation, fairness and balance are essential. Of course, recognizing all types of performance is also the right thing to do. An employee evaluation is a test in the eyes of the law as it reflects a decision that affects an individual's status in the organization (Zemke, 1991). The organization needs to be able to confidently assert that this test was nondiscriminatory and unbiased.

A variety of strategies are used for collecting and organizing evaluation data. Keep a log (DelPo, 2005), computerized or on paper, that details memorable incidents, patient care exemplars, projects, leadership activities, or other job-related occasions. Consider constructing a spreadsheet using Excel or some other software program that enables the user to quickly add and retrieve information (Shaneberger, 2008). Make certain to ask staff to share information about their involvement in professional organizations and continuing education activities. Take advantage of e-mail and request that staff periodically respond to requests for information related to their practice, education, and professional activities. Electronic responses are easily filed away in individual computer-based folders or printed in hard-copy form for traditional files.

In addition to logs, keeping paper-based files for each employee is also useful. Hanging files labeled with each employee's name are useful in preparation for the written evaluation. File letters from families, patients, colleagues, and administrators. Save flyers from in-service programs that the employee has presented or attended. Keep copies of documentation that demonstrates the employee's typical charting habits. Photocopies or computer printouts are easiest to save, but make certain to remove any patient identifiable data. Maintain records in a separate file detailing the origin of these materials in case chart retrieval is necessary.

There are times when the CNS notices either an exceptional effort or a troubling behavior. At these times, it is important to give immediate evaluative feedback. If oral feedback is offered, make certain to document the conversation in writing and place it in the employee's file. The facts of the event, positive or negative, are important to both the written annual evaluation or to possible disciplinary action at some point in the future (DelPo, 2005). Remember that there should be no surprises.

Make certain to document anecdotal information as close to the event's occurrence as possible. DelPo and Guerin (2003) noted that employees who fail to document workers' performance may be tempted to try to pass off these notations as having been made at the time of the incidents. Not only is this dishonest, but also if the true timing of the documentation is discovered, the CNS's credibility will diminish. In the event of a problem that involves human resources or a lawsuit, credibility is important.

It is important for performance appraisals to be consistent with job descriptions. Make certain to have copies of job descriptions and nursing department standards, guidelines, and protocols available for review. This is a good opportunity for both the staff and the CNS to become reacquainted with job expectations and professional development opportunities.

Documenting Appraisal Findings

It can be challenging to describe behaviors or expectations in written form. Employees expect that the evaluative comments are unique and pertinent to their individual contributions or practice patterns. Comments should relate to observable, measurable activities and outcomes. Developing a repertoire of varied comments and observations using a variety of wording and phrases emphasizes the individuality of the written evaluation and promotes an understanding that evaluations have been uniquely tailored for each nursing employee (Table 4-1). In other words, try to avoid a "cookbook" approach to written appraisals. Each written evaluation should be fairly unique. A variety of published resources provide helpful suggestions and templates for documenting a variety of behaviors. These resources may be helpful to the CNS, as well as to nurse managers.

Table 4-1 EXAMPLES OF EVALUATIVE FEEDBACK

Never misses details.

Hair is frequently unkempt and unwashed.

Dress and grooming are exceptional.

Wears inappropriate footwear inconsistent with dress code.

Wears necklines that are too low.

Never comes back late from lunch.

Called in sick the day before two holidays.

Gossips during shift report about nursing colleagues.

Uses profanity or vulgarity.

Properly plans staff workloads during periods of increased acuity.

Source: Adapted from Shepard, 2005.

Most nurses perform in an average fashion. This idea has important implications. The concept of average deserves consideration. In general, average performance is expected or typical performance. It satisfies job expectations, meets performance standards, and is a reasonable and usual level of employee performance. Job descriptions identify the employing institution's expectations of the nurse. Average performance is not always perceived as a flattering description; however, it is most common. Typical performance is more difficult to evaluate than atypical or extreme performance. As a result, ratings tend to be less accurate when they involve average work performance (Chandra, 2006).

In comparison, exceptional performance is an exception from the norm. It is unique. Exceptional behaviors may be positive or negative. Assisting staff to identify areas in which they are exceptional versus average is important to developing realistic self-appraisals and productive evaluation encounters. Shepard (2005, p. 4) noted, "There are superstars in the workforce, and there are derelicts. The vast majority of the workforce falls between these two extremes." This observation is true for the nursing workforce just as it is for the workforce at large.

Many institutions tie financial remuneration and incentives to job performance. If the CNS regards every employee as exceptional rather than most as average and some as underperforming, resource allocation can become unfair. In fact, associating financial incentives with performance evaluations is one area in which supervisors routinely cheat to make the system work to satisfy their own purposes (Zemke, 1991). These behaviors contribute to the skepticism that many employees have regarding the fairness of performance appraisals.

CNSs should have documentation available to support evaluative comments. When the CNS is contributing to a negative performance appraisal that may lead to employee suspension or termination, the CNS should seek the advice of human resource personnel before the actual appraisal session to make certain that the necessary documentation is in order and to ensure that the written evaluation is consistent with personnel policies, procedures, and practices.

Seeking preliminary support and feedback early may prevent litigation or grievances in the event of employee dissatisfaction with the appraisal.

Job descriptions and institutional goals and objectives should drive performance appraisals. It is important to compare the nurse to these standards and not necessarily to the level of peer group performance. There are times when CNSs evaluate nurses who are performing better than, consistent with, or less than the norm of the staff practicing on the unit. If an average nurse works within a group of high performers and exceptional practitioners, the written appraisal should reflect this average, but satisfactory, level of performance. Of course, it is reasonable to encourage the average nurse to increase his or her level of productivity and expertise and to use colleagues as mentors and supports. If pay incentives are linked to the appraisal outcomes, the financial rewards should be less for the average performing nurse than that awarded to the more productive peers.

Job Descriptions or Job Standards

Job descriptions typically have results standards and behavior standards. A results standard is a description of a result that is expected from any employee who holds a particular job (DelPo & Guerin, 2003). For example, an RN might be required to present two unit-based educational programs each year using a variety of presentation strategies and supplemented by a bulk pack of related readings.

A behavior standard is a description of how nurses should behave while getting their work done. For example, the healthcare institution might be prioritizing patient and family satisfaction. A behavior standard related to this value might be that a nurse will respond to all patient and family requests with courtesy and professionalism. Job description standards should be shared with nurses on hire and should be periodically reviewed with staff, particularly if there are revisions. Job standards are the foundation of the performance appraisal, in conjunction with job goals (DelPo & Guerin, 2003).

Job goals vary among employees. They are developed mutually and in relation to an employee's gifts and challenges. The goals are critically important to making certain that the performance evaluation is meaningful. Goals should be selected based on areas of the nurse's performance that require improvement, strengths that the employee should capitalize on and continue to enhance, and skills that the nurse should learn that will improve job performance and professionalism.

Types of Appraisal Forms and Processes

Performance appraisal processes vary by institution. Most systems are paper based but Web-based tools are available (SuccessFactors, 2008) and may become increasingly common given potential cost-savings and efficiencies. Hamilton et al. (2007) conducted a review of evidence and current practice specific to performance assessment in healthcare providers and found that there is a wide range of assessment methods, and each has its advantages and disadvantages with some having more rigorous underpinnings than others (Table 4-2). They recommend multimethod strategies for

---

Table 4-2   TYPES OF PERFORMANCE APPRAISAL METHODS

1. Appraisal review: composed of employer evaluation and self-evaluation
2. Reflection
3. Process review, including critical incident technique
4. Multisource feedback, including 360° assessments
5. Observation
6. Supervision
7. Standards

Source: Adapted from Hamilton et al., 2007.

clinical performance assessment in nursing, as well as midwifery; however, most CNSs are involved in performance appraisal processes that are institutionally defined with select instruments and procedures.

Setting the Tone for a Productive Evaluation: Arranging the Evaluation Interview

Employees should receive advance notice of the evaluation time, date, and setting to gather documentation and to have time for self-reflection. Conducting an evaluation session on the run is not conducive to productive goal setting or relationship building. The evaluation session should be in a private setting without distractions.

CNSs may be involved in these sessions as either the sole evaluator or as a partner to the nurse manager. Each party should be comfortably positioned, and if the CNS and nurse manager are evaluating together, efforts should be made to eliminate a possible impression that there are "two against one" during the evaluative session. It is usually more appropriate for the nurse manager to control the meeting with input offered by the CNS when requested by the manager.

Keeping It Real

There is an expression—"keeping it real"—that refers to the importance of keeping relationships authentic and honest. Authentic relationships are built on candor and mutual respect. If the CNS avoids sharing performance problems with a nurse or colleague, the individual will not know what is needed to improve. In this situation, there is no real opportunity to share perceptions and work through incorrect assumptions. The fundamental rule of performance appraisals is that they must be honest, even if this honesty contributes to discomfort.

Stick with the Facts, Not the Persona

Nursing is a people profession. Personality does count and affects key relationships, including patient, family, and coworkers. Many different communication styles and ways of work contribute to effective and efficient outcomes. Reflect on whether the employee's style is personally unappealing or if the employee's style is inappropriate within the confines of professional behavior.

Remember to evaluate performance and not personality (DelPo, 2005). If a performance problem is directly related to a nurse's conduct, focus on the behavior and offer specific details. As an example, consider, "You have made negative comments during taped shift reports specific to patients' weight, alcoholism, or family circumstances on at least five occasions in the past 6 months. This behavior is unacceptable and must stop." Focus on behaviors and the results of these behaviors.

Goal Setting   Goals must be specific, realistic, challenging, and measurable. When people are asked to do the best job possible, they rarely do so. The request is too arbitrary and intangible and can be satisfied by a wide range of acceptable performance levels (Locke & Latham, 2002). Goals should not be ambiguous; rather, they must be specific (DelPo, 2005). Focus on exactly what the nurse should do. For example, try "provide shift report without profanity or personal commentaries" or "start change of shift report at the correct time" rather than "give a better shift report."

When goals are individually determined, people with a strong belief that they are able to accomplish the task will set higher goals than people with lesser confidence in accomplishing the task. These same highly confident people are more committed to the assigned goals, use better strategies for reaching the goals, and are more receptive to negative feedback (Locke & Latham, 2002). These points are important to the context of goal setting (Table 4-3).

In other words, include the nurse in goal setting. Make goals specific. Goals should be attainable but should require effort and persistence. Research findings suggest that the most important agents of high and low productivity include employees themselves, immediate supervisors, and the organization's resources. If the performance appraisal is going to affect changes in practice patterns, it will do so via these agents.

Goals should also include deadlines. If there is a date by which a behavior, project, or assignment must be completed, say so. Goals must be realistic. Impossible goals discourage employees. Goals should not be so easy that they require little effort, but established goals should take into consideration the limitations and realities of the setting (DelPo, 2005). It may be worthwhile to purchase a book that offers creative phrases for performance reviews.

Once goals have been established, make certain to ask the nurse what he or she needs to be successful. Perhaps the nurse will set a goal of "certification in specialty area within 9 months." The nurse may need the CNS to share expertise or suggest resources that might be helpful. If this is the case, agree on a time frame and set deadlines.

Avoiding a Successful Wrongful Discharge Suit

Wrongful discharge is a common basis for litigation. Although employers have the right to fire employees, it is illegal to fire when the job termination is based on discrimination of protected classes; specifically, race, religion, sex, or age. Paper trails are absolutely essential to demonstrate that an employee has been treated fairly and has been afforded progressive discipline (DelPo & Guerin, 2003; Shepard, 2005).

The paper trail should accurately reflect the reality of the evaluation process. In other words, CNSs must be careful to offer evaluative input that is honest, reasonable,

---

Table 4-3   GOAL-SETTING TIPS

1. Include the employee. The nurse who participates in the goal-setting process will probably have more success.
2. Goals provide focus. Without established goals, nurses are distracted by less-important activities.
3. Goals are energizing. High goals lead to greater effort.
4. Nurses need the tools and strategies necessary for goal attainment.

and free of bias. Shepard (2005) offers 10 common evaluator errors. These errors include stereotyping, leniency bias with evaluative ratings inflation, severity bias with unreasonably harsh expectations, central tendency where everyone is rated as average, cluster tendency that fails to discriminate between distinct levels of performance, halo or horn effects that distort clear views of performance, and other types of biases. HRN Management Group (2004) has added other common errors made by evaluators when appraising employees (Table 4-4). Keep in mind that an appraisal session is not a disciplinary session (HRN Management Group, 2004). Corrective action should be addressed immediately following inappropriate behavior. Remember, there should be no surprises during a meeting scheduled to evaluate performance.

CNSs with an interest in improving their evaluation skills should seek direction and suggestions from the many printed resources on this subject. There are often education and training programs at work sites specific to performance evaluations. CNSs should take advantage of these opportunities if they will be regularly contributing to formal appraisal processes.

Evaluating the Unsatisfactory Performer

There are many types of employee problems, including low productivity, performance deficiencies including clinical practice incompetencies, insubordination, interpersonal problems that affect the work environment, excessive absenteeism, drugs and alcohol, theft and dishonesty, violence, and morality issues (DelPo & Guerin, 2003). Many CNSs are directly involved in addressing staff productivity and performance issues. They may be peripherally involved in reporting other employee problems as either a direct observer or as a confidant of staff.

CNSs are often involved with appraising the performance of a nurse or staff member who is practicing below expectations. CNSs are viewed as coaches and clinical experts. As a result, they are frequently asked to work with struggling nurses and to develop remediation plans to improve performance. Struggling nurses may be established practitioners who have transferred to a different practice area requiring new skills, nurses demonstrating performance deficiencies caused by difficult life circumstances, or new nurses having difficulty meeting the challenges of orientation programs (Figure 4-2). The nurse who is new to the clinical setting or new to practice is significantly different than the nurse who has experience but begins to demonstrate low performance in key areas.

The Struggling New Employee

Before beginning the written performance appraisal, CNSs should begin by meeting with the employee and discussing the nurse's perspective, including concerns, worries, and suggestions. Do not assume that the nurse has chosen to perform poorly. Care must be taken to avoid arguing or eliciting defensive posturing. In general, although the CNS and employee may have differing opinions on the quality of performance, examples of behaviors should be discussed in matter-of-fact language that includes the outcomes of these behaviors. Quotations, charting, medication administration records, and patient/family complaints and compliments should be reviewed.

Table 4-4   COMMON ERRORS MADE WHEN APPRAISING EMPLOYEE PERFORMANCE

1. The Halo Effect

Allowing one highly favorable, or unfavorable, employee behavior or characteristic to affect judgment about the entire appraisal ignores other employee strengths and weaknesses.

2. Bias or Prejudice

We all have our biases. However, allowing personal biases or prejudices to influence the appraisal process can make evaluations unfair and inconsistent. Know your biases.

3. Not Knowing Employees

Unfortunately, many supervisors don't really know their employees or the quality of their work. Such evaluations are not credible.

4. Overemphasis on Isolated Events

A particularly recent or significant event may skew overall judgment of an employee. Take informal notes about employees (both good and bad things) throughout the year to ensure your evaluation is based on the entire appraisal period—not just what happened last week.

5. Lenient or Inflated Appraisals

It is difficult for most managers to give employees poor ratings. However, not doing it simply avoids the problem and doesn't give the employee the opportunity to correct it. It is also difficult to later discipline or terminate an employee whose appraisals have always been good. It opens up risks of discrimination charges.

6. Appraisal of Potential Worth

When managing a new or inexperienced employee make sure to rate on actual job performance—not on what the employee may become. Evaluate based on current results and action. You can use comments to address potential worth.

7. Postponing or Skipping the Appraisal

Delays create the wrong impression. Employees begin to perceive that neither they nor the appraisals are important.

8. Poor Preparation

"Seat of the pants" meetings rarely produce effective results. It quickly becomes apparent that the appraiser is not well prepared. The employee may assume that the manager does not know what is going on or that he or she doesn't care enough to prepare.

(continues)

Table 4-4 (continued)

9. Using the Evaluation as Corrective Action

The appraisal meeting should not be a disciplinary session. Inappropriate behavior must be dealt with when first observed. Discipline and discussion of performance and goals don't work well together. Corrective action should have been addressed earlier. The evaluation is a time to discuss strengths and weaknesses, perhaps assessing how an employee has done in correcting past behavior. However, it isn't the place to raise new disciplinary actions.

10. Overemphasizing Good Performance

Praise and positive reinforcement are terrific. However, compliments quickly become meaningless if they aren't specific and substantive. They can also give an employee the false impression that you are completely pleased with everything he or she does. Be honest and direct.

11. Not Following Through

Most of the time and effort spent in planning for and conducting an effective interview is lost if you don't follow through with the actions and plans discussed in the evaluation. Performance management should be a daily (not annual) activity.

12. Avoiding the Tough Issues

Employee problems rarely correct themselves. Nearly everyone is uncomfortable raising sensitive issues or criticizing others. However, unless the tough issues are addressed, they inevitably get worse, the CNS and manager lose credibility, and the nurse may not ever know there is a problem.

13. Evaluating Attitude

While we all are forced to deal with employees' attitudes, attitudes are basically impossible to evaluate and even harder to change. Focus on results and objective, observable actions. They are easier to complete and much more readily justified.

14. Accepting Excuses

There may be legitimate reasons why an employee has been unable to complete assigned goals. However, don't immediately accept excuses for poor performance. Often they are simply not valid. If they are appropriate, then a solution and action plan should be developed to avoid such problems in the future.

15. Ignoring Employee Feedback

Asking employees for input only to ignore their comments can be very damaging. It makes evaluation meetings much less effective and communicates to employees that while their ideas may be asked for, they are not listened to or acted upon.

Source: Reprinted with modification from HRN Management Group at www.hrnonline.com.

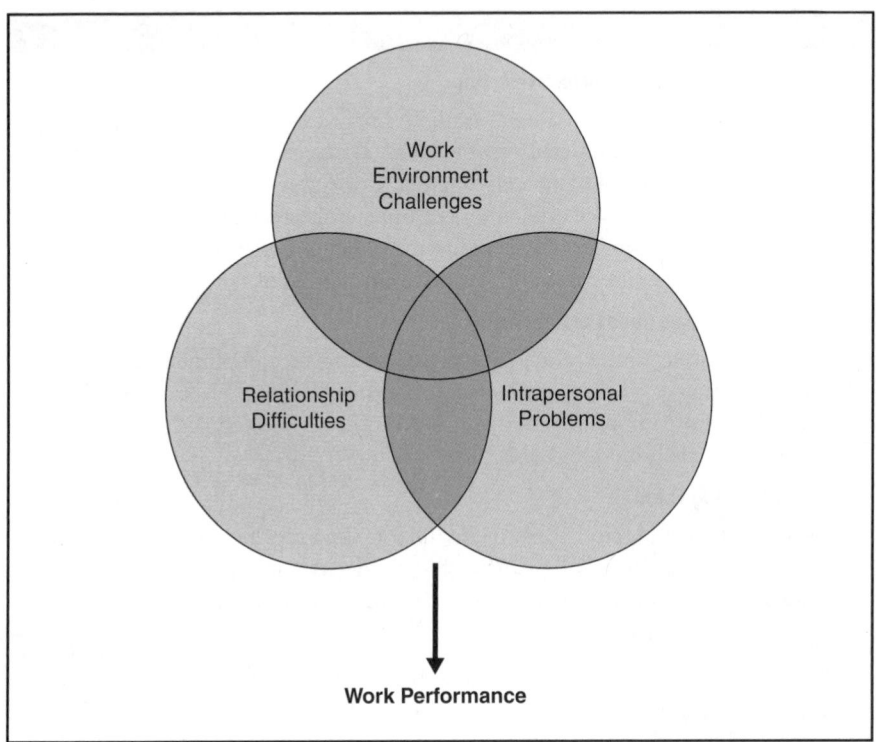

Figure 4-2   Intervening influences on work performance.

This reflective process should include discussion specific to the orientation structures and processes (Figure 4-3). Many institutions arrange preceptored experiences
to guide new employees. These arrangements may be referred to as orientations, unit-
based orientations, or mentorships. The basic structure and processes are the same
across programs: (1) develop a structured orientation program that includes behavioral objectives and opportunities to evaluate feedback; (2) assign one or more individuals to work with the new nurse; (3) gradually increase employee independence;
and (4) evaluate at probationary period end and make a decision on whether to continue the employment.

In this type of arrangement, the preceptor wields significant influence on the quality of the orientation and the outcomes of the experience. It is important to consider
the skill of the preceptor and the relationship between the new employee and the preceptor. In some cases, this relationship does not click, and as a direct result, the new
employee is unsuccessful. Research study findings reveal that conflict does exist in
nursing student/preceptor relationships (Mamchur & Myrick, 2003), and it makes
sense that this same conflict may manifest itself in new employee/preceptor relation-

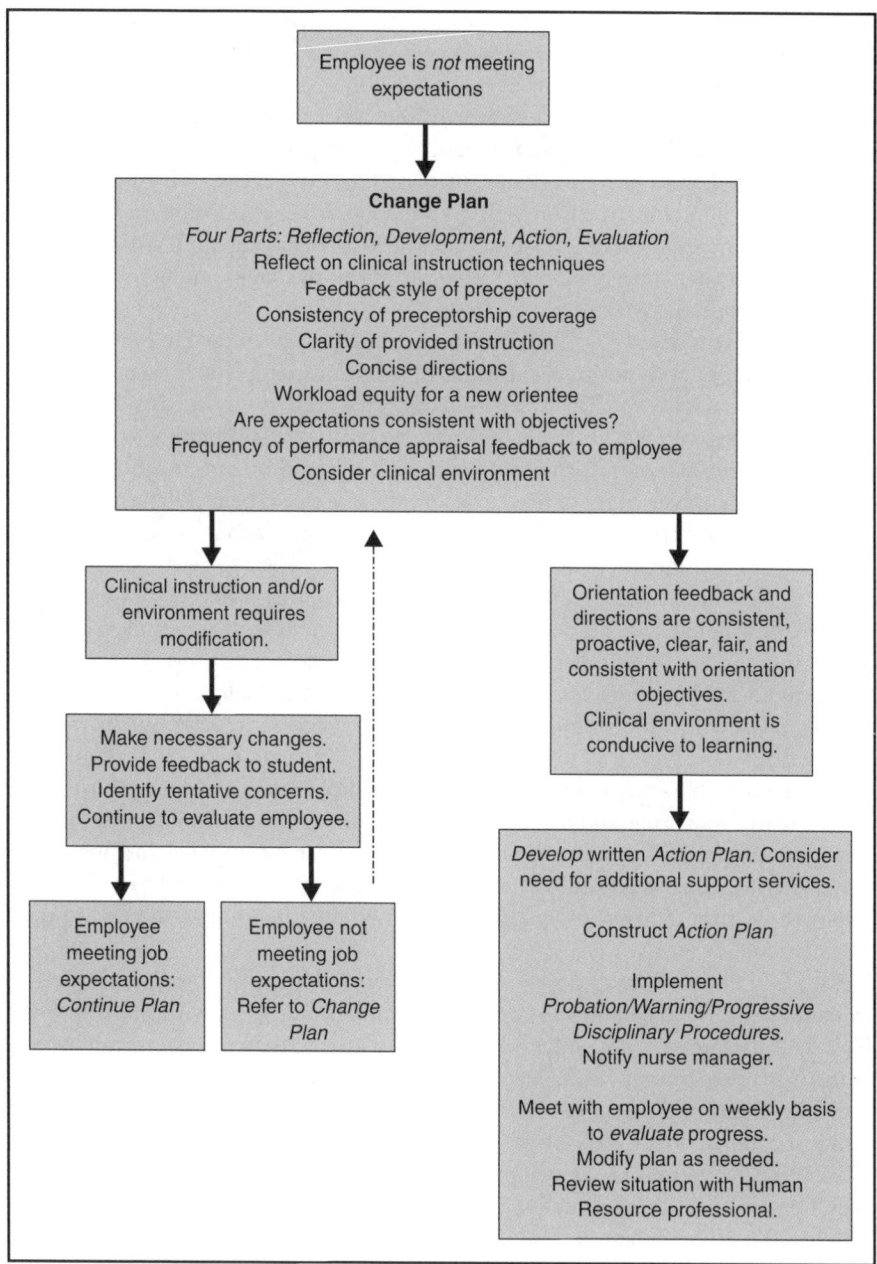

Figure 4-3   Struggling employee evaluation algorithm.

Source: © 2006 Patti R. Zuzelo. Reprinted with permission.

ships. The CNS must keep an open mind when considering this possibility and recognize that it is also possible that the preceptor is being wrongfully blamed for the lackluster performance of the new hire.

Workload equity may also be a concern. New hires should be able to anticipate a reasonable workload that provides for learning opportunities and guidance throughout the day. Perhaps a heavy workload, increased patient census, or high acuity have prevented the new employee from doing a good job. It is not uncommon for preceptors to juggle orientation responsibilities while also managing a full patient assignment. This divided attention may adversely affect the new employee's access to guidance through the system.

New employees deserve regular, objective feedback that is offered to them privately and that includes both positive and negative behavior exemplars. Preceptors should treat evaluative data as confidential, shared only on a need-to-know basis. If orientees are not receiving objective feedback, they have no legitimate opportunity to improve or succeed. If performance is discussed outside the preceptor–orientee relationship with employees who have no right or need to know, the orientee is being sabotaged with legitimate grounds for formal complaint. The preceptorship relationship should be based on trust and good intentions to encourage the new employee to share questions and concerns. New hires cannot identify clinical skill deficiencies if they do not feel safe.

The CNS should also critique the clinical environment with the employee. Make certain that the new hire feels comfortable and supported. If not, specific areas must be identified and behaviors must be addressed. If there are challenges or intimidating exchanges with other professionals, including the medical staff, these issues must also be remedied.

Another possible explanation for poor performance may be substance abuse. Employees who abuse drugs and alcohol may demonstrate diminished job performance, reduced productivity, lateness, or absenteeism. If the new employee demonstrates these behaviors, make certain that they are accurately documented and inform the employee that these behaviors will be brought to the attention of the appropriate administrator.

If the CNS notes slurred speech, alcohol on breath, changes in pupil size, or uncoordinated motor movements, document the findings and speak with the employee. The situation should be immediately addressed. Patient safety is the imperative obligation. There are times when behaviors are the result of prescribed medications, and as such, response options may be limited. Notify the administrator and follow through with institutional policy. Remember that the CNS needs to address the results of alcohol and drug-related behaviors, particularly if these behaviors are occurring after work but are affecting the quality of the employee's work performance (DelPo & Guerin, 2003) (Exemplar 4-1).

Responding to the Issues

After reflecting on the circumstances of the employee's unsatisfactory performance and speaking with both the orientee and the preceptor, the CNS must decide how to

---

Exemplar 4-1

The Case of the Partying Orientee

Josie is a newly hired RN on a medical–surgical nursing unit. The CNS is responsible for developing an orientation program and tracking the employee's progress through this program. The CNS arranges for a consistent preceptor to work with Josie. The preceptor is an experienced mentor. The preceptor informs the CNS that Josie frequently goes out following the 3–11 shift and "parties through the night." The preceptor is concerned that this lifestyle is destructive and that Josie appears fatigued and stressed. The CNS shares these same concerns but recognizes that Josie's lifestyle choice is outside the purview of the employee–employer relationship and to address this concern with Josie would be an intrusion into her personal life. However, the CNS is concerned about patient safety and job performance. If Josie demonstrates a pattern of lateness, poor performance, clinical errors, or absenteeism, the CNS will note the specifics and address the results of Josie's drinking and late nights with the nurse manager.

---

proceed. These assessments and discussions should be documented. Share the data and conclusions with the appropriate administrator.

If the problem lies with the work environment or the preceptorship arrangement, correct these problems and establish a date for performance reevaluation. Perhaps a new preceptor or targeted education will move the orientee back on track. If these changes correct the performance deficiencies, the orientation plan should continue with the revisions in place.

On the other hand, perhaps careful scrutinizing of the preceptorship relationship, work environment, and workload reveal that the system is not the problem. Rather, evaluation reveals that the performance deficiencies directly relate to the skill set, disposition, or motivation of the orientee. In this case, the CNS needs to participate in developing a remediation plan to address these issues or needs to support both the employee and the manager during the termination process.

Developing the Action Plan

Evidence suggests that the most effective remedy for poor performance is to focus on the future rather than the past. Focusing on the past is unproductive because performance cannot be undone and because such a discussion is likely to encourage arguments due to differing perceptions of past events (Zemke, 1991). Once it is clearly established that the new employee is performing at an unsatisfactory level, it is common for the CNS to participate in developing an action plan.

The action plan's intent is to specify the behaviors, target dates, and steps that the employee is required to fulfill to achieve required outcomes. The plan's focus is to provide opportunities for the employee to master requisite job expectations. The CNS must remember that this is a private event for the new employee. A remediation plan must be handled sensitively and in such a way that the employee receives needed support and learning experience opportunities without bearing the brunt of the curiosity and gossip of coworkers and members of the healthcare team.

The employee should clearly understand that if the established goals of the remediation plan are not met, the employee will be discharged. Remember to make certain to evaluate, remediate, and reevaluate within the time limits of the probationary period. If this is not enough time to give the employee a reasonable time for improvement, consider extending the probationary period in consultation with human resources.

After the Action Plan

Remediating the struggling employee can be a time-consuming activity. The CNS will probably work with an administrator, perhaps a nurse manager, when completing the initial written appraisal. Once this evaluation has been shared with the employee and an action plan has been developed, the CNS may be responsible for coordinating and monitoring the employee's progress. Good organizational skills and effective communication strategies are essential during this period.

The CNS should schedule interim meetings, preferably with the nurse manager in attendance. These interim meetings are intended to measure the progress the employee has made toward the action plan goals. Generally, probationary periods are short. Schedule the interim evaluations frequently enough that the employee receives feedback and suggestions in a timely fashion relative to the amount of time remaining in the probation. Meetings may be scheduled weekly or biweekly, depending on employee shift patterns.

Interim appraisal sessions are also good opportunities to "check in" and really listen to this new employee. Keep in mind that this process is anxiety producing for any employee and particularly for a new employee. Be ready to give specific feedback and practical suggestions. Have genuine dialogue about the expectations. If they require revision, do so. Make certain that the employee has early notification of the scheduled interim review sessions. Encourage the nurse to prepare for the review and to consider additional suggestions for strategies, supports, and resources that might be helpful to the employee as he or she continues to develop his or her skills.

Some institutions have formal mechanisms for documenting interim reviews, whereas others leave the format to the discretion of the evaluator. In general, it is wise to come to the interim review with written documentation. Share feedback that you have received from coworkers, patients, and families. If the employee has demonstrated improvement and goals appear attainable, make certain to share this positive feedback but do not offer guarantees of continued employment. Remember that the employee needs to demonstrate continual and consistent growth as measured against the agreed-upon goals.

If the employee continues to demonstrate an unsatisfactory level of performance, continue to provide objective examples of concerning behaviors and skill deficiencies. Offer assistance where appropriate while making certain that final responsibility for job performance lies with the employee. Remember that there are times when probationary periods should not be extended. There may be other viable alternatives for this struggling employee. As an example, perhaps the new employee is struggling in a high-acuity intensive care unit but may perform satisfactorily in an inpatient or out-patient area. This may be a reasonable suggestion if the employee's performance deficiencies relate to technical skills.

During the interim evaluation session, keep in mind that demeanor is important. It is not uncommon for the struggling employee to view these sessions as threatening. This is not an unreasonable perspective, given that continued employment requires a satisfactory level of performance. The CNS is obliged to treat the employee with respect. Hostility or frustration is inappropriate, and expressions of such may escalate into personal attacks.

When meeting with the employee, keep the door open but schedule the evaluative discussion in a reasonably private area. Ultimately, the decision to terminate a new employee is an administrative decision that is made by an administrator. CNS input is critical to the process and is usually an important consideration when making the determination of whether to continue the employment relationship.

The Struggling Established Employee

When a nurse has been practicing satisfactorily and then begins to demonstrate problems with productivity or practice quality, the CNS is often the first person to whom staff turns for advice. Losing a nurse is expensive in terms of both dollars and human cost, particularly a nurse who has previously practiced as an effective member of the healthcare team. The CNS should consider a variety of possible explanations for the performance deficiencies, including possible changes in the nurse's personal life or work environment (Table 4-5). As mentioned, substance abuse is always a concern and should be considered and ruled in or out early in the process.

The best initial strategy is to collect preliminary information before approaching the nurse. There is a possibility that the CNS has been misinformed about the employee's performance. Observe the nurse during clinical practice. Review charts and documentation and develop a clear sense of whether there is an actual performance issue.

After preliminary data review, approach the employee in a thoughtful and considerate fashion. If the CNS has an established relationship with the employee, having a private discussion in a relaxed environment over lunch or coffee may be an effective approach to this difficult conversation. Remember that patient safety is paramount. If the employee is providing safe care but care that is less organized or productive than usual, the performance problem is easier to address than if patient safety is at risk.

Consider the institutional resources that may be available to the nurse. Many healthcare systems have employee counseling programs that can assist staff with problem solving for a wide range of issues. Encourage the nurse to take advantage of available services. Consider including the nurse manager in a conversation to share possible changes in scheduling or shift rotations to accommodate the employee's issues. For example, there are times when nurses who are struggling with difficult

Table 4-5   POSSIBLE EXPLANATIONS FOR PERFORMANCE DEFICIENCIES
Work challenges
• Discrimination or harassment
• Overwhelming physical demands
• Fast-paced workload demands
• Changing technologies
Intrapersonal problems
• Substance abuse
• Changes in vision or hearing
• Alterations in physical health or stamina
• Mental health concerns
• Worries
• Crisis in faith
Relationship difficulties
• Divorce
• Death
• Conflicts with family, friends, coworkers, supervisors
• Fear of violence

family circumstances find that weekend 12-hour shifts or a permanent evening or night shift can help with financial worries or remedy a need for predictability. Again, keep the nurse manager informed and involved when appropriate from the beginning of the process.

Self-Regulation and Peer Review

Peer evaluation or peer review is associated with activities that require self-regulation within the context of professional practice. Self-regulation strengthens the nursing profession's credibility in society and builds a sense of personal and professional responsibility (McAllister & Osborne, 1997) within the nursing rank and file. Scholarly journals use blind peer-review processes to review manuscripts submitted for publication consideration. Peer review is also used for grant reviews, tenure and promotion decisions, conference abstract submissions (Dougherty, 2006), accreditation processes, and to supplement performance evaluations. Peer-review processes are also being used to facilitate student learning (McAllister & Osborne, 1997).

Peer-review processes place practice evaluation squarely in the hands of the professional. Professionals should be evaluated by their peers, specifically colleagues with similar competence and possessing clear understanding of practice demands and standards. Briggs, Heath, and Kelley (2005) reported that some states expect some form of peer review. Also, when peer-review processes are required for advanced practice nurses (APNs), some state boards of nursing stipulate that the review must be conducted by a similarly licensed APN practicing in the same clinical area. The peer-review process may also be statutorily required as part of fact-finding activities related to a nurse's conduct (Walters, 2000).

Peers should be evaluated against established, written standards (Briggs, Heath, & Kelley, 2005; McAllister & Osborne, 1997), regardless of the motivation for the peer review. Journals, foundations, organizations, accrediting agencies, universities, and employment settings have performance standards. Peer-review conflicts often relate to the interpretation and application of standards as well as conflicts that arise from contentious communications and perceived unfairness.

Connecting Evaluation Processes to CNS-Specific Job Descriptions

It is challenging to participate in valid performance appraisal processes if there is an absent or tenuous relationship between the performance evaluation system and the CNS job description. In fact, anecdotally, CNSs report that job descriptions are often inappropriate and may categorize CNSs as generic APRNs, staff nurses, staff development or clinical educators, or administrators. Such ambiguity presents challenges beyond the performance appraisal concern and may contribute to role strain and CNS job dissatisfaction. The performance appraisal process should directly relate to the job description that is informed by the needs of the organization as influenced by the larger healthcare environment (Figure 4-4).

CNSs should scrutinize their job description and ensure that the description accurately describes the role and its responsibilities. If the job description requires modification or needs to be crafted from scratch, the CNS should use any and all available resources that specifically relate to CNS practice (Table 4-6). CNSs need to keep in mind that articulating differences between nurse roles is imperative if patients, nurses, and systems are to reap the full benefit of CNS practice (Exemplar 4-2).

Peer-Review Performance Evaluations

Peer-review processes are useful to include in the performance appraisal of all categories of nursing staff members. Data sources that inform the processes should be selected based on the practice of the nurse. Traditional methods of performance evaluation can be problematic for APRNs, particularly when directors do not see CNSs practicing on a regular basis. Staff nurses have these same concerns regarding the legitimacy of appraisals. Devising a peer-review system may help alleviate some of these issues, although the very nature of peer review can stimulate nurses' anxieties as they worry about confidentiality protections and the potential for disparaging comments.

Canadian nurses are required to participate in continuing competence programs (CCPs) to ensure that nurses are current and competent in professional practice

External environment

↓

Work environment

↓

CNS JOB DESCRIPTION
Consider three spheres and applicability to specialty practice and/or
core competencies (selected activities—not exhaustive)

Patient/Client
1. Grand rounds
2. Outcomes management
3. Safety
4. Implement select conceptual framework

Nurses and Nursing Practice
1. Contribute to staff evaluation processes
2. Education
3. Professional development activities
4. Role modeling/change agent
5. Research and evidence-based practice

Organization and Systems
1. Strategic plan development, implementation, evaluation
2. Committee and task force efforts
3. Professional activites that represent the institution
4. Resource managment including product evaluation
5. Risk managment
6. Accreditation and recognition efforts

CNS PERFORMANCE APPRAISAL TOOL AND PROCESSES

Figure 4-4   Proposed template for CNS performance review: structure and process
model.

Table 4-6   SUGGESTED RESOURCES FOR CNS JOB DESCRIPTION DEVELOPMENT

1. Request copies of CNS specific job descriptions from networking colleagues accessible through listservs or discussion boards. The CNS-listserv found through the National Association of Clinical Nurse Specialists (NACNS) (www.nacns.org) is one option.

2. Connect with CNSs through specialty organizations and request copies of job descriptions relevant to the practice area and type of work setting.

3. Consider crafting a job description framed by the *Statement on Clinical Nurse Specialist Practice and Education* (NACNS, 2004) and incorporating specialty specific concepts, definitions, and theoretical frameworks.

4. Explore the literature for materials that differentiate CNS practice from other APRN practice models, and use this evidence to inform and support the CNS-specific job description.

5. Include CNS coworkers in the process. Consider that CNSs may have differing priorities and role expectations depending upon the department and specialty. Make certain to provide opportunities to validate and modify the job description using the input of CNSs, internal stakeholders, and, perhaps, outside experts.

Exemplar 4-2

Role Blurring: Misdirected Egalitarianism?

Gloria Jenkins is an experienced CNS recently hired to guide the staff of two intensive care units. She is certified as a critical care nurse specialist (CCNS). Gloria's position reports to the director of nursing education (DNE). Other positions reporting directly to the DNE are the clinical educators, employed to provide staff education, including employee orientation, critical care classes, new product updates, and programs mandated by accrediting agencies.

For many years, the nursing education department has struggled to meet the burgeoning educational programming needs of staff. Since much of this programming is considered mandatory as a result of written policies, the need for staffing the educational programs has been routinely prioritized over the more unit-based CNS work. Over time, CNS job responsibilities have become indistinguishable from clinical educator job responsibilities.

This role blurring has contributed to significant CNS turnover. By comparison, the clinical educator group has enjoyed much stability. While the CNSs are often required to assist the clinical educators with classes, education programs, and mandatory in-servicing requirements, the CNSs find that their unique work is often left undone. Over time, this work has assumed less and less importance leading to further CNS dissatisfaction. Notably, department projects are assigned to both CNSs and clinical educators without regards to role or credentials.

Gloria Jenkins is frustrated by this situation and is finding that she, too, is increasingly unhappy in her new role. Rather than developing evidence-based projects, working with nurses to improve point-of-care processes, or establishing programs to affect changes in outcomes as measured by National Data Nursing Quality Indicators (NDNQI), Gloria finds that she is teaching cardiopulmonary resuscitation classes, running critical care classes, in-servicing staff on new intravenous infusion devices, and pursuing updated copies of nurse licenses. She approaches her CNS colleagues to discuss the situation and, as a group, they decide to discuss their concerns with the DNE.

The DNE, in consultation with the chief nurse executive (CNE), recognizes that work processes require change. The CNE believes that there is a knowledge deficit specific to the role of the CNS and differences between CNSs and clinical educators. She asks Gloria to present a comparison and contrast of the two roles to members of the nursing education department as well as to the nursing management team.

Gloria investigates the roles of CNS and staff development/clinical educators and presents this information to the group. Following the presentation, there is much discussion. The CNSs are enthused and feel professionally validated by the shared information. The clinical educators are generally distressed. Comments ensue that suggest that "we're all in this together" and that the "drudgery tasks" should not belong only to the clinical educators. A few CNSs share that they would rather "pitch in" to help their colleagues rather than potentially contribute to animosities within the department.

Gloria is surprised by these reactions. She poses the following questions to the group for their consideration and requests to schedule a meeting in 2 weeks to continue the discussion:

1. Is the concept of equality as citizens/humans consistent with the idea that people have varying levels of education and expertise and this formal and informal expertise opens doors to opportunities that are unavailable to those without requisite credentials? Can job responsibilities reflect these differences while still promoting a sense of team spirit and collegiality?

2. Is egalitarianism used to justify leveling of work-related responsibilities so that those who are best prepared are compelled to participate in the daily work of those who are less formally prepared? Is guilt used to sabotage efforts made to distinguish educational, licensing, and certification differences between nurse groups?

3. Is it cost-effective to involve advanced practice nurses hired to perform as unit- or department-based CNSs in the daily routines of orientations, required in-service activities, and annual competencies when nurses in job categories with lower associated compensation packages can fulfill the responsibilities?

4. There are clinical educators that are prepared as CNSs but have chosen the clinical educator role despite the availability of vacant CNS positions. Should the DNE distribute work based on credentials or based on hired role?

5. How should this situation be best addressed? What strategies could be proposed that would maintain a team spirit and engender feelings of mutual appreciation and respect without limiting CNSs to nonadvanced practice activities or assigning clinical educators to projects that are not commensurate with their nonadvanced practice role?

(Mantesso, Petrucka, & Bassendowski, 2008). CCPs often integrate reflective practice as a vehicle for self-assessment. One aspect of reflective practice is peer feedback. Nurses are varyingly receptive to peer feedback depending upon locus of control, a personality variable. Giving and receiving peer feedback requires a conversation between colleagues that emphasizes dialogue and development. CNSs should consider working with staff to develop peer feedback opportunities that may enhance nursing practice. Locus of control may be an important variable to consider when planning continuing development programs for staff with both internal and external control foci since nurses with external locus of control may be more anxious during feedback processes when compared to the more assertive and confident internally controlled nurse (Mantesso et al., 2008).

Establishing peer-review processes takes planning. Review tools need to reflect job expectations, values, and required competencies. When developing a peer-review process, CNSs should solicit stakeholder input, establish the criteria against which the nurse will be evaluated, and create the process for reviewer selection (Briggs et al., 2005).

If a CNS is facilitating the development of a peer-review process for staff, it is important to have staff select appraisal items and develop guidelines. The guidelines should include the number of peer appraisals per staff member, role of self-evaluation, reviewer selection criteria, and confidentiality protections (Mathews, 2000).

When constructing an advanced-practice peer-review process, CNSs should incorporate indicators that are consistent with those of APN organizations. Several organizations offer CNS or CS (clinical specialist) certifications: Oncology Nursing Certification Corporation (ONCC), American Association of Critical-Care Nurses (AACN), and American Nurses Credentialing Center (ANCC) on Certification. These organizations invest considerable resources into establishing valid and reliable examinations. Test maps and APN-specific materials in electronic and print forms are useful tools to examine when constructing evaluation tools. Test maps build on job analyses and are realistic measures to use as comparators against job descriptions and evaluation criteria.

CNS peer-review tools should be consistent with the American Nurses Association (ANA) *Scope and Standards of Advanced Practice Nursing* (1996). Specialty organizations are useful as sources of standards, including AACN's *Scope of Practice and Standards of Professional Performance for the Acute and Critical Care Clinical Nurse Specialist* (2002), *Statement on Clinical Nurse Specialist Practice and Education* (NACNS, 2004), and *The Role of the Advanced Practice Nurse in Oncology Care* (Oncology Nursing Society [ONS], 2007).

There are numerous ways to structure peer-review processes and format evaluation tools. Some review systems are fairly unstructured, whereas others use guiding questions or very specific review criteria (Briggs et al., 2005). CNSs should examine a variety of structures and processes and choose a format that is best suited to the needs of the CNSs within the particular organization. Briggs et al. cautioned that peer review differs from traditional, annual performance evaluations. Often, peer review supplements the standard review process.

Identifying colleagues to serve as reviewers is an important activity. CNSs must also determine whether physicians should be included in the process. There are pros and cons to physician inclusion. Certainly, if physicians are included, they need to have an accurate understanding of the role of the CNS and how it differs from that of the nurse practitioner, physician, and RN. Reviewers need to be informed of the process and boundaries of the evaluation program and will require education and training.

When designing a peer-review process, CNSs need to have frank discussions about whether the reviewer should be anonymous or known. Anonymity may facilitate honest and candid feedback. At times anonymity can also allow for aggressive, mean-spirited reviews. Briggs et al. (2005) commented that individuals often express the belief that they have the right to know who is reviewing their work. There are times when the CNS might want additional information or clarification from the reviewer, and in an anonymous process, this option is not possible.

Peer review implemented as an open process with identified, known reviewers has different associated concerns. Reviewers may feel pressure to provide positive feedback. Some reviewers may worry about retribution when an honest review reveals performance deficiencies that are shared with the reviewed peer. These types of concerns should be openly discussed within the CNS group, guidelines should be established, and education should be provided.

When CNSs engage in peer-review processes as a supplement to performance evaluations, they should also conduct self-evaluation. Using peer-review feedback to manage personal performance assists the CNS and nursing staff members in reaching desired goals. Peer review is a legitimate source of data that facilitates self-development. Vuorinen, Tarkka, and Meretoja (2000) examined nurses' experiences with peer evaluation and its potential impact on professional development. RNs (N = 24) employed on an intensive care unit in Finland completed questionnaires with five open-ended questions pertaining to peer review. Content analysis revealed that peer review assisted nurses in better understanding their actions. Peer feedback offered the reviewed nurses alternative ways of looking at and conducting their work. The respondents evaluated peer evaluation as positive and collaborative.

CNSs may find appealing the perspective that the feedback from peer review offers alternative ways of viewing the work environment and the CNS practice patterns. Peer review fosters collaboration and facilitates the development of trust. CNSs can use the input from peers to develop further as an APN. To facilitate peer-review processes, CNSs should consider portfolios as an additional data source. Sharing an organized portfolio with up-to-date information is a good way to provide reviewers with supplemental information.

Peer Review: Abstracts and Manuscripts

Peer review is essential for high-quality scholarly work. It is usually conducted as a double-blind process. The reviewer is unfamiliar with the author of the submission, and the author receives feedback that is anonymous. Similar to the notion of double-blind research studies, the system protects the integrity of the decision making by divorcing the person from the quality of the work.

Double-blinded peer review is incorporated into selection processes for most types of professional activities and venues (Table 4-7). Many new CNSs find review procedures intimidating or confusing. Some would like to contribute as reviewers. Understanding the basic process is necessary to actively contribute to the scholarly work of CNSs and to disseminate information that may be useful to the profession and to practice.

There is a need for expert CNSs to serve as reviewers for nursing journals. CNS expertise may be in education, research, administration, or clinical practice. Many journals have requests for reviewers posted on their home page. Some journals prefer publishing experience. Reviewers volunteer their services. Most are acknowledged through some type of simple gesture, such as an annual published list of reviewers in the journal, a certificate of acknowledgment, or a thank-you letter on journal stationery. CNSs should make certain to include reviewer activities on their curriculum vitae or résumé as a professional activity or professional service. Usually, reviewers serve a predesignated time commitment. Manuscripts are presented in an unscheduled fashion, but there is a reasonable time period between manuscript review requests.

Manuscript reviews vary in format and process. Some reviews are submitted electronically, whereas other journals use hard-copy manuscripts with various options for review return. Reviewers are selected based on the manuscript topic and the reviewer's area of expertise. More than one reviewer is assigned to each manuscript.

Most journals provide verbatim feedback from reviewers to authors. Part of the peer-review process should be to provide constructive feedback in such a way that even when a manuscript is rejected, the author does not feel personally rejected or insulted. Most authors work very hard on manuscripts. This does not mean that all submissions are well written or even logical. Nonetheless, remember that the comments and criticisms written on the review page are going to be read by the author. If the

Table 4-7   SELECT ACTIVITIES INCORPORATING DOUBLE-BLIND, PEER-REVIEW PROCESSES

Manuscript review processes for journals

Podium abstracts for conference presentations

Poster abstracts

Dossier review by outside experts for tenure and promotion in university settings

Grant applications

Fellowship applications

Awards

review is too harsh or unkind, the writer may never submit another manuscript. Reviewers should be candid but should also be professional. Consider the review process as an opportunity to mentor and develop a colleague.

CNSs may also elect to participate in peer-review processes for conferences. Most popular or highly regarded conferences are competitive. A call for abstracts is issued for both paper and poster submissions. Reviewers are needed to select those abstracts that are suitable for podium presentations versus those that are more appropriately shared in poster form. A percentage of abstract submissions will be rejected based on reviewers' critiques. The number of rejections will depend on the number of submissions. Reviewers play a key role in this process. Many organizations solicit abstract reviewers during conferences. This is a good way to serve an organization and get involved at an entry level in regional, national, or international conference planning.

Conclusion

Participating in performance appraisal processes and working with nurses to address deficiencies or build on strengths are challenging aspects of CNS practice. Many supervisors cringe at the thought of giving honest feedback to employees, particularly if this feedback relates to performance deficiencies, disciplinary concerns, or the possibility of employment termination at the conclusion of a probationary period.

These are certainly stressful events; however, CNSs are wise to consider the benefits of the performance appraisal process. In general, CNSs are working with a nurse manager or other nurse administrator. The CNS may be able to offer the struggling employee a very real opportunity to improve performance. CNSs are typically regarded as an advocate for nurses, rather than as a threat to nurses. This rapport provides CNSs with the means to make a difference in the professional life of a nurse and the work life of a nursing team.

Performance evaluation may also be best viewed as a continuous quality improvement activity that has the potential to truly change practice. Verbal coaching, written kudos, reminders of practice expectations, and gentle nudging are interventions that can foster strong relationships between nursing staff and CNSs. Continuous evaluative feedback may elicit higher levels of professional practice and improved patient care outcomes. From this perspective, the CNS role in performance appraisal has the potential to be empowering and uplifting. Concrete skills, logistical and legal responsibilities, and documentation habits need to be developed, but resources are available and should be used as the CNS learns to contribute to an expert and fair appraisal process.

References

American Association of Critical-Care Nurses (AACN). (2002). *Scope of practice and standards of professional performance for the acute and critical care clinical nurse specialist.* Aliso Viego, CA: Author.

American Nurses Association (ANA). (1996). *Scope and standards of advanced practice nursing.* Washington, DC: American Nurses Publishing.

Briggs, L. A., Heath, J., & Kelley, J. (2005). Peer review for advanced practice nurses. What does it really mean? *AACN Clinical Issues, 16*(1), 3–15.

Chandra, A. (2006). Employee evaluation strategies for healthcare organizations—A general guide. *Hospital Topics, 84*(2), 34–38.

DelPo, A. (2005). *The performance appraisal handbook: Legal & practical rules for managers.* Berkeley, CA: Nolo.

DelPo, A., & Guerin, L. (2003). *Dealing with problem employees: A legal guide* (2nd ed.). Berkeley, CA: Nolo.

Dougherty, M. (2006). Editorial: The value of peer review. *Nursing Research, 55*(2), 73–74.

Hamilton, K., Coates, V., Kelly, B., Boore, J., Cundell, J., Gracey, J., et al. (2007). Performance assessment in health care providers: A critical review of evidence and current practice. *Journal of Nursing Management, 15,* 773-791.

HRN Management Group. (2004). *15 common errors managers make when appraising employees.* Retrieved September 29, 2008, from http://www.hrnonline.com/tryit/AppraisalTip-15CommonAppraisalMistakes.pdf

Locke, E., & Latham, G. (2002). Building a practically useful theory of goal setting and task motivation: A 35-year odyssey. *American Psychologist, 57*(9), 705–717.

Mamchur, C., & Myrick, F. (2003). Preceptorship and interpersonal conflict: A multidisciplinary study. *Journal of Advanced Nursing, 43*(2), 188–196.

Mantesso, J., Petrucka, P., & Bassendowski, S. (2008). Continuing professional competence: Peer feedback success from determination of nurse locus of control. *Journal of Continuing Education in Nursing, 39*(5), 200–205.

Mathews, D. (2000). Developing a perioperative peer performance appraisal system. *Association of PeriOperative Nurses, 72*(6), 1039–1042, 1044, 1046.

McAllister, M., & Osborne, Y. (1997). Peer review: A strategy to enhance cooperative student learning. *Nurse Educator, 22*(1), 40–44.

National Association of Clinical Nurse Specialists (NACNS). 2004 Statement Revision Task Force. (2004). *Statement on clinical nurse specialist practice and education* (2nd ed.). Harrisburg, PA: National Association of Clinical Nurse Specialists.

Oncology Nursing Society (ONS). (2007). *ONS position. The role of the advanced practice nurse in oncology care.* Retrieved October 6, 2008, from http://www.ons.org/Publications/positions/documents/pdfs/AdvancedPracticeNurseinOncologyCare.pdf

Shaneberger, K. (2008). Managing your staff's performance. *OR Manager, 24*(6), 23–24.

Shepard, G. (2005). *How to make performance evaluations really work.* Hoboken, NJ: Wiley.

SuccessFactors, Inc. (2008). *Performance and talent management.* Retrieved September 29, 2008, from http://www.successfactors.com/performance-management-software

Vuorinen, R., Tarkka, M. T., & Meretoja, R. (2000). Peer evaluation in nurses' professional development: A pilot study to investigate the issues. *Journal of Clinical Nursing, 9*(2), 273–281.

Walters, G. (2000). A checklist for better understanding of the peer review process. *RN Update, 31*(4), 4–5.

Zemke, R. (1991). Do performance appraisals change performance? *Training, 28*(5), 35–39.

Zuzelo, P. (2004). Clinical evaluation algorithm. Unpublished work.

Cnss and Difficult Clinician–Patient Situations: Strategies for Success

Zane Robinson Wolf, PhD, RN, FAAN

The categorization of patients as difficult or unpopular has emerged from the culture of nursing (English & Morse, 1988; Kus, 1990; Trexler, 1996) as well as other health-care disciplines. Most nurses acknowledge that difficult patients come with the territory of nursing practice. Few admit that the label "difficult" matches the social phenomenon of deviance; deviance refers to illegal or immoral actions (Trexler, 1996). Some consider the label and other characterizations to be derogatory (e.g., crocks, gomers) (Shahady, 1964) and stigmatizing (MacDonald, 2003; Rogge, Greenwald, & Golden, 2004). The label of "difficult" is not inherent, but conferred by those in contact with patients (Carveth, 1991). Moreover, the label used by healthcare providers represents various patient descriptions or behaviors (Table 5-1). The behaviors are considered dysfunctional (Carveth, 1995) and may implicitly recognize problems with nurse–patient communication.

Healthcare providers might admit they dislike difficult patients (Smith, 2006). Such negative opinions often spread throughout the staff, as they prejudge patients and family members before having contact (Carveth, 1995). Difficult patients are unpopular and marginalized; nursing staff distance themselves from patients and withdraw from their relatives (Maupin, 1995). They also separate themselves from patients' suffering, keeping the professional's pain internal and perhaps isolating patients (Arbore, Katz, & Johnson, 2007). This challenging clinician–patient relationship can be viewed as an unequal power structure influenced by the protection and maintenance of professional egos (Hart & Freeman, 2005; Henderson, 2003). Ultimately, the quality of care provided by nursing staff may decline as a consequence of avoidance, evident by reduced nursing visits (Carveth, 1995; Corley & Goren, 1998). Some contend that nursing may be seen as a distancing and avoidance relationship with patients (Flaskerud, Halloran, Janken, Lund, & Zetterlund, 1999).

The potential for unprofessional, unethical, or noncaring nurse–patient relationships exists in difficult clinician–patient situations. Because of this problem and their

Table 5-1   DIFFICULT PATIENT DESCRIPTIONS

Terminally ill	Moody
Chronically ill	Irrational
Suffering in pain	Uninsured
Dependent	Sexually provocative
Require complex nursing care	Easily agitated
Elderly	Has poor hygiene
Manipulative	Use more nursing time than reasonable
Demented	for condition
Abusive	Act helpless
Violent	Has unexplained symptoms
Assaultive	Multiple somatic complaints
Threatening	Adheres poorly to care regimens
Demanding	Dramatically different cultural orientation
Intimidating	Dramatically different values
Victim of gunshot wound	Dramatically different socioeconomic
Gay or lesbian	status
Racially or ethnically different	Health behaviors (e.g., smokes, obese)
"Own fault" diagnoses	Unable to interpret patient's verbal and
Homeless	nonverbal communication
Fail to cooperate with requests	Language barrier
Nonresponse to standard medical therapy	Different socioeconomic status
Noncompliance with treatment regimens	Schizophrenic
Ask for special privileges	Severe personality disorder
Play one staff against another (splitting)	Obsessive–compulsive disorders
Bullying	Alcoholic
Aggressive	Substance abuser (e.g., alcohol,
Recalcitrant	IV drug use)
Make insulting remarks	Anxiolytic abuser
Violate rules	Analgesics abuser
Lying	Sickle cell disease
Angry	Pancreatitis
Frightened	Musculoskeletal disease
Confused	Chronic fatigue syndrome
Seductive	Fibromyalgia

Source: Andersson, Hallberg, & Edberg, 2003; Asbring & Narvanen, 2002; Astrom, Furaker, & Norberg, 1995; Bowers, 2003; Carveth, 1995; Eriksson & Saveman, 2002; Gorman, 1996; Hinshelwood, 1999; Kestler, 1991; Kuritzky, 1996; Kus, 1990; Lerner, 1997; Morrison, Ramsey, & Snyder, 2000; Murdoch, 2004; Steinmetz & Tabenkin, 2001; Strandberg & Jansson, 2003; Swartz et al., 2003; Thomas & Ellis, 2000; White & Keller, 2000; Wileman, May, & Chew-Graham, 2002; Wilkes, Boxer, & White, 2003; Wolf et al., 1997.

scope of practice, CNSs might benefit from reading Goffman's (1963) perspectives on stigma and MacDonald's (2003) concept analysis of stigma and the difficult patient. Further, Rogge et al. (2004) typify relationships with overweight persons with the phrase *civilized oppression* (Bejciy-Spring, 2008; Harvey, 1999). These perspectives provide insights into this clinical dilemma and are a foundation for problem solving and leadership.

A serious challenge for CNSs arises from the likelihood that difficult patients may experience stigmatization (Asbring & Narvanen, 2002; MacDonald, 2003) and receive inadequate care (Nield-Anderson et al., 1999). When CNSs strategize to improve and resolve difficult patient situations, they must consider that the label "difficult" might also describe the status of healthcare professionals involved in these problematic situations. Healthcare professionals could be distressed, helpless, and frustrated when trying to manage difficult patient situations that persist despite best efforts (Brook, 1993).

Patients, family members, healthcare professionals, and changes in healthcare financing may all contribute to escalating difficult patient situations (Bowers, 2003; Gorman, Raines, & Sultan, 2002; Haas, Leiser, Magill, & Sanyer, 2005; Hinshelwood, 1999; White, Keller, & White, 1998). Furthermore, noncompliant or uncooperative behavior may not necessarily be a maladaptive response for patients, but serves to call attention to their suffering and need for alternative plans of care (Somboontanont et al., 2004). Healthcare providers, patients, and family members become enmeshed in situations that involve intense reactions (White & Keller, 2000; Wileman, May, & Chew-Graham, 2002).

CNSs demonstrate expert skills when managing difficult clinician–patient situations. They use their "influence to improve patient outcomes" (Darmody, 2005, p. 263). They often solve challenging patient situations that thwart less-seasoned, less-expert nurses, thus demonstrating their troubleshooting abilities (Wolf, 1994).

CNSs address patient problems directly and indirectly through other providers (Dabbs, Curran, & Lenz, 2000; Darmody, 2005). They serve as mediators in problematic situations and remind nurses and other providers of moral and professional obligations to provide care (Maupin, 1995). CNSs and other providers are required to resolve conflict (Davies & Hughes, 2002; Smith, Tutor, & Phillips, 2001), prevent violence, and create relationships with patients that involve communication and negotiation so that interventions patients desire, succeed (Browne, Dickson, & Van Der Wal, 2003). The safety of patients, nursing staff, and other providers is critical.

Coaching to Change Nursing Staff's Approach

It is likely that expert CNSs, who work chiefly in acute care hospitals, may frequently encounter difficult patient and family problems. CNSs might coach nursing staff when they recognize that problem clinician–patient situations have emerged on hospital units. They know how to advise staff to set reasonable limits on patients' behavior, adjust their unrealistic expectations of improved behavior, try patience, increase contacts with patients, and listen to patients (Ujhely, 1963).

CNSs could also propose that staff consider showing patients concern; providing explanations about treatments, procedures, and medications; teaching anxiety-reducing exercises; and encouraging patients to participate in their care (Butler, 1986). Additional recommendations consist of avoiding retaliation and holding preconceived ideas about patients, acknowledging patients' distress, and resolving conflicts early to avoid escalating situations (Harris, 1989).

CNSs may possibly encourage nursing staff to persist when patient care requires complex skill and extracts great emotional costs, such as the care demands of patients suffering from malignant, malodorous wounds (Wilkes, Boxer, & White, 2003). This example, taken from palliative care nursing practice, showed nurses comforting patients and family members alike. Although the nurses experienced distress at the suffering of patients and family members, they also supported the dignity of patients, interacted with patients as individuals, and attempted to reduce patients' isolation. Nurses relieved patients' pain and admired their indomitable spirits. They shared the workload with colleagues, discussed the challenges of care, and rotated assignments. The behaviors of the nurses serve as models for other clinicians. CNSs could post this study for nursing staff to peruse, conduct lunchtime discussion sessions, or contribute a class on difficult clinician–provider situations in new nurse graduates' orientation programs.

Building on a focus group study (Juliana et al., 1997), guidelines (Table 5-2) were created and implemented in the hope they would serve as a resource for caring for difficult patients (Wolf et al., 1997). A loose-leaf binder and poster (Table 5-2) were produced in which nine main color-coded categories and interventions that matched those main categories were compiled in the binder. The colors chosen for the categories matched the color of the specific interventions. The standard approach, provided by the poster and loose-leaf binder, helped staff use a more methodical set of interventions that was flexible as they cared for four "difficult" patients. Modest improvements were noted, patients' concerns were ascertained, and negotiation improved situations.

CNSs recognize that difficult clinician–patient situations vary widely. Therefore, coaching nursing staff with a backup reference such as the guidelines (Juliana et al., 1997) may help them carry on with care that is positive and strategic. CNSs might also develop and test protocols that resolve difficult clinician–patient situations and improve care outcomes, such as the protocol developed in the daily care of nursing home residents (Krichbaum, Pearson, & Hanscom, 2000).

Another program designed to assist in the treatment of substance abuse patients, those frequently associated with negative attitudes of healthcare professionals, resulted in increased knowledge of nurses regarding recognition and treatment of substance-abusing patients (Swenson-Britt, Carrougher, Martin, & Brackley, 2000). CNSs could propose that there are no difficult patients and encourage staff to debate this assertion and consider alternative explanations of patients' behavior, such as inquisitiveness and assertiveness (Roos, 2005).

Table 5-2 DIFFICULT PATIENT INTERVENTIONS

This chart will help the CNS to care for difficult patients. However, before using this chart, as a nurse you must **maintain personal safety and patient's safety** if violent behavior is present or seems imminent.

Definition of "difficult" patients: those who consume more nursing time than reasonable for their condition, those who act helpless, demand special privileges, make insulting remarks, violate rules, fail to cooperate with requests, play one staff against the other, fail to comply with regimens, or use threats or demonstrate assaultive behavior toward staff to get their needs met.

Establish, Develop Nurse–Patient/Family Relationship and Communicate Effectively

Core or Basic Nursing Interventions	Anticipatory Interventions	Fact-Giving/Teaching Interventions	Control-Giving Interventions	Negotiating Interventions	Individualized Nursing Interventions	Mobilizing Other Support Systems	Nurse-to-Nurse Support	Personal Characteristics of the Nurse
Demonstrate Courteous Behavior	Predict Patient Needs	Be Specific: Present Patient with Factual Information	Give Patient Control	Provide Alternative Choices	Identify the Sources of Patient's Concern or Anxiety	Enlist Support of Natural, Organized, and Professional Support Systems	Advocate for Nurses on Unit	Be Persistent
Establish Trusting Relationship		Teach Patient About Procedures and Tests		Make and Keep Contracts with Patients	Respond to Patient's Concern		Engage Nurses on the Unit to Act for the Welfare of the Patient	Be Resourceful
Treat Patient as a Unique Human Being				Set Limits		Try to Understand Patient's Point of View		Be Adaptable
Show Patience				Impose Control	Share Perceptions with the Patient About His/Her			Be Calm So Patient Mirrors Calm Behavior

(continues)

Table 5-2 (continued)

Core or Basic Nursing Interventions	Anticipatory Interventions	Fact-Giving/Teaching Interventions	Control-Giving Interventions	Negotiating Interventions	Individualized Nursing Interventions	Mobilizing Other Support Systems	Nurse-to-Nurse Support	Personal Characteristics of the Nurse
Show Caring					Behavior and How Behavior Affects Self and Others			Accept Humanness of the Nurse and the Patient/Family
Be Attentive					Do Extras for Patient			
Be Nonjudgmental								
Treat Patient as You Would Want Yourself or Your Loved Ones to Be Treated								
Maintain Physical Comfort								
Maintain Physiological Comfort								
Regulate Sensory Input								

Source: Reprinted from *MEDSURG Nursing*, 1997. Volume 6, Number 5, pp. 304-314. Reprinted with permission of the publisher, Jannetti Publications, Inc., East Holly Avenue, Box 56, Pitman, NJ 08071-0056. Phone (856) 256-2300; Fax (856) 589-7463. (For a sample issue of the journal, visit www.medsurgnurse.org.)

Table 5-2   (continued)

Difficult Patient/Family Intervention

Core or Basic Nursing Interventions

Demonstrate Courteous Behavior:

- Introduce yourself to patient and family, repeat name periodically
- Project a pleasant manner
- Provide privacy
- Demonstrate respect

Establish Trusting Relationship:

- Connect with patient through eye contact and touch
- Inquire about how he/she feels
- Uphold your promises
- Use a team approach when establishing routines with patient
- Allow patient to comfort you regarding work concerns
- Build rapport with patient over time

Treat Patient as a Unique Human Being:

- **REGARD EACH PATIENT AS A DISTINCTIVE INDIVIDUAL WITH A LIFELONG HISTORY**
- Make patient feel important by inquiring about his/her needs

Show Patience:

- Take your time with patient
- Allow patient the time to respond

Show Caring:

- Act kindly and tenderly
- Listen to the needs of the patient
- Ask how you can be helpful to him/her
- Show patient how he/she can call for you

Be Attentive:

- Fulfill his/her stated needs in a timely fashion
- Remind patient that you or your replacement are available to help him/her
- Spend a few extra minutes with him/her
- Position yourself close to him/her when communicating

(continues)

Table 5-2   (continued)

- Check on him/her frequently, especially when difficult behaviors are apparent
- Stay with patient if situation warrants it
- Apologize about unit events that may have interfered with care

Be Nonjudgmental:
- **AVOID LABELS**
- Be open-minded

Treat Patient as You Would Want Yourself or Your Loved Ones to Be Treated:
- Provide care as if you or your family member were the patient
- Show concern for his/her feelings

Maintain Physical Comfort:
- Assess and treat pain
- Provide sedatives as needed
- Keep patient warm and dry

Maintain Physiological Comfort:
- Monitor airway and breathing
- Monitor vital signs
- Assess fluid and electrolyte balance
- Evaluate medication regimen (consider adverse reactions)
- Observe for complications associated with any illness

Regulate Sensory Input:
- Explain sensory stimuli
- Balance noise and activity level
- Decrease sensory input
- Use distraction measures

Difficult Patient/Family Intervention

Anticipatory Interventions

Predict Patient Needs:
- Assist with activities of daily living
- Orient to environment
- Explain all procedures including sensations likely to be experienced by him/her

Table 5-2   (continued)

Difficult Patient/Family Intervention

Fact-Giving/Teaching Interventions

Be Specific: Present Patient with Factual Information:

- Present the difficult patient with specific information about the interventions that are to be performed
- Give the patient explanations using a positive approach
- Avoid supplying the patient with information during times of agitation, stress, low energy, or low tolerance; he/she will not be able to focus on the information
- Be direct; reorient the patient; for example, remind the patient of his/her daily activities
- Tell the patient what you plan to do
- Confront the patient with nurses' perception that behavior is not acceptable
- Present the patient with distorted facts, as sometimes this will accomplish therapeutic outcomes. For example, tell the patient it is applesauce when it is medication and applesauce

Teach Patient about Procedures and Tests:

- Give the patient information about the tests and procedures that he/she will be receiving

Difficult Patient/Family Intervention

Control-Giving Interventions

Give Patient Control:

- Enable the patient to control the situation
- Encourage the patient to make decisions
- Carry out or respond to specific requests made by the patient
- Go along with the patient's decision; this shows the patient that you support him/her
- Act on the patient's preferences, he/she wants things done a certain way because that is his/her routine; **MAINTAIN THE ROUTINE**
- Defer to the patient by giving him/her a say in his/her own care as this allows him/her to feel in control of the situation

(continues)

Table 5-2   (continued)

Difficult Patient/Family Intervention

Negotiating Interventions

Provide Alternative Choices:
- Give the patient options and choices of how and when things are done
- Assure the patient that he/she will not be forced to go through with things

Make and Keep Contracts with the Patients:
- Take the time to write a schedule and make a contract
- Institute behavior modification techniques

Set Limits:
- Enforce agreed-upon limits
- Apply institutional policies

Impose Control:
- Assess precursors to impending/actual aggressive episode
- Apply verbal, chemical, and physical restraints as appropriate for aggressive behavior

Difficult Patient/Family Intervention

Individualized Nursing Interventions

Identify the Sources of the Patient's Concern/Anxiety:
- Listen to the patient and observe his/her body language
- Try to understand his/her point of view
- Stop periodically to see the patient rather than waiting for him/her to ring for something: this will indicate that you are thinking about him/her
- Encourage the patient to tell you his/her feelings
- Get what he/she is really asking for, what truly concerns him/her; ask wide-ranged, open-ended questions so complaints become more specific

Respond to the Patient's Concerns:
- Ask the patient what you can do to help
- Meet his/her topmost priority and work on that one goal
- Change the focus of the patient's behavior to the problem that is most troubling right now

Table 5-2 (continued)

Try to Understand the Patient's Point of View:
- Remember that the patient reflects what is happening in his/her family's life
- Be sensitive to the patient's situation
- Listen attentively to the patient's views
- Acknowledge the patient's point of view
- Confirm what you think the patient is saying by describing what you hear him/her say
- Choose the appropriate time
- Assess the patient's physical, emotional, and psychological state
- Avoid talking to the patient at times of great agitation, stress, low energy, or low tolerance
- Be empathetic
- Be sympathetic
- Remember that the patient is sick and at his/her all-time low

Share Perceptions with the Patient about His/Her Behavior and How Behavior Affects Self and Others:
- Use direct questions and ask for an explanation if you think that someone is being short with you or he/she doesn't want to be bothered with your questions/assessment
- Give the patient feedback by describing his/her behavior and its effect
- Be open; allow the patient to see you as another human being so that you are no longer the object of his/her anger

Do Extras for the Patient:
- Do little things or out of the ordinary things for him/her

Difficult Patient/Family Intervention

Mobilizing Other Support Systems

Enlist Support of Natural, Organized, and Professional Support Systems:
- Enlist family involvement, as patient's behavior may reflect what is happening in his/her family life
- Mobilize support systems, such as friends and clergy, to provide immediate help
- Seek assistance of other healthcare providers and hold interdisciplinary meetings at a time convenient for the patient

(continues)

Table 5-2   (continued)

- Consult with psychiatry; at times a psychopathological process can underlie the patient's behavior
- Make referrals to other agencies and support groups for postdischarge needs

Difficult Patient/Family Intervention

Nurse-to-Nurse Support

Advocate for Nurses on the Unit:

- Be a source of unconditional support for each other. If you do not agree with the way that someone has handled a difficult patient/family situation, do not belittle him/her in public. Rather, discuss concerns in a private, nonthreatening, professional way. **Be part of the solution**.
- Approach your manager regarding the possibility of conducting problem-solving sessions about difficult patients/families. This may allow for the resolution of concerns before they become more complex. Due to decreased length of stay, these meetings would need to be scheduled on short notice and have support of nursing management. **Be part of the solution**.

Engage Nurses on the Unit to Act for the Welfare of the Patient:

- Don't lose sight of why we are here
- Point out that the perception of a difficult patient/family may only be based on hearsay from another colleague. Formulate your decision based on your own assessment of the situation
- Don't be too quick to judge, as the difficult patient/family label is hard to eliminate. Reinforce how these labels can "stick" and may cause someone who is just having a stressful time to be burdened with a negative title
- Practice consciousness-raising with each other: Informally monitor each other for signs of overreacting that may be related to burnout, a need for some time off, or too much overtime. Perhaps have a "buddy system" so two colleagues can constructively support each other with feedback when an objective opinion is needed
- Be flexible and support each other: Switch assignments if a colleague has been assigned to a difficult patient for an extended period of time and interventions are not producing a positive change in nurse/patient/family interactions
- Expect professional behavior from yourself and each other: You will hold yourself to a higher standard, and your colleagues may mirror your behavior
- Share successful and unsuccessful strategies that were used with the patient/family

Table 5-2   (continued)

Difficult Patient/Family Intervention

Personal Characteristics of the Nurse

Be Persistent:
- Learn more about the patient's situation
- Look for and expect to find a solution
- Remember that there are many ways to solve a difficult situation

Be Resourceful:
- Know how and when to ask for help. Become familiar with the options available to you when you need to tap outside resources (e.g., psychiatric CNS, Social Service)
- Encourage patient/family to become part of the solution by encouraging him/her to suggest options that are mutually acceptable

Be Adaptable:
- Keep an open mind. Try the unconventional if conventional interventions do not work
- Be willing to relinquish control to the patient/family as appropriate
- Tailor your interventions to patient's/family's cultural background/values
- Realize that his/her anger is not targeted toward you

Be Calm So Patient Mirrors Calm Behavior:
- Avoid displaying frustrated or angry behaviors that may be mirrored by others
- Be prepared to stay calm when the unexpected happens

Accept Humanness of the Nurse and the Patient/Family:
- Reconcile the desire to please with the appropriateness of setting reasonable limits
- Remember that cordial, reasonable people can become difficult when dealing with the loss of control associated with acute or chronic illness
- Acknowledge your own culture and values and how these can affect your perceptions about the patient/family
- Be aware of the natural "fight-or-flight response" that can occur when you are threatened or frustrated, as this may cause avoidance and distancing
- Be prepared to respond to difficult behaviors. ACT, DON'T REACT
- Be aware of tendencies to blow things out of proportion. This response can result in labeling a person or situation "difficult"

(continues)

Table 5-2 (continued)
• Remember that nurses prefer order over chaos and may consider order their responsibility
• Don't take the difficult behavior personally
• **KNOW WHEN TO WALK AWAY**

Source: Wolf, Z.R., et al. (1996). Difficult Patient/Family Interventions. (Unpublished manuscript). Graduate Nursing Programs, La Salle University, 1900 West Olney Avenue, Philadelphia, PA 19141. Reprinted with permission.

Education and Supervision: Helping Staff Avoid the Dark Side of Nursing

A model representation of the "dark side" of nursing (Corley & Goren, 1998) illustrates a sequence of factors leading to patient stigmatization and marginalization. The model provides CNSs a position at which to intervene in difficult patient–clinician scenarios. Specifically, CNSs might act by exploring nurses' perceptions of patient stigma and nurses' responses to stigma by presenting periodic in-service education sessions that foster the development of individual consciousness and improved care. An example of objectives and content that may be included in teaching plans for educational sessions is found in Tables 5-3 and 5-4. Because nurses are often frustrated and angry when interacting with difficult patients and family members, educational sessions conducted by CNSs might assist nursing staff to interact with patients and families, avoid conflict, and move toward positive resolutions of difficulties (Bland & Rossen, 2005; Podrasky & Sexton, 1988).

Other educational programs might be created for caregivers of patients with dementia, often classified as difficult patients. In one study, assaultive behaviors (hitting, hitting attempt, kicking, kicking attempt, biting, biting attempt, throwing things, and spitting) during showers in nursing homes were associated with caregiver behaviors more than environmental conditions (Somboontanont et al., 2004). Incorporating caregiver behaviors during bathing or other interventions may assist in preventing the physical assault of staff by patients. Preventive behaviors are avoiding confrontational communication, avoiding restraints, alerting residents or patients to an impending action, using respectful speech, and avoiding startling residents or patients. Creating ongoing educational sessions based on these behaviors with staff in acute and long-term care settings may protect staff from physical assault and calm patients.

Psychiatric–mental health CNSs assist nursing staff to care for difficult patients, specifically those diagnosed with borderline personality disorder (Bland & Rossen, 2005). Clinical supervision of nurses, recommended for many years in the psychiatric nursing literature, has not been implemented consistently for nursing staff. Nursing staff might benefit from education provided by CNSs on patient dynamics, staff

Table 5-3	DIFFICULT FAMILY/PATIENT INTERVENTIONS TEACHING PLAN 1

Suggested objectives and content. CNSs should use creative teaching methods and select appropriate evaluation strategies.

Objectives	Content
1. List patient/family characteristics that might elicit the "difficult" patient/family label.	1. Definitions of "difficult" patient/family 2. Characteristics of difficult patient/family situations 3. Expected patient norms: physical, behavioral, attitudinal, demographic, diagnostic 4. Perceptions of "valuable" patients
2. Compare patient/family situations that might lead to escalating situations.	*Examples of Escalating Situations:* 1. Patient dependency on nursing care 2. Demented patients in acute care settings 3. Challenging physical care 4. Fear of injury by combative patients 5. Inability to interpret patients' verbal and nonverbal communication
3. Describe attributes of the difficult patient.	1. Behavioral characteristics that conflict with expected patient role 2. Presence of certain personal characteristics that conflict with beliefs and values of nurses 3. Presence of patient behaviors that nurses perceive as challenging their competence and control
4. Analyze the potential of teamwork and inter-disciplinary collaboration in caring for difficult clinician-patient situations.	Teamwork to avoid dehumanization and punitive responses 1. Referral 2. Consultation 3. Collaboration

5. Identify interventions aimed at resolving difficult clinician-patient situations.	*Interventions:*
	1. Demonstrate courteous behavior
	   a. Introduce yourself to patient
	   b. Show courtesy to patient
	2. Show regard for patient's dignity
	   a. Respect patient's dignity
	   b. Provide privacy

(continues)

Table 5-3 (continued)	
Objectives	**Content**

	3. Treat patient as a unique human being
	   a. Treat patient as an individual
	   b. Treat person as a whole person with a life history
	   c. Exert yourself in attempt to know patient
	   d. Make patient feel important
	4. Identify source of patient's concern or anxiety
	   a. Listen to patient
	   b. Allow patient to ventilate feelings
	   c. Get to patient's concern
	   d. Get to patient's hidden agenda
	   e. Ask patient what he/she wants
	   f. Attend to the patient's nonverbal communication
	   g. Ask patient to tell you how he/she feels
	   h. Assess patient's pain level
	5. Respond to patient's concern
	   a. Work on one concern at a time
	   b. Change the focus of the patient's behavior
	6. Try to understand patient's point of view
	   a. Be sensitive to patient's situation
	   b. Validate patient's perceptions
	   c. Respond to the patient in the moment
	   d. Show patient that you are empathetic
	   e. Show patient that you are sympathetic
	   f. Remember that patient is sick
	7. Predict patient's needs
	   a. Anticipate patient's needs
	8. Present patient with factual information
	   a. Present patient with the facts
	   b. Give information about tests, procedures (teach)
	   c. Tell patient your plans

Table 5-3   (continued)

Objectives	Content

    d. Tell patient how you feel

    e. Remind patient that nurses checked on him/her

    f. Apologize about unit events

    g. Repeat your name

    h. Confront patient with nurse's perception that behavior is not acceptable

9. Show patience

    a. Give patient time to respond

    b. Take your time with patient

10. Develop relationship

    a. Connect as human being with patient

    b. Develop relationship with patient

    c. Take time needed to develop relationship

    d. Involve yourself as teammate

    e. Allow patient to comfort you

11. Show caring

    a. Be kind

    b. Show patient that you care

12. Be attentive to patient

    a. Be available

    b. Be present

    c. Communicate attentiveness to patient through physical proximity

    d. Touch patient, if acceptable

    e. Reassure patient you are there to help

    f. Spend time with patient

    g. Move quickly to meet patient's requests

    h. Check on patient frequently

    i. Watch over patient more frequently

    j. "Patient"-sit patient

    k. Cover the patient and the nurse

13. Be nonjudgmental

    a. Be nonjudgmental

    b. Give the patient a chance

(continues)

Table 5-3   (continued)

Objectives	Content
	14. Make patient temporary member of nurse's family
	a. Treat patient as family
	15. Care for family members
	a. Treat family as patient
	b. Help family
	c. Show consideration to family members
	16. Make and keep contracts with patients
	a. Make contract with patient
	b. Institute behavior modification techniques
	17. Establish trusting relationship
	a. Cultivate patient's trust
	b. Be prompt and return as scheduled
	18. Impose control
	a. Set limits
	b. Put patient into restraints
	19. Exert effort on behalf of patient
	a. Do extras for patient
	b. Exert efforts to turn situation around
	c. Persist no matter how difficult the situation
	20. Be adaptable
	a. Be flexible
	b. Try different strategies
	21. Maintain physical and physiological comfort
	a. Keep patient warm and dry
	b. Give sedative to patient
	c. Change patient's medications
	d. Treat pain
	e. Provide quiet environment for rest and sleep
	22. Provide alternative choices
	a. Give patient choices
	b. Make suggestions to patient

Table 5-3 (continued)	
Objectives	**Content**
	23. Enable patient to control situation
	a. Give patient control
	b. Respond to specific requests of patient
	c. Go along with patient's decision
	d. Act on patient preferences
	e. Defer to patient
	f. Maintain the routine
	g. Try to follow patient's schedule
	24. Regulate sensory input
	a. Provide sensory information (teach)
	b. Decrease sensory input
	c. Distract patient
	d. Balance noise and activity level
	25. Enlist support of natural, organized, and professional support systems
	a. Enlist family members' help
	b. Mobilize support systems
	c. Seek help of other providers for assistance with schedule that is more beneficial to patient
	d. Consult with psychiatric/mental health CNS or psychiatrist
	e. Consult with clergy or spiritual advisor
	f. Make referrals to other agencies and support groups
	26. Engage nurses on unit to act for welfare of patient
	a. Change the situation on the unit
	b. Influence other nurse's perceptions of patient
	c. Enlist nurses' help to work together
	d. Share what you know about caring for patient with fellow nurses
	e. Assign same nurse to patient
	f. Switch assignments with other nurses

(continues)

Table 5-3 (continued)	
Objectives	**Content**
	g. Schedule additional personnel
	27. Accept nurse's humanness
	a. Recognize nurse's limits
	b. Take time out to reflect before acting
	28. Be calm so patient mirrors calmness in turn
	29. Be alert to patient's anger and potential for violence
	a. Identify source of anger and help patient to resolve it
	b. Be on guard in case of violence
6. Describe interventions effective in managing challenging behavior.	1. Effective interventions
	a. Give confirming messages (positive social or task oriented)
	b. Allow personal control by allowing the expression of anger or resentment
	c. Describe staff feelings by speaking honestly
	d. Point out patient's choice by providing face-saving alternatives
	e. Use structure (set limits ahead of time about accepted behavior) to make independent decisions
	f. Facilitisitive to nonverbal cues of patient and provider
	g. Monitor situation on unit by anticipating impending difficulties
	h. Allow time to calm down or talk through problem
	i. Be sensitive to nonverbal cues of patient and provider

Source: © 1996 by R. Brennan, L. Ferchau, M. Magee, S. Miller-Samuel, L. Nicolay, D. Paschal, J. Ring, A. Sweeney, & Z. Wolf.

Table 5-4	DIFFICULT PATIENT/FAMILY INTERVENTIONS TEACHING PLAN 2

Suggested objectives and content. CNSs should use creative teaching methods and select appropriate evaluation strategies.

Objectives	Content
1. Explore stigmatization theory.	1. Goffman: Physical deformities; blemishes of individual character; Tribal: race, nation, religion 2. Victimization 3. Secondary gain 4. Discredited persons 5. In groups and out groups
2. Examine the impact of stigmatizing responses on patients.	1. Enmeshment 2. Escalation 3. Conflict 4. Anger 5. Fear 6. Frustration 7. Isolation 8. Humiliation
3. Identify nursing staff behaviors that might be interpreted as stigmatizing.	1. "Dark side of nursing" 2. Nurse behavior: controlling, manipulating, hostile, angry, interpersonally distancing, minimizing or avoiding patient contact, failing to provide patient needs, providing more care than patient wants 3. Situations of force, abuse, and neglect 4. Absence of caring 5. Retaliation 6. Fight or flight

4. Evaluate patient behavioral cues that indicate positive resolution of difficult patient situation.	1. Cues indicating difficult patient behavior changing:
	  a. Mental status improves
	  b. Remembers nurse from previou contact

(continues)

Table 5-4 (continued)	
Objectives	**Content**
	c. Verbal communication
	i. Tone of voice more pleasant
	ii. Stops yelling
	d. Nonverbal communication
	i. Listens to nurse
	ii. Makes eye contact
	iii. Smiles
	e. Self-esteem improves
	f. Controls personal situation
	g. Easier to care for
	h. Takes on more responsibility for self-care
	i. Appreciative
	j. Pleasant
	k. Secure
	l. More relaxed
	m. Less angry
	n. Less tense
	o. Less anxious
	p. Less fearful
	q. Vital signs improve
	r. Cooperative
	s. Better outlook
	t. Positive attitude
	u. Less combative
	v. Follows instructions
	w. Complies with regimen
	x. Focuses on healing
	y. Puts light on less frequently
	z. Complaints decrease
	aa. Fewer complaints about self
	bb. Complaints become more specific
	cc. Demands decrease
	dd. Makes requests of nurse

Table 5-4 (continued)	
Objectives	**Content**
	ee. Shows courtesy
	ff. Interacts with roommate
	2. Interacts positively with staff
	3. Understands others
	4. Mutual understandings achieved with providers
	5. Establishes rapport with one nurse
	6. Trusts nurse
	7. Recognizes nurse not hostile
	8. Shows confidence in nurse
	9. Seeks out nurse
	10. Stops blaming others
	11. Is open to negotiation

responses, and the effect of treatment decisions. Nurses require ongoing education and training, including how to stabilize interpersonal relationships and moods as well as manage manipulation, splitting, transference, and countertransference. Improved knowledge and attitudes toward patients with borderline personality disorder and strategies to improve skills in developing therapeutic relationships and better management may result from the supervision and education provided by CNSs.

Emotional support for nurses within formal and informal systems of individual and/or group supervision has also been connected with improved patient care and job satisfaction and possibly staff retention. In addition to CNSs, other mentors might be called on to assist nurses caring for cancer patients involved in ethically difficult care situations (Astrom, Furaker, & Norberg, 1995).

Case Studies: Practicing De-escalation Techniques

Helping nursing staff rehearse positive, de-escalating responses to difficult patient/ family member situations has the potential of preventing difficult clinician–patient conflicts. CNSs might hold brown-bag lunches during which case studies are presented and positive, de-escalating solutions are demonstrated through role playing. They can collect case studies from staff ahead of time, print them, or send them through e-mail to prepare nursing staff for the discussion. CNSs should ensure that Health Insurance Portability and Accountability Act (HIPAA) 1996 guidelines are followed in the case presentations.

Expert nurses skilled in de-escalating escalating patients are recognized by their colleagues. Little-known practices were uncovered in a study on psychiatric nurses' calming practices (Johnson & Hauser, 2001). Patterns of action were disclosed. Nurses noticed patients, read situations and patients, knew where patients were on the continuum of escalation, understood the meaning of their behavior, knew what patients needed at the moment, connected with patients, and matched interventions with patients' needs. Noticing escalating patient behaviors involved detecting early verbal and other behavioral signs of increasing agitation. Nurses interpreted patients' cues in the context of their specific knowledge about patients and knowledge of psychopathology. They were very skilled at reading the dangerousness of situations and assessing the impact of situations on others. By listening, empathizing, and understanding patients, nurses initially connected and stayed connected with patients. Nurses matched interventions with patients' need for de-escalation. CNSs might apply the patterns of action to case studies.

Nursing staff members may possibly develop increased confidence and self-esteem as they role-play different case studies. The risks of impending aggression and violence can be reduced by ongoing practice as nurses rehearse strategies through role playing. Recognition and treatment of trigger behaviors must be identified during case presentations. An instrument that lists 84 aggressive behaviors, including three scales (precursor, defensive, and acting out), could also be reviewed to sensitize staff to serious patient behaviors (Haber & Allen, 1997). CNSs who support and prepare staff to manage future, likely difficult clinician–patient situations will affect the incidence of crises, including violent episodes. Practice in recognizing conflict and escalating situations as well as identification of the techniques of de-escalation help staff to reduce risks and may promote retention (Rew & Ferns, 2005).

Knowledge and skill of de-escalation techniques have benefited mental health settings when aggression and violence surface (Cowin et al., 2003). CNSs and nursing staff would benefit from education sessions that explore how to gradually resolve potentially violent or aggressive situations, such as those that emerge in difficult clinician–provider relationships. For example, de-escalation strategies include approaching patients with caution, not startling them; avoiding provocations; being aware of providers' facial expressions and posture; using calm, respectful language and open-ended sentences; avoiding challenges and promises; removing dangerous objects from providers' persons; being aware of exits; avoiding vulnerable positions; using distraction and redirection, and being firm and compassionate (Cowin et al., p. 65). Including these techniques in education sessions for CNSs and staff might avoid crises when applied to escalating situations.

Furthermore, ongoing sessions and a published plan that is shared with all staff would benefit providers and patients alike should the knowledge and skills be needed (Cowin et al., 1996). Additionally, alerting staff to indicators of increasing agitation, such as pacing and excessive body movement and increased voice volume and tempo, may also assist CNSs and staff to intervene early when difficult clinician–patient situations surface.

Referral, Collaboration, and Behavioral Contracts

CNSs must develop referral processes and consultation practices with each other (France, 2005). Deriving a formal network of referral among CNSs working in the same institution and healthcare system as well as the region facilitates CNS access to nursing staff who share their expertise.

CNSs skilled in psychiatric–mental health nursing practice can be called on by nursing staff and other CNSs when difficult psychiatric patients or complex behavioral situations confound their plans of care. Referral to such experts helps to isolate and define patient problems and advantages staff through the creation of individualized plans of care. Referral to psychiatric–mental health specialists benefits staff before situations escalate, as expert CNSs manage patients' behavioral issues and issues with complex physical care following consultations (Williams, 2003).

The nature of the conflict, the patients' healthcare concerns, their discomfort, complexity, involvement in the plan of care, and situational urgency all converge on the hospitalization trajectory. Staff education incorporates recommendations documented by CNSs on consultation forms, and the consultant checks in periodically to determine progress. Staff is encouraged to demonstrate caring; at the same time, it is hoped they feel the caring support of CNSs who urge them to institute positive plans of care. Staff will feel supported as they change behavior and succeed; their determination to improve the situation sets the stage for future, challenging, difficult patient situations.

The perceptions of patients and family members might be dramatically improved following successful consultations with CNSs. Consultation guidelines may possibly improve the skills of the nursing staff and influence the caring and concern shown for patients and family members. Teamwork to coordinate a plan of care, based on consultant recommendations aimed at reducing conflict and improving the situation, can improve patient satisfaction. Ideally, the care experienced by patients and family is as good as or better than expected.

Behavioral contracts or patient care agreements developed by CNSs and nursing staff may be useful when other interventions do not improve difficult clinician–provider situations (Campbell & Anderson, 1999; Morrison, Ramsey, & Snyder, 2000). Contracts ultimately prevent staff from being sidetracked from their work. The contract is initiated following communication and collaboration with the multidisciplinary team and risk management personnel. Successful implementation of a patient care agreement requires a cohesive team in 24-hour communication about patient progress (Morrison et al., 2000). Patients who continue to display extreme behavior (violence, criminal) may be discharged.

Patient care agreements specify the patients' and caregivers' obligations and the consequences of not performing these expectations. Agreements may include positive reinforcement (Campbell & Anderson, 1999). Although a patient's perspective is included at the beginning of the plan, health care is the goal just as dangerous behavior is nonnegotiable. A CNS functions as liaison among caregivers on the team. Patient care agreements include the hospital's commitment to provide the best possible care, the patient's responsibility to follow treatment guidelines, the patient's right to open communication from the healthcare team, the conditions the patient has to meet to continue receiving treatment at the hospital, actions the patient must take to comply with the treatment plan, consequences of not meeting the conditions, and signatures of patient, nurse, and physician (Campbell & Anderson, 1999; Morrison et al., 2000).

Interdisciplinary Rounds

CNSs have used interdisciplinary rounds to improve discharge planning (Halm et al., 2003). Rounds illustrate the interdependence of healthcare teams. Interdisciplinary rounds address the planning and evaluation of patient status, needs, and problems as they are discussed by all healthcare team members. They are linked to improved patient outcomes (Curley, McEachern, & Speroff, 1998).

In one example of interdisciplinary rounds, staff nurses presented and discussed an individual patient's needs and progress, revealing the details of the patient's care and family circumstances. When evaluating the practice of a clinical nurse specialist regarding rounds (Halm et al., 2003), this clinical expert served as a link to the multidisciplinary team. Opportunities for group education, collaboration, conflict resolution, and care coordination emerged as the benefits of rounds were analyzed. Ethical dilemmas and other problems, such as difficult provider–patient situations, can be worked out as a result of the coordinated plan of care emerging from interdisciplinary rounds.

CNS participation during rounds with physicians and other providers could foster shared decision making, cooperation, joint planning, and open communication (Vazirani, Hays, Shapiro, & Cowan, 2005), thus preventing crises. An observational pilot study categorized CNS activities within three spheres of influence or practice domains (patient/client, nursing, and organization/system) (Darmody, 2005). Interdisciplinary patient rounds, a patient/client practice domain, represented one of the CNS activities that consumed a good amount of time. This activity was defined as multidisciplinary care conferences involving planning and evaluating patient care (Halm et al., 2003). Key activities are:

> Summarizing pertinent health data, identifying patient/family problems, defining goals, identifying interventions, discussing patient/family responses to interventions, discussing progress toward goals, revising goals and plans as necessary, generating referrals, reviewing discharge plans, and clarifying responsibilities related to implementation of the plan. (p. 134)

Interdisciplinary rounds and the interdisciplinary care that results may affect the outcomes of difficult patients, potentially keeping them safe (Stapleton, 2005). Difficult clinician–provider situations might be reduced or eliminated on units in which interdisciplinary rounds affect nurse and physician collaboration.

Therapeutic Communication

Nursing is often described as a stressful occupation. Since the emotional demands of patients and families result in stress that can ultimately lead to depression, it is imperative that CNSs assist nursing staff to avoid emotion-focused coping strategies, such as escape avoidance and distancing strategies (McCleave, 1993). Instead, they could note the effect that the social support they provide staff as advanced practice registered nurses can potentially reduce nurses' depression, a consequence of sustained stress.

The "overwhelming emotional expressions" (Pergert, Ekblad, Enskär, & Björk, 2008, p. 651), including indicators of grief and anger displayed by patients, parents, and relatives may threaten nurses' professional composure. Whether confronted by screaming, cursing, and threats or crying and howling, nurses react to unexpected situations by feeling fearful and being intimidated. CNSs can assist nursing staff to develop cultural competence and prepare to maintain their professional composure and manage care situations. Transcultural education assists nurses to learn differences in cultural expressions displayed during emergencies and illness events. Rather than responding with a power display, nurses can maintain a professional facade through a controlled expression that calms the situation. Their strategic behavior, although not representative of classic therapeutic communication techniques, nevertheless needs to be acknowledged as part of the nursing culture. These nursing strategies are most likely learned activities that are worth labeling and sharing so that other nurses can reflect on them and apply them more consciously to difficult patient and family situations.

CNSs can assist nursing staff to avoid group conformity or collective socialization when nurses join together in their dissatisfaction with difficult patients and consequently avoid them. Patient care may be uncaring and can diffuse among members of the group (Duxbury, 2000). In contrast, preparing and maintaining a therapeutic nurse–patient relationship can reduce the occurrence of difficult clinician–patient situations. CNSs might review the phases of the nurse–patient relationship: preinteraction phase, orientation or introductory phase, maintenance or working phase, and termination phase. During the transpersonal relationship, patients' need for protection and self-determination and independence must be honored (Duxbury). Nurses must listen to and comprehend their perceptions of their healthcare needs. The working phase of the relationship calls for practical solutions, and CNSs offer and sustain them.

CNSs support nursing staff involved in difficult clinician–provider relationships. They encourage partnerships between nurses and patients and attempt to reduce conflict. They are often viewed as clinical experts. To examine frequently used and priority strategies ranked by CNSs on the Clinical Nurse Specialist-Difficult Clinician–Provider instrument, a randomly selected sample of members of the National Association of Clinical Nurses specialists were surveyed (Wolf & Robinson-Smith, 2007). Respect for the patients was ranked highest for the most frequently used and highest priority strategies. The complexities of the CNSs' troubleshooting abilities were revealed in the study results. Table 5-5 includes frequently used strategies on the survey arranged in clusters: direct care strategies (assessing, deescalating, and setting limits) and indirect care (engaging in team strategies, planning care, teaching and supporting nursing staff, documenting the plan of care, and consulting the literature) strategies.

Table 5-5	STRATEGIES FREQUENTLY USED BY CNSs WHEN WORKING WITH DIFFICULT PATIENTS/FAMILIES

Direct Care Strategies

Assessing

Assess underlying behavioral problems.

Attempt to learn the meaning of illness for a patient/family member.

Try to understand how the patient copes with illness.

Ask the patient what he or she wants.

Listen carefully to understand the patient's or family member's agenda.

Check for understanding by naming the patient's or family member's issues.

Pay attention to the needs of the family members.

Attempt to allay fears and concerns of the patient/family member.

Assess the patient's mental status through chart and interview.

Pay attention to the patient's nonverbal communication, such as grimaces.

Try to understand the patient's experience in this situation.

Evaluate patient's behavior over time to gauge treatment plan effectiveness.

De-escalating

Approach the patient and family with respect, openness, and sincerity.

Respect the patient's dignity.

Show the patient and family that they are respected.

Act empathetically.

Be patient when communicating with the patient/family.

Maintain control over your emotions.

Use appropriate humor to defuse the situation.

Spend additional time to determine the root causes of the situation.

Focus on the issue at hand.

State and restate the problem.

Protect the patient from conflict.

Apologize to the family member for errors and conflicts if appropriate.

Apologize to the patient for errors and conflicts if appropriate.

Attempt to defuse the emotionality of the situation.

Share factual information with the patient.

Share factual information with the family member.

Help the patient to control the situation.

Attempt to calm the patient.

Provide the patient face-saving alternatives.

Share knowledge of patient's diagnosis and treatment with him or her.

Table 5-5 (continued)

Provide the patient with improved comfort and pain relief.

Comply with certain family members' demands.

Comply with certain patient's demands.

Administer medication to control patient behaviors as needed.

Apply physical restraints following correct procedures and consistent with policies.

Check on the patient periodically.

Setting Limits

Describe the constraints of the healthcare agency.

Point out some of the stresses of the healthcare system.

Identify the patient's or family member's responsibilities in the difficult situation.

Help the patient and family member acknowledge the mutuality and reciprocity of the nurse–patient relationship.

Share decision-making power with the patient.

Share ways to improve the nurse–patient–family relationship with the patient and family.

Persuade the patient to change his or her aggressive behavior.

Set firm limits by enforcing institutional policies.

Enforce a "zero tolerance" rule for physically threatening behavior.

Terminate relationship with patient/family.

Indirect Care Strategies

Engaging in Team Strategies

Clarify factors that may be the root of the situation with patient, family, and nursing staff.

Consult with interdisciplinary specialists to improve the plan of care.

Consult with psychiatric/mental health professional to evaluate the patient's potential psychological problems.

Communicate the details of the problem to other colleagues consistent with HIPAA.

Work with team members to understand the meaning of behavior perceived as difficult.

Help team members consistently follow the treatment plan.

Conduct in-service programs that address behaviors that stigmatize patients.

Planning Care

Meet with interdisciplinary team members to create the treatment plan.

Establish a plan of care in consultation with the patient/family.

(continues)

Table 5-5 (continued)

Explore the plan of care from the cultural orientation of the patient.

Propose alternative treatment options consistent with plan of care.

Develop a patient care agreement, including expectations, plans, and responsibilities of the patient.

Teaching and Supporting Nursing Staff

Review noncaring nurse behaviors with nursing staff.

Teach nursing staff conflict resolution strategies.

Teach nursing staff strategies to de-escalate problem situations.

Share information with the nurses about how to care for the patient.

Encourage nurses to reflect on patient's care before acting.

Help the nursing staff acknowledge the mutuality and reciprocity of the nurse–patient relationship.

Support nursing staff as they verbalize the emotional toll that the patient's suffering takes.

Discuss expectations of nurses regarding the patient.

Explain the patient's situation to nursing staff.

Review ethical principles with nursing staff.

Encourage nursing staff to express conflicts with the patient/family member.

Request that the nursing staff consider the effect that the situation is having on their feelings.

Provide emotional support to nursing staff.

Teach nursing staff strategies to care for the difficult patient.

Enlist involved nurses' help to work together to resolve the situation.

Change the nursing staff's assignment to the patient/family.

Increase the attention of the nursing staff on improving patient care.

Help nursing staff care for complex, challenging patients.

Meet with nursing staff after the situation is defused so that lessons are learned for the future.

Documenting the Plan of Care

Document the plan created by the team.

Document the new plan of care.

Document responses to the new plan of care.

Consulting Literature

Consult the literature for strategies to improve the plan of care.

Difficult clinician–patient situations call for CNSs to use their clinical expertise and decision-making abilities, critical thinking skills, and other competencies (Davies & Hughes, 2002) as they mobilize nursing staff and other providers to affect positive patient and family outcomes. Proactive strategies instituted in these situations before they escalate assist all stakeholders to achieve quality care.

References

Andersson, E. M., Hallberg, I. R., & Edberg, A. K. (2003). Nurses' experiences of the encounter with elderly patients in acute confusional state in orthopaedic care. *International Journal of Nursing Studies, 40*, 437–448.

Arbore, P., Katz, T. S., & Johnson, T. A. (2007). When professionals weep: Suffering and care providers. *Aging Today, 28*(4), 5.

Asbring, P., & Narvanen, A. (2002). Women's experiences of stigma in relation to chronic fatigue syndrome and fibromyalgia. *Qualitative Health Research, 12*(2), 148–160.

Astrom, G., Furaker, C., & Norberg, A. (1995). Nurses' skills in managing ethically difficult care situations: Interpretation of nurses' narratives. *Journal of Advanced Nursing, 21*, 1073–1080.

Bejciy-Spring, S. M. (2008). R-E-S-P-E-C-T: A model for the sensitive treatment of the bariatric patient. *Bariatric Nursing and Surgical Patient Care, 3*(1), 47–56.

Bland, A. R., & Rossen, E. K. (2005). Clinical supervision of nurses working with patients with borderline personality disorder. *Issues in Mental Health Nursing, 26*, 507–517.

Bowers, L. (2003). Manipulation: Description, identification and ambiguity. *Journal of Psychiatric and Mental Health Nursing, 10*, 323–328.

Brook, A. (1993). Emotional minefield. *Nursing Times, 20*(89), 48–49.

Browne, A., Dickson, B., & Van Der Wal, R. (2003). The ethical management of the noncompliant patient. *Cambridge Quarterly of Healthcare Ethics, 12*, 289–299.

Butler, B. M. (1986). When nurse and patient battle for control. *American Journal of Nursing, 49*(9), 67–68.

Campbell, D. B., & Anderson, B. J. (1999). Setting behavioral limits. *American Journal of Nursing, 99*(12), 40–42.

Carroll, D. W. (2008). Perspectives in psychiatric consultation liaison nursing: Care of the wounded soldier by a PCLN team. *Perspectives in Psychiatric Care, 44*, 211–215.

Carveth, J. A. (1991). *An investigation of perceived patient deviance and avoidance/distancing by nurses*. School of Nursing, University of Pennsylvania. AAT 9125608.

Carveth, J. A. (1995). Perceived patient deviance and avoidance by nurses. *Nursing Research, 44*(3), 173–178.

Corley, M. C., & Goren, S. (1998). The dark side of nursing: Impact of stigmatizing responses on patients. *Scholarly Inquiry for Nursing Practice: An International Journal, 12*(2), 99–118.

Cowin, L., Davies, R., Estall, G., Berlin, T., Fitzgerald, M., & Hoot, S. (2003). De-escalating aggression and violence in the mental health setting. *International Journal of Mental Health Nursing, 12*, 64–73.

Curley, C., McEachern, J. E., & Speroff, T. (1998). A firm trial of interdisciplinary rounds on the inpatient medical wards. An intervention designed using continuous quality improvement. *Medical Care, 36,* AS4–AS12.

Dabbs, A. D., Curran, C. R., & Lenz, E. R. (2000). A database to describe the practice component of the CNS role. *Clinical Nurse Specialist, 14*(4), 174–183.

Darmody, J. V. (2005). Observing the work of the clinical nurse specialist. *Clinical Nurse Specialist, 19*(5), 260–268.

Davies, B., & Hughes, A. M. (2002). Clarification of advanced nursing practice: Characteristics and competencies. *Clinical Nurse Specialist, 16*(3), 147–152.

Duxbury, J. (2000). *Difficult patients.* Oxford, UK: Butterworth Heinemann.

English, J., & Morse, J. M. (1988). The "difficult" elderly patient: Adjustment or maladjustment? *International Journal of Nursing Studies, 25*(1), 23–39.

Eriksson, C., & Saveman, B. (2002). Nurses' experiences of abusive/non-abusive caring for demented patients in acute care settings. *Scandinavian Journal of Caring Sciences, 16*(1), 79–85.

Flaskerud, J. H., Halloran, E. J., Janken, J., Lund, M., & Zetterlund, J. (1999). Avoidance and distancing: A descriptive view of nursing. *Nursing Forum, 34*(2), 29–35.

France, N. E. M. (2005). Strengthening clinical nurse specialist role socialization. *Clinical Nurse Specialist, 19*(6), 294–295.

Goffman, E. (1963). *Stigma: Notes on the management of spoiled identity.* Englewood Cliffs, NJ: Prentice-Hall.

Gorman, L. M., Raines, M. L., & Sultan, D. F. (2002). Nurses' responses to difficult patient behaviors. In L. M. Gorman, M. Luna-Raines, & D. Sultan (Eds.), *Psychosocial nursing for general patient care* (2nd ed., pp. 29–38). Philadelphia, PA: F. A. Davis.

Gorman, M. (1996). Culture clash: Working with a difficult patient. *American Journal of Nursing, 96*(11), 58.

Haas, L. J., Leiser, J. P., Magill, M. K., & Sanyer, O. N. (2005). Management of the difficult patient. *American Family Physician, 72*(10), 2063–2068.

Haber, L. C., & Allen, M. (1997). Comparison of registered nurses' and nursing assistants' choices of intervention for aggressive behaviors. *Issues in Mental Health Nursing, 18,* 113–124.

Halm, M. A., Gagner, S., Goering, M., Sabo, J., Smith, M., & Zaccagnini, M. (2003). Interdisciplinary rounds: Impact on patients, families, and staff. *Clinical Nurse Specialist, 17*(3), 133–142.

Harris, L. (1989). Bedside manners. *RN, 1,* 15–17.

Hart, A., & Freeman, M. (2005). Health "care" interventions: Making health inequalities worse, not better. *Journal of Advanced Nursing, 49*(5), 502–512.

Harvey, J. (1999). *Civilized oppression.* Lanham, MD: Bowman & Litttlefield.

Henderson, S. (2003). Power imbalance between nurses and patients: A potential inhibitor of partnership in care. *Journal of Clinical Nursing, 12,* 501–508.

Hinshelwood, R. D. (1999). The difficult patient. *British Journal of Psychiatry, 174,* 187–190.

Johnson, M. E., & Hauser, P. M. (2001). The practices of expert psychiatric nurses: Accompanying the patient to a calmer personal space. *Issues in Mental Health Nursing, 22,* 651–668.

Juliana, C. A., Orehowsky, S., Smith-Regojo, P., Sikora, S. M., Smith, P. A., Stein, D. K., et al. (1997). Interventions used by staff nurses to manage "difficult" patients. *Holistic Nursing Practice, 11*(4), 1–26.

Kestler, V. (1991). Limit setting: Dealing with difficult patients. *Orthopaedic Nursing, 10*(6), 19–23.

Krichbaum, K. E., Pearson, V., & Hanscom, J. (2000). Better care in nursing homes: Advanced practice nurses' strategies for improving staff use of protocols. *Clinical Nurse Specialist, 14*(1), 40–46.

Kupfer, Y., & Tessler, S. (2001). Weaning the difficult patient: The evolution from art to science. *Chest, 119*, 7–9.

Kuritzky, L. (1996). Practical tips for dealing with difficult patients. *Family Practice Recertification, 18*(2), 21–24, 27–28, 33–34, 36.

Kus, R. J. (1990). Nurses and unpopular patients. *American Journal of Nursing, 6*(90), 62–66.

Lerner, B. H. (1997). *The difficult patient: Ambulatory care syllabus.* Retrieved February 4, 2006, from http://cpmcnet.columbia.edu/texts/ambulatory/34DIFPAT.html

MacDonald, M. (2003). Stigma and its potential to inform the concept of the difficult patient. *Clinical Nurse Specialist, 17*(6), 305–310.

Maupin, C. R. (1995). The potential for noncaring when dealing with difficult patients: Strategies for moral decision making. *Journal of Cardiovascular Nursing, 9*(3), 11–22.

McCleave, K. J. (1993). An examination of the relationship between personal and contextual variables and occupational stress-related depression in nurses. Dissertation. University of Arizona. Ann Arbor, MI: UMI. 9333318

Morrison, E. F., Ramsey, A., & Snyder, B. A. (2000). Managing the care of complex, difficult patients in the medical–surgical setting. *MEDSURG Nursing, 9*(1), 21–26.

Murdoch, J. (2004). Assessing pain in cognitively impaired older adults. *Nursing Standard, 18*(38), 33–39.

Nield-Anderson, L., Minarik, P. A., Dilworth, J. M., Jones, J., Nash, P. K., O'Donnell, K. L., et al. (1999). Responding to "difficult" patients. *American Journal of Nursing, 99*(12), 26–34.

Pergert, P., Ekblad, S., Enskär, K., & Björk, O. (2008). Protecting professional composure in transcultural pediatric nursing. *Qualitative Health Research, 18*, 647–657.

Podrasky, D. L., & Sexton, D. L. (1988). Nurses' reactions to difficult patients. *Image: Journal of Nursing Scholarship, 20*(1), 16–20.

Reeves, R. R., Douglas, S. P., Garner, R. T., Reynolds, M. D., & Silver, A. (2007). The individual rights of the difficult patient: Commentary. *Hastings Center Report, 37*(2), 13–15.

Rew, M., & Ferns, T. (2005). A balanced approach to dealing with violence and aggression at work. *British Journal of Nursing, 14*(4), 227–232.

Rogge, M. M., Greenwald, M., & Golden, A. (2004). Obesity, stigma, and civilized oppression. *Advances in Nursing Science, 27*(4), 301–315.

Roos, J. H. (2005). Nurses' perceptions of difficult patients. *Health Sa Gesondheid, 10*(1), 52–61.

Shahady, E. J. (1964). Difficult patients: Uncovering the real problems of "crocks" and "gomers." *Consultant, 24*(4), 33–43.

Smith, R. C. (2006). *The difficult patient.* UpToDate. Retrieved February 16, 2006, from http://www.utdol.com/application/topic/print.asp?file=genr[BL]med/21732&type=A&selected

Smith, S. B., Tutor, R. S., & Phillips, M. L. (2001). Resolving conflict realistically in today's health care environment. *Journal of Psychosocial Nursing & Mental Health Services, 39*(11), 36–47.

Somboontanont, W., Sloane, P. D., Floyd, F. J., Holditch-Davis, D., Hogue, C. C., & Mitchell, C. M. (2004). Assaultive behavior in Alzheimer's disease: Identifying immediate antecedents during bathing. *Journal of Gerontological Nursing, 30*(9), 22–29.

Stapleton, J. (2005). Nurse staffing and outcomes: Differentiating care delivery by education preparation. *Journal of Nursing Administration, 35*(1), 7.

Steinmetz, D., & Tabenkin, H. (2001). The "difficult patient" as perceived by family physicians. *Family Practice, 18*(5), 495–500.

Strandberg, G., & Jansson, L. (2003). Meaning of dependency on care as narrated by nurses. *Scandinavian Journal of Caring Sciences, 17*(1), 84–91.

Swartz, M. K., Grey, M., Allan, J. D., Ridenour, N., Korner, C., Walker, P. H., et al. (2003). A day in the lives of APNs in the U.S. *Nurse Practitioner, 28*(10), 32–39.

Swenson-Britt, E., Carrougher, G., Martin, B. W., & Brackley, M. (2000). Project Hope: Changing care delivery for the substance abuse patient. *Clinical Nurse Specialist, 14*(2), 92–100.

Thomas, V. N., & Ellis, C. (2000). Support for A&E nurses caring for patients with sickle cell disease. *Nursing Standard, 15*(5), 35–39.

Trexler, J. C. (1996). Reformulation of deviance and labeling theory for nursing. *Image: Journal of Nursing Scholarship, 28*(2), 131–135.

Ujhely, G. B. (1963). *The nurse and her problem patients.* New York: Springer.

Vazirani, S., Hays, R. D., Shapiro, M. F., & Cowan, M. (2005). Effect of a multidisciplinary intervention on communication and collaborations among physicians and nurses. *American Journal of Critical Care, 14*(1), 71–76.

Wheeler, E. A. (2001). *Advanced practice nurses' provision of care to lesbian clients: Creating safe space.* Ann Arbor, MI: Bell & Howell Information and Learning Company. UMI Number 3023642.

White, M. K., & Keller, V. F. (2000). Difficult clinician–patient relationships. *Forum, 20*(6). Retrieved February 4, 2006, from http://www.rmf.harvard,edu/risklibrary/articles/f_v20n6-p4-diffult-pt-md-incP.asp

Wileman, L., May, C., & Chew-Graham, C. (2002). Medically unexplained symptoms and the problem of power in the primary care consultation: A qualitative study. *Family Practice, 19*(2), 178–182.

Wilkes, L. M., Boxer, E., & White, K. (2003). The hidden side of nursing: Why caring for patients with malignant malodorous wounds is so difficult. *Journal of Wound Care, 12*(2), 76–80.

Williams, M. L. (2003). A qualitative study of CNSs' views on depression in palliative care patients. *Palliative Medicine, 17,* 334–338.

Wolf, Z. R. (Ed.). (1994). *The experience of the expert advanced practice nurse.* Philadelphia, PA: La Salle University.

Wolf, Z. R., Brennan, R., Ferchau, L., Magee, M., Miller-Samuel, S., Nicolay, L., et al. (1996). Difficult patient/family interventions. Unpublished Manuscript.

Wolf, Z. R., Brennan, R., Ferchau, L., Magee, M., Miller-Samuel, S., Nicolay, L., et al. (1997). Creating and implementing guidelines on caring for difficult patients: A research utilization project. *MEDSURG Nursing, 6*(3), 137–143.

Wolf, Z. R., & Robinson-Smith, G. (2007). Strategies used by clinical nurse specialists to care for "difficult" clinician-patient situations: A descriptive study. *Clinical Nurse Specialist, 21*(2), 74–84.

The Clinical Nurse Specialist Consultant Role: Issues and Pragmatics

Janice M. Beitz, PhD, RN, ACNS-BC, CNOR, CWOCN, CRNP

Contemporary health care affords many opportunities for clinical nurse specialists (CNSs) to serve as consultants. Major societal forces are driving these opportunities (Table 6-1). The evolving shortages of nurses and nursing faculty, aging of the population, profound increases in chronic illnesses, and the increased usage of unlicensed support personnel, for example, are contributing to opportunities wherein CNSs can share their expertise in brief, informal encounters or through more formal contractually based relationships. In some instances, CNS consultation allows organizations to move services out of acute care, reducing expenses but preserving the level of services (Roggenkamp & White, 1998).

The U.S. economy promotes (and needs) healthcare consulting opportunities even while other economic sectors have faltered. Healthcare consulting in all its forms has grown by 8% to 10% in recent years (Evans, 2005). By helping struggling systems or distressed units within suprasystems, consultants can help overcome bad management effects such as financial losses and bankruptcy. The latter scenario has unfortunately become more commonplace in modern health systems.

The current healthcare milieu provides a glorious opportunity for CNS consultants in a variety of specialties. As of October 2008, the Centers for Medicare/Medicaid Services (CMS) no longer reimburse hospitals (acute care) for substandard care situations such as nosocomial pressure ulcers, surgical site infections, bloodstream infections related to venous access devices, wrong site surgery, and so on. Consultants can be integral to helping hospitals "take care of patients" while they "take care of business" (Cesta & Cunningham, 2008; Start Preparing, 2008). Consultants can identify key indicators, look for trends, and, most importantly, benchmark how organizations are performing. Combining standards of care and benchmarking is a powerful process by which consultants can determine if patients are receiving the best and most cost-effective care.

The literature provides support for the efficacy of CNS consultants' promotion of cost savings and improved patient outcomes (Bedell, Bradley, & Pupiales, 2003; Jones,

Table 6-1   HEALTH CARE AND SOCIETAL TRENDS PROMOTING CNS CONSULTATION

Trends	
• Continued technology explosion	• Continued nursing shortage
• Outsourcing for specialized services	• Continued nursing faculty shortage
• Demographic changes, especially aging	• Continued limitation of resources
• Information economy	• Continued patient safety concerns
• Increases in biotechnology	• Creation of new healthcare jobs
• Constant emphasis on cost control	• Insurance industry pressure for affordability
• Evidence-based practice movement	• Increasing federal oversight in healthcare industry
• Increasing collaboration among specialties	• Demand for more holistic services
• Emphasis on health promotion	• Increasing physician substitution
• Increasing proliferation of specialties	• Continued replacement phenomenon across health disciplines as clinicians age
• Continued focus on outcomes assessment	• Increased use of nonprofessional support staff
• Explosion of chronic disease	• Mounting ethical dilemmas for healthcare clinicians
• Care delivery across multiple settings	• Increasing litigations in all aspects of health care
• Increasing focus on performance measurement	
• Linking of performance measurement to reimbursement	
• Legislation permitting CNS reimbursement	

Sources: Anderson-Shaw, Ahrens, & Fetzer, 2007; Johnson, 2007; Kowal, 1998; LaSala et al., 2007; Norwood, 2003; Roggenkamp & White, 1998; Scott, 1999; Start Preparing, 2008.

2005; Kaufman, 2000; Kerstein, van Rijswijk, & Beitz, 1998; LaSala, Connors, Pedro, & Phipps, 2007; Manley, 2000b; McSherry, Mudd, & Campbell, 2007). Consistent themes are higher quality of care, improved continuity of care, and augmented consistency in therapeutic interventions.

How a CNS structures the consulting relationship is up to the individual. Basic questions that need to be answered include (1) What is nursing consultation? (2) What skills does it take to implement CNS consultation? (3) How does the CNS get started providing consultation services? and (4) What can the CNS offer to this consulting person, organization, or system? The effective CNS consultant must also be cognizant of the business aspects and legal ramifications of, and common barriers to, effective consultation.

The CNS as Consultant

CNSs are well suited to the consultant role because its parameters and functions are major components of CNS education, and the area is tested in clinical nurse specialist certification examinations. For example, the Gerontological Clinical Nurse Specialist Exam has five "domains of practice": practice, education, consultation, research, and administration/management (American Nurses Credentialing Center [ANCC], 2005). Clearly, consultant activities are central to contemporary CNS practice.

Some authors envision advanced practice nursing in a manner different from role dimensions. They emphasize competencies. Advanced practice nurse (APN) CNSs have clinical expertise; critical thinking and analytic skills; clinical judgment; decision-making, leadership, and management abilities; communication and problem-solving ability; and talents in collaborative education and research and program development (Davies & Hughes, 2002; Rose, All, & Gresham, 2003). These talents can be brought to bear on patient care.

Though often presented as an opportunity that is a "new'" role option, ironically consultation is not a new venture for nurses. Nightingale consulted with the British Army medical establishment to drastically decrease mortality and morbidity in the Crimean War (Norwood, 1998).

What Is Nursing Consultation?

Norwood (1998) suggested that nursing consultation is "the process of working with individuals or groups to help them resolve actual or potential problems related to the health status of clients or to health care delivery" (p. 16). Consulting in some settings and roles is mostly an indirect nursing intervention; that is, an activity performed away from the patient but on behalf of improved care for patients.

However, some consultant positions involve substantial direct patient care services in addition to "hands-off" actions. One example of this direct involvement is the wound, ostomy, continence (WOC) CNS consultant who is engaged to assess and institute expert nursing care for patients with complex wounds or skin, ostomy, and/or continence issues. Direct care is a major component of WOC consultation, at least for the initial consultation.

Conversely, CNSs may function in entirely hands-off roles. One increasingly active opportunity is the legal nurse consultant. Working for law firms or as independent entrepreneurs, legal nurse consultants combine their knowledge of the law with healthcare expertise to assist with both defense and plaintiff attorney endeavors. They may even be employed by boards of nursing to review complaints against nurses. (Albee, 2007; Burroughs, Dmytrow, & Lewis, 2007; Castellana & Sanchez, 2006; DiCecco, 2007; Zimmerman, 2008).

A CNS functions differently in consultant roles given the circumstances of patients' needs and organizational demands (Hurlimann, Hofer, & Hirter, 2001). As a direct caregiver, the CNS may provide individualized patient services such as teaching at the bedside, providing case management in a critical care unit, or participating in multidisciplinary rounds to share clinical judgment on selected groups of patients with complex conditions (Cohen, Crego, Cuming, & Smyth, 2002). As an indirect care provider, the CNS may manage a staff development department that educates nursing and other ancillary staff to provide care. As an educator, the CNS may develop and implement community-wide education programs for healthy living or hypertension control. This public education role component is increasing in importance, given the current emphasis on health promotion and disease prevention.

The CNS educator consultant has gained profound importance in light of recent up-regulation by the CMS for patient care standards. This intensification of scrutiny has occurred at the same time that staff development departments have been downsized to the point of eradication. Deficiencies in federal/state surveys (e.g., F. Tag deficiencies) can be targeted by consultants specifically hired to address staff development lapses (Legg, 2007). The long-term care industry is in special need of these services.

As a researcher, the CNS incorporates, via research utilization, the components for evidence-based practice to improve patient care. With the advent of the Internet and electronic desktop and handheld access, utilization of state-of-the-art care guidelines is available and easier than ever in healthcare history.

For example, a WOC CNS consultant can be instrumental in clarifying and overseeing use of pressure ulcer guidelines in organizations so that federal and state regulatory sanctions can be avoided and litigious events minimized (Boxer & Taylor, 2007; Kaufman, 2000; Youngberg, 2007). As an administrator or manager, the CNS has access to statistical data that can be used to improve patient care, direct needed changes, and provide evidence of one's effectiveness in the CNS role. A critical aspect of this latter activity is scrutinizing patient outcomes vis-à-vis CNS intervention.

As a consultant, the CNS functions in a variety of ways, depending on the nature of the employment relationship and employer expectations. One point is noteworthy. Research suggests that CNS roles will constantly overlap in practice, but expert clinical activities usually are the heaviest, eclipsing other activities, with research generation usually occurring least (Gibson & Bamford, 2001; Scott, 1999).

Norwood (2003) conceptualized nursing consultation roles in a different way. She described these roles as three "clusters": task or technical-oriented roles, process-oriented roles, and "universal" roles. Task or technical roles include such things as fact-finding and data gathering, advocacy, education, coordination, and diagnosis. Process-oriented roles include counseling and joint problem solving. She also noted "universal" consultant roles such as providing expertise, presenting information, role modeling, and providing leadership. Task roles are more directive, whereas process roles are more facilitative and nondirective. Universal roles are used throughout the consultative process.

CNSs have opportunities to engage in consultations through a variety of roles, including psychiatric liaison nurse, forensic nurse consultant, corporate wellness consultant, research consultant (an enlarging role given the magnet hospital movement), pain specialist, patient advocate, diabetic disease management, individual and family counseling, media consultant, ethics consultant, and WOC nursing consultant (Bernis, 2007; Kowal, 1998). If they choose, CNSs can develop the consultation role into a business activity and become entrepreneurs (Vollman, 2004), or they can work directly for a healthcare organization, such as a hospital, subacute facility, or long-term care center. Given the right set of circumstances, a CNS can develop a consultation service in most areas of the advanced practice nursing specialties either as an internal employee or contractual fee-based external consultant (Table 6-2).

Table 6-2	CONTRASTING INTERNAL VERSUS EXTERNAL CONSULTATION	
Component or Characteristic	**Internal Consultation**	**External Consultation**
Definition	CNS works as an employee for a healthcare facility; provides services within the organization as per job description and/or request; most common type of CNS consultation	Contracted by a facility or system to provide selected fee-based nursing services; usually not an employee of the organization; less-common CNS role but becoming more frequent
Role Examples	Psychiatric liaison nurse, perioperative CNS, critical care CNS, nursing education specialist, research specialist, WOC specialist	Nurse administrator consultant, WOC nurse consultant, legal nurse consultant, educational consultant
Advantages	Known to system employees; usually easier to develop a mutual trust
Expertise more evident over time
Knows "players" in interdisciplinary care team
More aware of "politics" and "games"
Can develop and implement systems of care and evaluate results over time
Usually does not need to market services extensively, but must create visibility in the organization	May be very well received if expertise makes improvements immediately
Can get balanced picture by talking to all parties without preconceived biases
May be able to command a higher salary because costs are time limited
May be able to convince system of need to continue contractual relationship
Tracking of outcomes written into paid services (budgeted for in advance)

(continues)

Table 6-2 (continued)

Component or Characteristic	Internal Consultation	External Consultation
Disadvantages	May not have respect of the system if not supported by administrators	Not known to system employees
	Familiarity may breed contempt	Have to develop trusting work relationship quickly
	Continuing employee cost (fixed cost)	Have to meet mutually agreeable goals in time frame
	May become a target for cost cutting by "bean counters"	May be viewed hostilely as "outsider" or "spy"
	May be hampered by traditional organizational culture	May be perceived as threat to the status quo
	May be pulled into other activities not part of CNS consultant role	Have to learn how the system works and does not work
	Legislative/regulatory mechanisms may hinder full practice of CNS role	Less aware of politics and power struggles in organization
	More susceptible to role strain as employer may have unrealistic expectations	Must "market" services provided by brochure, Web page, letter of introduction, etc.
	New consultant role may have been designed to be solution for problem rather than a well-designed plan	Cannot control follow through and follow-up to consultant recommendations
	Possible inadequate resources to track the CNS consultant effect (baseline vs. after intervention)	May suffer from lack of acceptance by stakeholders
		Legislative/regulatory mechanisms may hinder full practice of CNS role
		Not a continuing role; when it's over, the income stops (variable cost to consultee)

What Skills Does It Take to Implement CNS Consultation?

Internal scrutiny can help a nurse to decide if the CNS consultant role is attractive. Whether the CNS works within a healthcare system or is an independent entrepreneur contracting with a facility, several questions need to be answered. The potential CNS consultant should audit personal and professional attributes and reflect on whether personal abilities allow the CNS to do the following:

- Manage conflict constructively and come to effective resolutions.
- Develop good interpersonal skills.
- Manage and value diversity (of patients, staff, organizations).
- Be culturally competent.
- Be autonomous, independent, and accountable.
- Develop the self into a collaborative colleague.
- Work with or possibly disagree with other healthcare disciplines such as physicians, allied health therapists, and organizations administrators.
- Be comfortable with power.
- Use power to create win–win situations.

If the answers to this mental exercise are yes, then consultation may be a profoundly satisfying activity for the APN. Evolving into the role is easier if the practitioner really wants the new challenge.

CNS consultants require a significant and substantive skill set. CNS consultants need to have good time management and prioritization skills, presentation and public speaking capacities, networking talents, interpersonal skills, organizational skills, self-discipline, marketing talents, leadership traits, teaching and training capacities, research abilities, administrative abilities, mathematical skills, resourcefulness, and motivation (Dayhoff & Moore, 2003; Mattern, 2005). Jones (2005) suggested that confidence, adaptability, stamina, assertiveness, flexibility, negotiating skills, change agency, motivation, creativity, consistency, good marketing skills, and political savvy are imperative for successful APN consultation and practice. Schulmeister (1999) emphasized that the CNS must be enthusiastic, flexible, self-directed, and persevering. These skills do not appear miraculously. They must be planned for and developed (Table 6-3).

Dayhoff and Moore (2003) suggested that a good way to conduct a follow-up to one's self-assessment is to ask three people who will be honest with the requester to identify whether the CNS really has the characteristics associated with a successful entrepreneurial consultant. If not, the reviewers should assist the CNS in ascertaining what attributes and skills need to be developed and nurtured.

An alternative contemporary approach is to incorporate the concept of "branding." A brand embodies thoughts and perceptions on the part of the consumer. It is what differentiates the "product" (you, the consultant) from the competitors in the area

Table 6-3   PREPARATION CHECKLIST FOR CONSULTATION ACTIVITIES

Being a CNS consultant can be one of the most stimulating and exciting activities an advanced practice nurse can enact. However, the role requires a checklist of required activities if one is to be prepared as possible.

1. Obtain crucial advanced practice (master's level) nursing education and earn good grades. Employers like to know they are hiring a solid academic and clinician. To this end, have transcripts, licenses, and other documentation available for review.

2. Create a "stunning" resume; use high-quality paper, an eye-catching appearance, and have absolutely no typos or misspellings. To help with this, resume templates are contained within common software such as Microsoft Word.

3. Create a "brand"; develop a noteworthy professional hook and be consistent in its delivery. Do not try to "fake it till you make it."

4. Be aware of emerging trends by continuously reading professional journals. Seek out new educational opportunities positioning one to meet critical future needs (e.g., geriatric care, wound care, chronic illness case management, mental health care especially geropsychiatry, legal nurse consulting). Obtain national board certifications as necessary.

5. Become technologically savvy. Take a computer or communications course focusing on all aspects of technology including digital photography and use of unique project management software (e.g., Visio). Very important to learn PowerPoint. It is needed to teach others and to market effectively.

6. Consult knowledgeable people about financial (business) and legal aspects of consulting. Carry personal malpractice insurance even if working for a facility as an employee. These steps are critical if functioning as a self-employed consultant.

7. Continuously polish one's writing and speaking abilities. Take a course in either topic or both as necessary. An alternative is to purchase tapes or videos addressing these areas.

8. Dress for success; wear attire befitting an educated professional. The old adage, "Dress like a slob, don't get the job" is absolutely true. If personally deficient in this area, look at and study magazines and copy positive role models at work.

9. Seek a mentor in the new area if possible. An experienced preceptor or guide can get you up to speed quickly.

10. Research relevant states' nurse practice act and function within the legally accepted parameters of advanced practice abilities; do not exceed them at any time.

(continues)

Table 6-3   (continued)

11. Write a desired job description. Ask yourself if it is better to:
    a. Consult full- or part-time?
    b. Start a personal business or work for someone else?
    c. Stay local or be willing to travel?
12. Write a small business plan. Not sure how to do this? Check out the Internet and business textbooks. Many resources are available. At the least, write yearly goals for the consultation venture.

Sources: Bryant-Lukosius, DiCenso, Browne, & Dinelli, 2004; Hogue, 2007; Mattern, 2005; Norwood, 1998; Puetz & Shinn, 1997; Schulmeister, 1999; Stensrud, 2007.

(Perler, 2008; Sills, 2008; Zahaluk, 2008a, 2008b). In other words it is the professional identity one creates in the minds of others (Sills, 2008). For example, WOC nurse specialists are not the only clinicians offering wound care consultation. The question is: What about *your* brand raises *you* to the top of the list to be selected? What makes *you* the Disney, Cadillac, or IBM of consultants?

Branding means creating marketability, visibility, and recognition as the expert. Sills (2008) suggests that consultants develop their own "professional hook." One might be (the author's hook) "Jance loves healing wounds, and it shows." The résumé one creates summarizes accomplishments but "a brand shouts louder" (p. 63).

How Does a CNS Consultant Get Started?

Engaging in the consulting process requires multidirectional analyses. First, the CNS must direct assessment inwardly by asking, "What does one need to know to be an effective consultant?" The neophyte consultant should ponder, "What will be the context of the consultation?" The CNS also needs to ask, "What are my clinical strengths?" "What are my character strengths?" and "What sacrifices are worth the effort required to become a consultant?" (Schulmeister, 1999).

The fastest way to acquire the demanding skills required of the CNS consultant is for a nurse to obtain formal academic grounding in consultation concepts and processes. Attendance in a graduate program for CNS APN education is a great launching process (Norwood, 1998). Threaded throughout the curriculum are the theoretical and pragmatic skills that are integral to optimal consultation prowess. Once skills are acquired and the decision to consult has been reached, a neophyte consultant can take advice from consulting experts on how to engage in the process.

Norwood (1998) suggested that consultation is a five-step process: (1) gaining entry, (2) problem identification, (3) action planning, (4) evaluation, and (5) disengagement. Problem identification is based on high-quality comprehensive assessment of the client system. It is critical to clearly identify the cause(s) of the problem and factors potentially helping or hindering the resolution of the problem.

Norwood (2003) suggested preliminary questions needing to be asked regarding critical assessment issues, including:

1. What is the consultee experiencing as a result of the problem?
2. What stakeholders and players have been affected by the problem?
3. What has happened to these stakeholders and players as a result of the problem?
4. What about the consultee environment might be contributing to or worsening improvement of the problem?
5. What issues or conditions in the larger community or society may help or hinder the problem?
6. Who and what will gain or lose as part of the problem?

Assessment is critical during the problem identification phase. It also occurs throughout the entire consultation process. Formative assessment focuses on the status of the problem while it is in the process of improvement. Summative assessment permits the consultant and consultee to scrutinize how conditions were at the beginning of the relationship and how they have (it is hoped) resolved or at least improved substantially (Table 6-4).

A clinical exemplar of external consultation shows how this process is enacted in a realistic situation (Exemplar 6-1).

Table 6-4	FORMATIVE AND SUMMATIVE QUESTIONS IN NURSING CONSULTATION
Formative	**Summative**
1. What activities and objectives have been accomplished to this point?	1. What is the final status of the action plan or project?
2. Are project goals progressing according to timetable?	2. Has the project achieved targeted purposes?
3. What are the greatest roadblocks? How can we reduce them or remove them?	3. What factors helped and hindered the project's success?
4. What new challenges have arisen?	4. Was the consultant helpful?
5. What factors have occurred that are helping the project?	5. Was the consultee system helpful?
6. Are there any system components especially resistant to change?	6. Would both sides hire or work with each other again?
7. What alterations need to be made (if any) in the way the project is being enacted?	7. What is next (if anything)?

Exemplar 6-1

Clinical Exemplar of External Consultation: A Consultee Organization in Crisis

Elizabeth Smith, MSN, RN, CS, CWOCN, has a private wound, ostomy, continence (WOC) nursing consulting business. She is contracted by a local nursing home chain (three LTC facilities) that has been cited for substandard wound and continence care based on new Medicare reviewer guidelines (CMS F314 and F315 tags).

The director of nursing and Elizabeth meet and discuss the citations and the director's views on the whole system. No WOC consultant has ever worked with or within the chain of facilities. The facilities have "low levels" of established policies and substantial changeover of personnel. The director would like to have a staff advanced practice nurse in each facility, but that has not yet been approved. The director asks Elizabeth to help her and the whole system.

In preparing to enact needed changes, Elizabeth performs an analysis of the situation. What should she do? She began by initiating the following analytic activities:

1. Obtaining current policy and procedure manuals of the facilities.
2. Visiting each of the three facilities to assess documentation on current patients with wound and skin issues vis-à-vis care actually delivered.
3. Obtaining the formulary of skin and wound care products available at each organization.
4. Obtaining latest versions of federal long-term care tags and standards of practice from WOCN Society, AAWC (Association for the Advancement of Wound Care), and AMDA (American Medical Directors Association) organizations.
5. Meeting with the medical director of the chain to obtain a physician's perspective on the situation across facilities.
6. Meeting with the nursing, allied health, and ancillary staff of each facility for their perspectives on system challenges.
7. Obtaining available records on staff development activities at three facilities, including any medical or nursing "grand rounds" that have occurred.

Given her findings, Elizabeth instituted multiple initiatives to rapidly address the deficiencies.

A. Met again with all chief nurses (nurse executives) of each facility and the systemwide medical director to share her plans and ask for feedback/suggestions and support.
B. Developed systemwide policies and procedures for wound and skin and continence care based on documented standards of care.
C. Streamlined wound, skin care, and ostomy/continence products purchased for all three facilities. By working with the purchasing agent and the executive team, she was able to purchase higher-quality products at lesser cost.
D. Mandated a systemwide incidence and prevalence study related to wound care and incontinence to obtain a baseline level in the three facilities.
E. Instituted comprehensive staff development sessions for nursing staff on all shifts at all facilities.

F. Created Web-based learning activities on the nursing home chain's intranet to permit "24-7" learning.

G. Provided medical grand rounds sessions for medical staff and allied health personnel on wound healing, topical therapy of wounds, and federal legislative oversight of quality care in long-term care.

The following comments relate to how the consultant in the exemplar enacted the process:

1. *Gaining entry*: Elizabeth was initially contacted by a person of authority within the system. The director of nursing knew to contact her because Elizabeth had marketed herself with a brochure about her services, had developed a Web page about her business, and made available testimonials from previous satisfied clients.

2. *Problem identification*: The obvious problem on system entry was the cited deficiency in skin and wound care. System analysis and data gathered from personnel revealed a severe lack of systemwide thinking, planning, and purchasing acumen.

3. *Action planning*: Elizabeth attacked the consultee's problems on several fronts. She set up an infrastructure (wound, skin, and continence policies and procedures), garnered support of the highest level of administration (especially with an interdisciplinary flair), and arranged for one system of wound and skin and continence products. She then in-serviced the nursing staff and held medical grand rounds for the physicians on moist wound healing and contemporary topical wound and skin care therapy.

4. *Evaluation*: Elizabeth wisely analyzed the baseline of the problem as she commenced her consultant relationship. Following 3 months of interventions, she initiated a systemwide incidence and prevalence study. This was repeated again at 6 months. She was able to statistically and visually demonstrate the efficacy of her consultation activity via a PowerPoint presentation to her consultee.

5. *Disengagement*: Contractually, Elizabeth had agreed to provide consultation for 6 months. Her services proved so effective that reevaluation by the site visitors showed total eradication of the deficient criteria. The consulting organization was so pleased that they asked Elizabeth to continue as a consultant for their most complex patients and to set up a program addressing improvement in urinary incontinence rates. Given her successes, Elizabeth agreed to continue but at an increased consultant remuneration rate.

Another clinical scenario with discussion is presented in Exemplar 6-2.

The realistic scenario in Exemplar 6-2 depicts an example of internal consultation processes and how the consultant used the consultation process. The following comments relate to that process:

Exemplar 6-2

Clinical Exemplar of Internal Consultation: A Family in Crisis

Jackie is an adult health CNS who is also specially educated and credentialed in palliative care. She is consulted by a staff nurse of the intensive care unit (ICU), who is upset about family issues surrounding a patient's care in the ICU. The patient is a 25-year-old Hispanic male who was admitted to the ER with a sudden decrease in consciousness, subsequent transport to the hospital, and is now status post multiple tests for neurological functioning. Initial assessment demonstrated severe hypertension. Neurological testing reveals a massive intracranial bleed secondary to malignant hypertension. Brain scanning and other examinations suggest brain death and extremely poor prognosis. He is totally unresponsive to any stimulating triggers during physical examination.

The patient's family is hysterical, angry, and accusatory about the patient's care. His mother is refusing to allow any physical care by the nursing staff and sits and holds his hand. The physicians and the staff nurses are frustrated and trying to comfort the family while being therapeutic but realistic. Using the five-step process of Norwood (1998), what should Jackie do? How should she approach the consultation situation?

In preparing to intervene, Jackie analyzed the situation and:

1. Read the patient's chart thoroughly and discussed the case with the ICU and attending physicians.
2. Met with all pertinent nursing staff and managers to gain their perspectives.
3. Discussed the case with the hospital chaplain, who has been involved with the family but with only limited success.
4. Met with family members who were more approachable to ascertain their views on how to help.

Following a thorough analysis, Jackie intervened in the following ways:

A. Alerted the hospital hospice team that their help would likely be needed at some point.
B. Met with the patient's mother and the family members the mother selected to hear their voiced concerns.
C. Contacted the family's clergy to meet with the hospital chaplain to work together on helping the family.
D. Shared the family concerns with physicians, nurses, and other staff.

1. *Gaining entry*: Jackie was consulted by the nursing staff in her facility in recognition of her organizational position and special expertise as a palliative care specialist point person. This entry was smooth and welcomed, given the fact that Jackie was a full-time employee. However, she had previously communicated to staff via hospital e-mail and intranet regarding her availability so staff nurses were well aware of her presence and her contact number and e-mail address.

2. *Problem identification:* The problem was identified by the staff regarding the patient and the family. The challenge was especially acute, given the dismal prognosis and youth of the patient.

3. *Action planning:* Jackie attacked the problem on several fronts. She gathered critical data to find out what were real and what were perceived issues. Using internal and external resources, she targeted the problems identified by the family regarding perceived poor patient care and other staff and family interactions. She met with all parties to disseminate information and to serve as an impartial negotiator.

4. *Evaluation:* Following the patient's discharge to hospice and subsequent demise, Jackie asked the physicians and nursing staff how she performed and solicited suggestions on how to improve her services and assistance. Jackie also surveyed (by phone and mail) the family several months later asking for their input and how she could better serve future patients and families.

5. *Disengagement:* Jackie disengaged herself with the patient when the time was appropriate and then maintained contacted with the staff and family until summative evaluation processes were complete. Jackie was so successful that she became increasingly contacted to assist with palliative care patient and family scenarios.

What Can the CNS Consultant Offer the Consulting Person, Organization, or System?

The nature of the CNS consultant role directs the skills and knowledge provided by the individual. Usually, the support delivered is mutually determined by the consultant and consultee. There are a variety of consultation approaches, and the approach used in a particular situation depends on the nature of the problem being addressed, characteristics of the consultee, resources, constraints within the client system, and the skills of the nurse consultant (Norwood, 1998; Schulmeister, 1999).

For example, the author has provided wound, ostomy, continence (WOC) nursing services for multiple organizations. Though the knowledge and abilities required of the WOC nurse are acquired through postbaccalaureate specialty education, how this skill set is enacted differs depending on the consulting relationship with the organization. For instance, one organization required the author (who was considered an employee) to write comprehensive assessments in a style similar to that of physicians (Exemplar 6-3). In another more traditional setting, the author was considered an independent consultant and was required to write only abridged consultation notes (Exemplar 6-4).

In both settings, options in treatment were called recommendations only because the author was not permitted to write prescriptive orders nor to contact physicians via the telephone. Physicians had ultimate responsibility to accept or reject the consultant's advice. More recently, some healthcare organizations are supporting advanced practice WOC nurse practitioners' use of prescriptive privileges to avoid delaying or possibly disrupting needed services.

Sample Comprehensive Consultation

Date: ———————————   Patient's Name: ———————————
Time: ———————————   Identifying Information: ———————————
Consult Form

WOC Nursing Consult

58-year-old African American female admitted with nonhealing midline vertical abdominal wound with enterocutaneous fistula. HPI: Transferred from acute care hospital S/P perforated ruptured diverticular repair; currently NPO and receiving TPN; developed abdominal pain and symptoms of shock 1 month PTA; had emergency surgery; developed wound dehiscence and fistulous output within 7 days postop; had respiratory failure—was intubated and mechanically ventilated for 2 weeks. PMH: NKDA; multiple medical issues: HTN (diuretic controlled); COPD 2° to heavy smoking (2PPD); also heavy ETOH use (1/2 fifth of whiskey daily); Labs: Albumin 1.5; Prealbumin 12; WBC ↑ to 18,000; HGB 10.5 HCT; 30

Assessment: Not presently on pressure reduction mattress; Limited mobility due to abdominal discomfort and deconditioning; labs as above; receiving nothing orally; on TPN; Multiple skin issues evident; (1) has bilateral heel breakdown L 2×1 cm and R 2×3 cm—both are Stage I pressure ulcers; reddened skin that is not blanchable need protection and offloading; (2) Sacrum—2×3 cm Stage II pressure ulcer; 100% pink granulation tissue; cleansed and applied Tegasorb; surrounding skin intact; (−) drainage or odor; perineal and perirectal skin currently intact; (3) vertical midline full thickness surgical, wound 15×5 cm × 2 cm deep; wound base is 70% pink muscle and fascia, 15% tan slough and 15% visible "stoma" at top of wound (E-C fistula).

Fistula draining semiliquid brown fecal mildly odorous stool; surrounding skin intact; cleansed with copious amount of normal saline; given size of fistula (4×4 cm stoma) dubious about spontaneous closing of fistula; likely need surgical repair in future. Applied large-size Hollister wound manager connected to urinary catheter bag; protected surrounding skin with 3-M No–Sting and achieved good seal. Demonstrated whole procedure to primary nurse and nurse manager; directions at bedside; discussed ordering of supplies and order number. Other pressure points and remainder of skin intact except for noted areas. Photodocumentation of affected areas obtained for baseline.

Recommendations: Please Order

1. Place on Pro 2000 mattress immediately.
2. Check prealbumin and albumin levels.
3. Elevate heels on two pillows; keep positioned 30° side to side and off back.
4. Proshield ointment TID to heels.
5. Tegasorb hydrocolloid to sacral ulcer; change q 5–7 days and PRN.
6. Apply Hollister large-size wound manager to abdominal wound; cleanse wound bed and replace 4×4 dressings q8H and PRN. Change entire system q 3 days and PRN if leaking. Protect surrounding skin with 3M No-Sting at every wound manager change.
7. Order Hollister large-size wound managers from storeroom (serial # xxxx).

Discussed care with primary nurse, Nancy Nurse. Will follow. Elizabeth Smith, MSN, RN, CWOCN

Exemplar 6-4

Sample Abridged Consultation

Patient's Name: ———————————— Date/Time: ————————————

Identifying Information: ————————————————————————————————

Progress Notes

Wound, Ostomy, Continence Nursing Consult:

Consulted by attending physician to assess skin integrity and preventive care issues. Admitted 2 days ago; *no noted allergies*. Not currently on pressure support surface; has limited mobility due to recent left sided CVA; Braden Score 10; Current albumin level 2.5. No prealbumin ordered; protein supplements on order. Skin currently intact on all pressure points including heels, except for sacrum and perineum. Has 2×3 cm stage III sacral pressure ulcer, 100% pink granulation tissue, surrounding skin intact; no drainage or odor. Has mild perirectal and perineal skin breakdown likely due to fecal and urinary incontinence; consists of light red rash; likely not fungal in nature; no satellite lesions. Not itchy.

Recommendations: Please Order:

1. Place on Accucair mattress immediately.
2. Hydrocolloid dressing (Duoderm) to sacral ulcer; change q 5–7 days and PRN.
3. Proshield ointment TID and PRN to perineal/perirectal skin breakdown; do *not* use diapers.
4. Keep turned side to side q2 hours; keep off back!
5. Elevate heels on two pillows.
6. Check prealbumin level.

Will follow—Elizabeth Smith, MSN, RN, CWOCN

Whether internal or external, the CNS consultant can help improve patient outcomes in a variety of organizational settings by doing the following:

1. Implementing research findings in daily practice by incorporating new products and processes of care.
2. Evaluating the outcomes of these interventions before making them systemwide via unit-based pilot studies.
3. Educating nurses and others in the area of focus (cardiac care, wound management, etc.) by presenting courses and in-services and seminars within the healthcare organization and possibly regionally and nationally.
4. Developing guidelines for patient care whether they are called critical pathways, policies, standards, or whatever.
5. Counseling nurses and other staff members about patient care issues.
6. Offering specific care advice about selected patient scenarios.
7. Managing patients' cases depending on whether this is a component of the CNS's consultant role.
8. Understanding reimbursement issues.

9. Conducting outcomes and cost-efficiency research.
10. Establishing continuing relationships with patients and their families.
11. Advocating for patients while motivating them to be active partners in their own care.
12. Knowing patients' stories and advocating for their care.
13. Assessing patient progress and recommending plan of care changes to physicians and other healthcare providers.
14. Applying advanced knowledge about pathophysiology, healing processes, patient education, and behavioral change.
15. Instituting timely individualized recommendations for treatment to effect more positive outcomes (Bedell et al., 2003; Hurlimann et al., 2001; Kerstein et al., 1998).

A particularly "hot" topic in patient outcomes assessment is analysis of patient care performance measures. For example, multiple validated wound care clinical guidelines are available for use by clinicians (www.guidelines.gov) targeting care of pressure, arterial, venous, and neuropathic ulcers. Consultants can help develop benchmarking systems by which wound care/patient care documentation can be measured for completeness/currency (Table 6-5).

Research findings support that consultation effects of the CNS do not happen quickly. Effective consultation takes time until clinical credibility is recognized and interventions start to generate real changes (Gibson & Bamford, 2001; Jones, 2005).

An interesting update to wound care consultation opportunities has evolved in response to technology. Particularly for patients in long-term care facilities, WOC consultants may be providing services via remote consultation that is Web-based (telemedicine) (Hammett, Harvath, Flaherty-Robb, Sawyer, & Olson 2007). Using digital photos, consultants may be offering a plan of care for patients many miles distant. Such systems may prove invaluable to rural facilities.

Forms of Business Association for CNS Consultation

The most common form of CNS consultation is full-time work within a healthcare system facility. Sometimes the CNS stays in one facility or covers several buildings in the system. This format is sometimes described as intrapreneurship (Leong, 2005; Roggenkamp & White, 1998). This arrangement requires no special business acumen. It is similar to being a full-time employee, such as a staff nurse, a role familiar to nurses. The CNS is expected, however, to know how to move across multiple units at a single facility or at various locations and facilitate change. This role is very demanding in "people" acumen (Cohen et al., 2002).

However, CNS consultant positions within hospitals have decreased since the 1990s. Many CNS consultants decided to embark on new ventures when they were downsized out of hospitals. They have chosen roles as independent nurse consultants functioning as a sole proprietor of a business that does not exist apart from the owner (Dayhoff & Moore, 2003; Schulmeister, 1999).

Table 6-5	BENCHMARKING PARAMETERS: WOUND CARE PERFORMANCE MEASURES		
Generic Wound Care Indices			
Comprehensive assessment	Yes ___	No ___	
Admission	Yes ___	No ___	
Ongoing	Yes ___	No ___	
Documented plan of care/goals identified	Yes ___	No ___	
Anthropometrics (height, weight, BMI)	Yes ___	No ___	
History and physical completed	Yes ___	No ___	
Specified medications affecting wound healing (steroids, chemotherapy, etc.)	Yes ___	No ___	
Nutritional indices (albumin, prealbumin, transferrin, etc.)	Yes ___	No ___	
Admission	Yes ___	No ___	
Ongoing	Yes ___	No ___	
Risk assessment (pressure ulcer)	Yes ___	No ___	
Pain management	Yes ___	No ___	
Appropriate biopsy/culture technique (as necessary) (Avoiding superficial swab)	Yes ___	No ___	
Pressure Ulcer			
Pressure redistribution surface/specialty bed	Yes ___	No ___	
Topical therapy (dressings) (avoidance saline W-D)	Yes ___	No ___	
Debridement as appropriate	Yes ___	No ___	
Preventive repositioning	Yes ___	No ___	
Continence care as appropriate	Yes ___	No ___	
Control of infection (as needed)	Yes ___	No ___	
Patient/caregiver education: Pressure ulcer	Yes ___	No ___	
Venous Ulcer			
Topical therapy (dressings) (avoidance saline W-D)	Yes ___	No ___	
Compression therapy (method identified)	Yes ___	No ___	
Debridement as appropriate	Yes ___	No ___	
Control of infection (as needed)	Yes ___	No ___	
Patient/caregiver education: Venous ulcer	Yes ___	No ___	
Arterial Ulcer			
Topical therapy (dressings) (avoidance saline W-D)	Yes ___	No ___	
Protection of affected area (limb)	Yes ___	No ___	

Table 6-5 (continued)		
Revascularization as appropriate	Yes ___	No ___
Circulation assistance (pharmacologic, device) as appropriate	Yes ___	No ___
Control of infection (as needed)	Yes ___	No ___
Patient/caregiver education: Arterial ulcer	Yes ___	No ___
Neuropathic Ulcer		
Topical therapy (dressings) (avoidance saline W-D)	Yes ___	No ___
Offloading (as appropriate)	Yes ___	No ___
Insensate limb protection (as appropriate)	Yes ___	No ___
Debridement as appropriate	Yes ___	No ___
Control of infection (as needed)	Yes ___	No ___
Patient/caregiver education: Neuropathic ulcer	Yes ___	No ___
Diabetes surveillance (FBS, HgB AIC, microalbuminuria)	Yes ___	No ___
Surgical Wound/Other Wound Types		
Etiology ascertained	Yes ___	No ___
Topical therapy (dressings) (avoidance saline W-D)	Yes ___	No ___
Advanced modalities (NPWT, biologic tissues)	Yes ___	No ___
Control of infection (as needed)	Yes ___	No ___
Patient/caregiver education: Surgical wound	Yes ___	No ___

A CNS consultant may also form a collaborative practice with a physician. These are called general partnerships. Usually the parties have a written agreement specifying responsibilities and earnings distributions (Schulmeister, 1999). A psychiatric clinical nurse specialist, for example, may bill Medicare for psychiatric services provided he or she has a physician collaborator and it is acceptable in that state's nurse practice act. The physician need not be present while the services are rendered (Baradell & Buppert, 2003). Diabetic educator CNSs, with a physician collaborator, can bill Medicare directly for their consultation services. Some have opened private businesses in the form of an S-corporation company, similar to a limited liability corporation (LLC) (Dayhoff & Moore, 2003).

The third possibility is some form of an LLC. This structure provides protection from both personal liability for debts and for a formal legal structure for the entrepreneurship (Dayhoff & Moore, 2003). Talking to a lawyer and accountant may elucidate the best arrangement for the neophyte CNS consultant. The reader is referred to the literature to read and learn more about establishing entrepreneurial businesses.

Legal Implications of Nurse Consultation

Though it is uncommon for nurse consultants to be involved in legal actions (Norwood, 2003), the CNS consultant must be conscious of the need to be legally astute and to protect both personal and professional integrity, especially if functioning as an independent consultant. Among human service consultants, the most common cause of malpractice is lack of skill. It is also possible to bring legal action against a consultant related to his or her behaviors associated with the conduct of the consultation business (Norwood, 2003). Selected possible causes of legal action include breach of contract, breach of confidentiality, giving poor advice, poor record keeping, failure to consult others about difficult situations, and fraud or misrepresentation about one's skills or credentials for consulting (Exemplar 6-5).

Though most consultation processes proceed smoothly, it is possible for misunderstandings or disappointments to occur in the consultee–consultant relationship. The CNS consultant needs to secure protection by talking to legal counsel, carrying liability insurance, and using "preventive" measures. Preventive measures include having open communication and recognition of one's limitations. Before any contract is signed or if a consultant is in negotiations, it is wise to secure legal counsel. A letter of understanding may be generated that serves as a form of contract (Exemplar 6-6).

Lastly, a CNS consultant should carry personal liability insurance, whether working internally or externally. Because the litigious nature of health care is increasing, the CNS consultant needs strenuous protection from potential legal actions.

Barriers to Effective Consultation

The literature suggests that certain factors can act as barriers to quality CNS consultation: feelings of inadequacy, lack of confidence, fears of being supervised by the consultee or employer, lack of support networks, and feelings of insecurity related to differing educational backgrounds between the CNS with a master of science in nursing and doctorally prepared colleagues (Jones, 2005).

Exemplar 6-5

An Ineffective Implementation of Nursing Consultation

A CNS consultant accepts a contract from a long-term care agency to develop a protocol for the assessment and management of clients with urinary and fecal incontinence. At the time of relationship, the agency employed two nurses who were "continence" certified. The consultant devised the protocol without consulting the F315 tag in the CMS Guidelines for long-term care expectations. The consultant herself was wound certified but not continence certified. In the interim, the two continence nurses left the agency. The protocol required continence nurses to see patient consults. When the protocol could not be followed, the agency was displeased with the consultant because she did not have full information on the topic, did not fully communicate with agency personnel, and authored a protocol that could not be immediately implemented. As a result, the agency was placed in a potentially litigious situation, and the consultant could potentially be held liable for unsatisfactory project quality.

Exemplar 6-6

Sample Letter of Understanding

Janice L. Smith, PhD, RN
Research Consultant
Philadelphia, PA
215-222-4444

Jane Brown, MSN, RN, CS
Director, Patient Care Services
John K. Jones Medical Center
222 Large Street
Philadelphia, PA 11111

Dear Ms. Brown:

This correspondence serves as a letter of understanding about the nursing research consultation services I will be providing for John K. Jones Medical Center.

The purpose of this consultative activity is to help nursing employees develop a plan for and implement a program of nursing research as part of the Medical Center's plan to achieve "magnet hospital" designation. I will be conducting focus groups with nursing staff across the organization to ascertain their interests and abilities. I will compile the results and present them to the nursing administrative staff along with a plan for a research program.

My understanding is that this project will proceed for 12 months and that I will be working for the agency 16 hours weekly. As we discussed, I will receive $75.00 per hour plus expenses for materials. At the end of the project, a potential for continued relationship may be negotiated at that time. Staff will be released from their regular duties with pay to participate in focus groups and pertinent committee meetings during their regular work hours.

As we agreed, I will report directly to you and will have triweekly progress meetings. All staff input will be recorded anonymously and reported as aggregate data only.

Would you please sign this letter and return it to me and indicate your acceptance of this project and its terms? Thank you for the opportunity to be involved with this exciting project.

Sincerely,

Janice L. Smith, PhD, RN

Accepted:
Name: _____
Title: _____
Date: _____

One of the most difficult barriers to overcome is the need to be a good girl or good boy. The CNS consultant role entails a change in relationships and demeanor. The consultant may have to share challenging messages or confront problematic aspects of a system. This transformation from the traditional role of the staff nurse to assertive, confident consultant may be an uncomfortable trip, but it is an indispensable component of consulting.

Healthcare systems may not yet be designed to accommodate the roles of the CNS consultant, whether the CNS functions internally in an employing organization or as an external fee-based consultant. The influence of organizational culture is powerful in helping or hindering the consultant (Manley, 2000a, 2000b). A lack of office space and clerical support; unavailable or inadequate communication technologies such as a computer, Internet access, and fax; and varying opportunities for education are common role problems. Administrative inattention to these supports severely hampers the CNS consultant and communicates the unspoken message that the CNS consultant is not truly valued (Bryant-Lukosius, DiCensa, Browne, & Dinelli, 2004).

Another major hurdle is the knowledge deficiencies of other healthcare providers specific to the CNS role. Often physicians, fellow nurses, physical therapists, and others are unfamiliar with advanced practice nursing. The CNS consultant may have to expend much time and effort to educate others about the role. Resistance from others such as physicians and bureaucratic inhibitors can severely constrain optimal CNS consultation in either internal or external forms (Leong, 2005).

Another barrier to effective utilization of the CNS consultant is the limited amount of evidence regarding the efficacy and efficiency of the role. Some studies (Manley, 2000a, 2000b) support the enormous benefit of CNS or APN consultation on improving organizational culture, improving patient outcomes, and decreasing nursing staff turnover. The magnet hospital movement, for example, strongly incorporates the usage of expert APN CNS consultation.

A recent research study of four highly successful nurse entrepreneurs found three major themes associated with their success. The major instigating factor to enter entrepreneurship was a love of nursing, the major business concern was overcoming the lack of business skills, and the personal factor was a commitment to their personal mission (Roggenkamp & White, 1998).

The CNS consultant must continually try to hone the craft of consulting by reading and learning from others. *Tips of the Trade for the Entrepreneur Consultant* (Table 6-6) offers suggestions that are based on wisdom acquired by the author through personal experiences, reading the literature, attending professional conferences, networking with colleagues, and observing and copying wise mentors. In addition to the *Tips of the Trade*, potential consultants should reflect on a few select real-life consulting challenges and work through possible solutions (Exemplar 6-7).

Conclusion

CNS consultants can affect patient care in significantly positive ways. Whether providing direct care or affecting patient services indirectly through policy development, education, staff counseling, or legal review, CNSs can influence a variety of outcomes that demonstrate quality nursing care. As health care shifts to nontraditional settings

Table 6-6	TIPS OF THE TRADE FOR THE ENTREPRENEURIAL CNS CONSULTANT

1. The best job security one can have is the trust of the consulting organization (the employer in any form). The consultee should feel cared for and like doing "business" with the consultant.

2. Be available when needed. The consultee should value the consultant's input and feel it's available when needed.

3. Be honest always; never lie or dissemble on an invoice. Never lose personal integrity; it is hard to reassemble once shattered.

4. Take credit for the honest work done; don't give "freebies" to impress potential customers.

5. Detail the tasks performed for the consultee; whether it's patients' names and positive outcomes, policies, or standards, SHOW what has been accomplished.

6. Use technology to track billing and consultee payments; accounting systems exist that can help.

7. Communicate clearly and well and continue to develop this skill throughout one's career.

8. The way to be financially successful is to help the consultee to do the same. If it is a nonprofit entity, help it to be financially wise.

9. Educate oneself in an ongoing fashion; always improve clinical or business skills. Strive for daily excellence.

10. Ask for feedback about personal performance from the consulting organization or facility, and LEARN from it.

11. Increase one's cultural awareness in an ongoing fashion; expect diverse clientele, research and respect ethnic/religious practices as possible.

12. Recognize that as a consultant one's advice may not be taken and that the CONSULTANT alone cannot make it happen. Changes must be implemented by persons within the larger system. This is especially true if one is an independent consultant.

13. If a consulting relationship ends, ask for a reference from a consultee for one's files for future usage.

14. Never act entitled to a consultant position; consider it a privilege and honor to consult for the organization.

15. Never, ever disrespect the consultee or its employees or anything like it; never be off color in any form.

Critical Thinking Application Exercises

Using the five-step consultation process previously described, how would a CNS consultant address the following challenges?

1. A perioperative CNS works for a major urban tertiary care facility. The operating room suite consists of 14 rooms. The facility purchases two other facilities, a surgical center and a local community hospital in the nearby suburbs. The CNS is called into the vice president of nursing's office and is interviewed for the new systemwide position of perioperative clinical consultant. The major goal is to streamline OR services across the three settings and to develop an "OR educational institute" to train new staff.

2. A CNS is a new full-time hire into an adult critical care division that has been cited by The Joint Commission visitor as substandard in care. A major hospital administrative shake-up occurred, and all high-level nursing administrators and the CEO were replaced. The critical care CNS is responsible for SICU, MICU, and neurological ICU.

3. A nationally respected CNS consultant on decreasing errors in health care is hired contractually by a troubled hospital system in which the rate of medication errors is very high. Several deaths have occurred in the system, and very bad publicity has been published in several newspapers. Unfortunately, wrong site surgery has been recently reported in one hospital of the system. A patient needing a gallbladder removal was switched with a patient needing a parathyroidectomy. The latter procedure was almost half completed before the error was detected.

4. A geriatric CNS consultant employed by a local community hospital is asked by the CEO to work with community leaders and a local home care agency and nursing home to set up a "seamless system" of geriatric care. Its goal is to keep elders at home while well and ease their entry into and through the healthcare continuum (hospital to nursing home to home care to previous state, as possible).

5. A major hospital system consisting of five acute care facilities experiences bankruptcy related to poor management at the highest executive levels. A CNS administrative consultant is contracted to work with the chief nursing officer of each hospital to "think out of the box" regarding restructuring of the system and likely consolidation of services.

6. A CNS consultant is hired by a surgical group to develop a total system of wound care involving surgeons, nurse practitioners, and nurses. The system involves one hospital, a wound center, and 15 affiliated nursing homes. The venture is entirely new. The consultant has been asked to be "creative but pragmatic." The goal is for the care team to become designated as a wound care center of excellence.

7. A legal nurse consultant with an extensive perioperative background is hired to address identified risk management challenges in a hospital's perioperative suite. Several "near misses" have occurred, nurse management is perceived as "weak and ineffective," and multiple new lawsuits are threatening. Documentation is also substandard.

and patients demand high-quality services with measurable outcomes, CNS consultants will continue to have new opportunities, providing they develop the skills required for success.

References

Albee, T. (2007). The legal nurse consultant as a board of nursing expert witness. *Journal of Legal Nurse Consulting, 18*(11), 11–14.

American Nurses Credentialing Center (ANCC). (2005). Clinical specialist is gerontological nursing board certification exam content outline. Retrieved from http://www.nursingworld.org/ancc/certificate/cert/exams

Anderson-Shaw, L., Ahrens, W., & Fetzer, M. (2007). Ethics consultation in the emergency department. *JONA's Healthcare Law, Ethics, and Regulation, 9*(11), 32–35.

Baradell, J. G., & Buppert, C. (2003). Billing for psychiatric clinical nurse specialist services within the Medicare program. *Topics in Advanced Practice E Journal, 3*(1). Retrieved February 10, 2006, from http://www.medscape.com/viewarticle/449180

Bedell, B., Bradley, M., & Pupiales, M. (2003). How a wound resource team saved expenses and improved outcomes. *Home Healthcare Nurse, 21*(6), 397–403.

Bernis, P. (2007). The time is right! Nurse entrepreneur and the forensic nurse. *On the Edge, 13*(4). Retrieved December 23, 2007, from http://www.Iafn.org/publications/ote/otewinter2007.cfm

Boxer, B. A., & Taylor, E. M. (2007). In-house consulting helps disseminate EBP. *Nursing Management, 38*(9), 41–45.

Bryant-Lukosius, D., DiCenso, A., Browne, G., & Dinelli, J. (2004). Advanced practice nursing roles: Development, implementation, and evaluation. *Journal of Advanced Nursing, 48*(5), 519–529.

Burroughs, R., Dmytrow, B., & Lewis, H. (2007). Trends in nurse practitioner professional liability: An analysis of claims with risk management recommendations. *Journal of Nursing Law, 11*(1), 53–60.

Castellana, V., & Sanchez, R. (2006). *Legal nurse consulting: The LNC marketing handbook.* Tampa, FL: Zoey.

Cesta, T., & Cunningham, B. (2008). Taking care of patients also means taking care of business. *Hospital Case Management, 16*(3), 33–36.

Cohen, S., Crego, N., Cuming, R., & Smyth, M. (2002). The Synergy Model and the role of clinical nurse specialists in a multihospital system. *American Journal of Critical Care, 11*(5), 436–447.

Davies, B., & Hughes, A. M. (2002). Clarification of advanced nursing practice: Characteristics and competencies. *Clinical Nurse Specialist, 16*(3), 147–152.

Dayhoff, N. E., & Moore, P. S. (2003). Entrepreneurship start up questions. *Clinical Nurse Specialist, 17*(2), 86–88.

DiCecco, K. L. (2007). Medical literature as evidence and expert witness: Considerations for the legal nurse consultant. *Journal of Legal Nurse Consulting, 18*(1), 3–9.

Evans, M. (2005). Consultants cutting in. *Modern Healthcare, 35*(35), 6–9.

Gibson, F., & Bamford, D. (2001). Focus group interviews to examine the role and development of the clinical nurse specialist. *Journal of Nursing Management, 9*(6), 331–342.

Hammett, L., Harvath, T. A., Flaherty-Robb, M., Sawyer, G., & Olson, D. (2007). Remote wound care consultation for nursing homes: Using a web-based assessment and care planning tool. *Journal of Gerontological Nursing, 33*(11), 27–35.

Hogue, E. (2007). Determining fair market value of consulting services. *Hospital Home Health, 24*(10), 112–114.

Hurlimann, B., Hofer, S., & Hirter, K. (2001). The role of the clinical nurse specialist. *International Nursing Review, 48,* 58–64.

Johnson, L. W. (2007). Lessons in conducting an ethics consult. *JONA's Healthcare Law, Ethics, and Regulation, 9*(3), 97–99.

Jones, L. (2005). Role development and effective practice in specialist and advanced practice roles in acute hospital settings: Systematic review and meta-synthesis. *Journal of Advanced Nursing, 49*(2), 191–209.

Kaufman, M. W. (2000). The WOC nurse: Economic, quality of life, and legal benefits. *Nursing Economics, 18*(6), 298–303.

Kerstein, M. D., van Rijswijk, L., & Beitz, J. M. (1998). Improved coordination: The wound care specialist. *Ostomy/Wound Management, 44*(5), 42–53.

Kowal, N. (1998). Specialty practice entrepreneur: The advanced practice nurse. *Nursing Economics, 16*(5), 277–278.

LaSala, C. A., Connors, P., Pedro, J. T., & Phipps, M. (2007). The role of the clinical nurse specialist in promoting evidence-based practice and effecting positive patient outcomes. *Journal of Continuing Education in Nursing, 38*(6), 262–270.

Legg, T. (2007). Staff development: The neglected discipline. *Nursing Home Magazine,* March, 28–35. Retrieved May 25, 2008, from http://www.nursinghomemagazine.com

Leong, S. L. (2005). Clinical nurse specialist entrepreneurship. *Internet Journal of Advanced Nursing Practice, 7*(1). Retrieved February 10, 2006, from http://www.ispub.com/ostia/index.php?xmlFilePath=journals/ijanp/vol7n1/entrepreneur.xml

Manley, K. (2000a). Organizational culture and consultant nurse outcomes: Part I—Organizational culture. *Nursing in Critical Care, 5*(4), 179–184.

Manley, K. (2000b). Organizational culture and consultant nurse outcomes: Part 2—Nurse outcomes. *Nursing Standard, 14*(37), 34–40.

Mattern, A. (2005). How to become a consultant. Retrieved November 25, 2005, from http://www.consulting.about.com/howtobecomeconsultant.htm

McSherry, R., Mudd, D., & Campbell, S. (2007). Evaluating the perceived role of the nurse consultant through the lived experience of healthcare professionals. *Journal of Clinical Nursing, 16*(11), 2066–2080.

Norwood, S. L. (1998). A course in nursing consultation: Promoting indirect nursing activities. *Nurse Education, 23*(5), 16–20.

Norwood, S. L. (2003). *Nursing consultation: A framework for working with communities* (2nd ed.). Upper Saddle River, NJ: Prentice-Hall.

Perler, B. A. (2008). Branding of vascular surgery. *Perspectives in Vascular Surgery and Endovascular Therapy, 20*(1), 6–8.

Puetz, B., & Shinn, L. J. (1997). *The nurse consultant's handbook.* New York: Springer.

Roggenkamp, S. D., & White, K. R. (1998). Four nurse entrepreneurs: What motivated them to start their own business. *Health Care Management Review, 23*(3), 67–75.

Rose, S. B., All, A. C., & Gresham, D. (2003). Role preservation of the clinical nurse specialist and the nurse practitioner. *Internet Journal of Advanced Nursing Practice, 5*(2). Retrieved February 10, 2006, from http://www.ispub.com/ostia/index.php?xmlFilePath=journals/ijanp/vol5n2/role.xml

Schulmeister, L. (1999). Starting a nursing consultation practice. *Clinical Nurse Specialist, 13*(2), 94–100.

Scott, R. A. (1999). A description of the roles, activities, and skills of clinical nurse specialists in the United States. *Clinical Nurse Specialist, 13*(4), 183–190.

Sills, J. (2008). Becoming your own brand. *Psychology Today,* January/February, 62–63.

Start preparing for October when reimbursement rules change. (2008). *Hospital Case Management, 15*(7), 97–99.

Stensrud, R. (2007). Developing relationships with employers means considering the competitive business environment and the risks it produces. *Rehabilitation Counseling Bulletin, 50*(4), 226–237.

Vollman, K. M. (2004). Nurse entrepreneurship: Taking an invention from birth to the marketplace. *Clinical Nurse Specialist, 18*(2), 68–71.

Youngberg, D. M. (2007). Wound, ostomy, continence nurse consulting. *Home Healthcare Management & Practice, 19*(4), 245–254.

Zahaluk, D. (2008a). What's so special about you? Part 2. *Podiatry Management,* 229–230.

Zahaluk, D. (2008b). MIP consulting group—multiple articles on building physician practice. Retrieved July 13, 2008, from http://www.ultimatepracticebuilder.com

Zimmerman, P. G. (2008). Providing expert witness testimony: Lessons learned. *Journal of Legal Nurse Consulting, 19*(2), 15–17.

Recommended Resources

Becoming a lactation consultant. Retrieved July 18, 2006, from http://www.lactationeducationconsultants.com/becominglc.html

How to become a consultant. *About Business.* Retrieved July 18, 2006, from http://www.consulting.about.com

National Association of Healthcare Consultants. Retrieved July 18, 2006, from http://www.healthcon.org

CHAPTER SEVEN

Workplace Violence: Creating and Sustaining a Healthy Place to Work

Patti Rager Zuzelo, EdD, RN, MSN, ACNS-BC

A healthy work environment is essential for quality patient care. Environments that are highly stressed, morally uninhabitable (Peter, Macfarlane, & O'Brien-Pallas, 2004), demoralizing, and abusive are associated with high RN turnover rates (Hayes et al., 2006; Way & MacNeil, 2006) and an increased number of errors (American Association of Critical-Care Nurses [AACN], 2005). Many factors encourage a sick organizational dynamic. These factors include opportunities and triggers for both physical and verbal assaults, heavy workloads with long hours, and poor, ineffective work relationships.

CNSs have opportunities to positively influence these concerns by working to reduce opportunities for workplace violence (WPV) of all types, establishing positive communication processes, and enhancing efforts to address workload concerns. This chapter offers information, strategies, and resource suggestions that will be useful to CNSs working toward healthy work environments through creative and comprehensive violence reduction strategies.

Workplace Violence

As society becomes more violent, WPV becomes more commonplace. WPV is recognized as an occupational hazard for healthcare providers, including nurses. The Health Care and Social Assistance occupation category identified a total of 129 fatalities (Bureau of Labor Statistics [BLS], 2006a) with 25 fatalities resulting from homicide, including 13 fatalities resulting from shooting (BLS, 2006b). Women were victims of workplace homicide at a rate over three times that of men (BLS, 2008b). In 2006, 13% of workplace fatalities were the result of assaults and violent acts (BLS, 2008a) although workplace homicides have decreased by 50% since 1994 (BLS, 2008b).

Factors that have led to the reduction in workplace homicide events are not clearly understood; however, identifying the positive influences is necessary if such factors are to be replicated and reinforced (National Institute for Occupational Safety and

Health [NIOSH], 2006). People are increasingly desensitized to violent behaviors while systems of work have become more complex and highly stressful with outsourcing and new management efficiencies contributing to increased employment destabilization and worker stress (NIOSH, 2002a).

The violence problem is serious and insidious yet remains unregulated. Only a few states have enacted WPV laws, although 48 bills were introduced in state legislatures during 2006 (Trossman, 2006). Compounding the problem, WPV is inconsistently defined, differences between violence and aggression are not established (Rippon, 2000), and there is a dearth of intervention studies (McPhaul & Lipscomb, 2004) examining the effectiveness of implemented programs, policies, and procedures designed to reduce the incidence or severity of violent behaviors. The healthcare culture is resistant to recognizing that nurses are at risk and demonstrates complacency related to accepting the idea that violence is simply part of the job of nursing.

CNSs are uniquely positioned to address all types of WPV and to promote healthy work environments. This chapter addresses the spectrum of violent behaviors in health care, including violence directed horizontally or vertically between healthcare providers or violence focused on nurses from patients, families, and visitors.

Background Information

The National Institute for Occupational Safety and Health (NIOSH) is a research agency of the Centers for Disease Control and Prevention (CDC) in the U.S. Department of Health and Human Services (DHHS) (NIOSH, 1996, 2002b). It is easy to confuse NIOSH with OSHA (the Occupational Safety and Health Administration), but they are different. OSHA is a regulatory agency in the U.S. Department of Labor that is responsible for ensuring the safety and health of American workers. NIOSH is an excellent resource for CNSs intrigued by the science of WPV and interested in possible risk reduction strategies.

There are many definitions of WPV and varying types of violence ranging from offensive language to homicide. NIOSH defines WPV as "violent acts, including physical assaults and threats of assault, directed toward persons at work or on duty (1996, p. 1). WPV includes physical and psychological violence, abuse, mobbing or bullying, racial harassment, and sexual harassment. Violent behaviors include interactions that occur between coworkers, supervisors, patients, families, visitors, and others (McPhaul & Lipscomb, 2004). Recent research findings suggest that nonphysical violence is highly associated with physical violence and should be seriously addressed as part of comprehensive WPV prevention plans (Lanza, Zeiss, & Rierdan, 2006).

Established typologies are helpful organizing frameworks and provide a context for developing interventions and researching the effectiveness of these interventions. Capozzoli and McVey (1996) described three types of WPV:

Type 1: Violence originates in the workplace and occurs in the workplace.
Type 2: Violence originates in the workplace and occurs outside the workplace.
Type 3: Violence originates outside the workplace but occurs in the workplace.

An example of Type 1 violence is when a hospital worker perceives that he or she has been victimized by an arbitrary evaluation that has led to a suspension. The employee comes to the work setting looking for retribution and directs this hostility toward the manager or to anyone else in the hospital. Type 2 violence is exemplified by the nurse who has a disagreement with a nursing assistant. The nursing assistant learns the nurse's home address and spray paints the nurse's automobile. Property destruction is considered a violent act, although many people might first think of murder or physical assault as examples for this type of violence. Type 3 violence may be illustrated by the shooting death of a nurse in the parking lot of the hospital by her estranged spouse.

The University of Iowa Injury Prevention Research Center (IPRC) (2001) offers four categories of violence that were developed to facilitate research and policy development. The four types of violence include:

Type I: Criminal intent
Type II: Customer/client
Type III: Worker-on-worker
Type IV: Personal relationship

This violence typology is consistent with the four violence categories of the Federal Bureau of Investigation's (FBI) National Center for the Analysis of Violent Crime (NCAVC), Critical Incidence Response Group (CIRG) (Federal Bureau of Investigation, 2004) and is also the typology used by NIOSH (2006). Type I violence occurs when an act is perpetrated during the commission of a crime, as when a person is victimized during an armed robbery. Type II violence is exemplified by violence directed toward a nurse by a patient. The majority of threats and assaults against care providers come from patients, families, and visitors (McPhaul & Lipscomb, 2004) and are reflective of this type of violence. Type III violence occurs when a perioperative nurse is verbally threatened by a surgeon, and Type IV violence may be illustrated by a violent act directed toward an individual by a person with whom the victim has had a personal relationship, such as an ex-boyfriend or ex-girlfriend.

Although these two typologies differ, there are similarities. Capozzoli and McVey (1996) have developed a typology that relates to the etiology of the violent relationship and the setting in which the violent behavior occurs, whereas the IPRC typology is grounded in the nature of the relationship, not where the violent act occurs. Both typologies are useful because they organize complicated events, WPV, into manageable, meaningful categories. Such typologies also facilitate pattern recognition when attempting to research the effectiveness of interventions based on type of violence. The typologies suggest differing preventive strategies for each category of violence.

Causative Factors of Violence

In the general public, approximately one-third of violent events are caused by personality conflicts and related stressors (Capozzoli & McVey, 1996). The healthcare sector experiences violent behaviors across all types of settings (NIOSH, 2002b; Trossman,

2006) but most frequently from patients, visitors, and patients' family members in emergency departments and psychiatric facilities (McPhaul & Lipscomb, 2004; NIOSH). Ascertaining an accurate count of the frequency and types of violent incidences in healthcare settings is not currently possible, as there is no system in place for collecting this data.

The National Traumatic Occupational Fatality Database reported a mean of 10 RN homicides annually between 1983 and 1989 (Love & Morrison, 2003). Healthcare workers are frequently assaulted by patients, particularly those with dementia or schizophrenia (Denenberg & Braverman, 1999; McGill, 2006). Hospitals rarely volunteer the extent of violence that occurs in their facilities and consider the costs of violence as the cost of doing business (Love & Morrison, 2003).

Although causes of violence vary, it is not uncommon for healthcare workers to unintentionally aggravate stressful situations (Duxbury & Whittington, 2005; Hollinworth, Clark, Harland, Johnson, & Partington, 2005). When work environments are stressed and highly charged, nurses, physicians, or other healthcare workers may escalate aggressive behaviors by responding rudely, callously, or impatiently to patients, families, or coworkers. Duxbury and Whittington (2005) found that patients from inpatient mental health units perceived poor communication to be a significant precursor to aggressive behaviors. One of the most common types of WPV occurs when the verbalization or behavior of another employee, a patient, or a visitor is perceived as threatening (Clements, DeRanieri, Clark, Manno, & Kuhn, 2005).

In addition, interacting with patients or family members who are under the influence of drugs or alcohol can require a level of finesse and communication expertise that may be in short supply when staffing levels are inadequate and staff is fatigued. Significant and chronic staff shortages, high acuities, and more violence-prone patients, including elders with dementia and patients with substance abuse or metabolic issues, increase the likelihood of violent encounters (McPhaul & Lipscomb, 2004).

Besides personality conflicts, violence perpetrated by employees is often related to a threat to job, threat to person, and extended working hours (Capozzoli & McVey, 1996). Job threats trigger employee worries about meeting basic needs for survival. Many employees live check by check without the means to afford housing, food, or family expenses during a period of unemployment. Although most people solve their needs using socially acceptable methods, when an employee believes that these acceptable methods are ineffective, he or she may resort to unacceptable tactics. Even people who are usually balanced and reasonable may reach a breaking point (Capozzoli & McVey, 1996).

When employees perceive that they have been victims of unfair or capricious treatment, they may respond violently. Capozzoli and McVey (1996) noted that in most cases of employee or ex-employee violence, the event was preceded by an event or sequential events in which the individual perceived that he or she was treated unfairly by superiors. Extended working hours can also be stressful and may trigger helplessness. If other employees do not mind the extra hours, the stressed employee may also feel isolated and ostracized, worsening the potential for violent behavior (Capozzoli & McVey, 1996).

Behavioral Typologies of Violent People

The history of violent events in the workplace suggests that some individuals are more likely to be perpetrators of violence than others. The challenge is to recognize these characteristics and consider them without stereotyping or further disenfranchising individuals, thereby exacerbating the problems that lead to violence. Past violent events have been more likely attributed to white males between the ages of 30 to 50 years of age. Although women have been known to behave violently in the work setting, they do not seem as likely to act violently in the workplace (Capozzoli & McVey, 1996).

There are three categories of males who behave violently but differently (Capozzoli & McVey, 1996). Asocial males are generally uncomfortable around other people. They are introverted, lack social skills, and internalize interpersonal conflict. These individuals tend to reach an explosion point. Their immediate families are stressful, and they are hypersensitive to criticism of any type. Their coping abilities are minimal, and they are quite territorial and controlling. Many men in this group are gun collectors or have access to firearms. They often have a violent past (Capozzoli & McVey, 1996).

Dysocial men are more outwardly aggressive and resentful of any authority (Capozzoli & McVey, 1996). They become selfish and argumentative without much impetus. Bullying and intimidation are common behaviors that may be influenced by alcohol and drug use. These individuals are more likely to abuse substances while at work. Mental illness characterizes the third category of men. They may have a variety of personality disorders, and neuroses and psychoses may contribute to these issues.

It is important to remember that the work context within which these individuals are employed does have bearing on displayed behaviors. The perpetrator of the violent act must be examined in the context of the system in which the behavior is occurring (Denenberg & Braverman, 1999). For example, supervisors' behaviors may contribute to the potential for violence. Managers who operate from a Theory X perspective, viewing employees as inherently lazy, poorly motivated, and requiring close supervision, may have poor relationships with subordinates and create highly stressful performance evaluation situations. This type of work milieu may also be associated with a lack of social support, little shared decision making, increased ambiguity, and role conflict. These issues increase the likelihood of WPV (Capozzoli & McVey, 1996).

Behavioral categories of potentially violent people relate to descriptions of people who, in the right circumstances, have increased potential for violence manifested by assault or even homicide. Women are not typical offenders. However, some data suggest that both women and men verbally intimidate and threateningly posture in the workplace during encounters with other healthcare professionals (Institute for Safe Medication Practices [ISMP], 2004a).

Conceptual Frameworks for Understanding Violence

Conceptual frameworks have been developed to explain the theoretical underpinnings of WPV. Models grounded in injury epidemiology, occupational psychology, and criminal justice (McPhaul & Lipscomb, 2004) include the Haddon Matrix, NIOSH/ National Occupational Research Agenda Organization (NORA) of Work Framework, and the Broken Windows Theory. Each theory offers a different way to view the phenomenon of WPV.

The Haddon Matrix, developed by William Haddon, Jr., over two decades ago, connects public health domains to WPV (Runyan, 1998). Host, agent, and disease are applied to primary, secondary, and tertiary injury factors. The host is the victim, whereas the agent or vehicle is a combination of the perpetrator, weapon, and force of the assault. The environment is split into the physical and social environment. The matrix is a tool that is useful when selecting strategies for injury prevention measures.

The matrix is constructed with four columns and three rows combining the concepts of pre-event, event, and postevent phases (rows) to the factors (columns). The factors, host, agent/vehicle, physical environment, and social environment interact with each other. Injuries are usually the result of sequential events rather than a discrete moment in time (Runyan, 1998).

A simple example of the Haddon Matrix is when a patient fall is the culmination of a pain experience requiring narcotic analgesia with a call bell out of reach and side rails in the up position. The patient, or host, may have urinary urgency and impulsivity concerns related to a previous stroke. The floor may be slippery, and the patient may be barefoot. The patient's room may be situated far from the nurses' station. In addition, other patients' family members heard the patient yell for help prior to climbing out of bed and falling but do not know how to alert staff and are uncomfortable going into the patient's room. These factors, if more fully developed on a Haddon matrix, would provide insight into interventions that would fit into each cell, thereby generating a variety of strategies for addressing this particular problem.

The NIOSH NORA of Work Framework (National Occupational Research Agenda, 1999) considers management and supervisory practices as well as production processes and their influence on the ways that work is conducted. This framework theorizes that work organization affects occupational illness and injury through the availability of occupational health services and activities and by exposure to psychosocial and physical hazards. Since 1996, NORA has recognized work organization as a priority research topic given that safety and the changing workplace are critical social concerns but relatively unexplored (National Occupational Research Agenda, 1999).

A third theory, the Broken Windows Theory (Kelling & Wilson, 1982), is a popular criminal justice theory that has had significant influence on law enforcement and local activism (McPhaul & Lipscomb, 2004). The theory asserts that when low-level crime is tolerated or ignored, the environment becomes increasingly conducive to more serious crime. In other words, environments with broken windows, stripped vehicles, and graffiti-clad buildings will have more serious crime than a neighborhood with clean walls, well-maintained yards, and no visible debris or destruction.

This theory may not be uniquely relevant to health care, but perhaps it offers insight into the possible influence of environment on patient and family behaviors. For example a dirty, trash-strewn waiting room area without windows and no magazines or toys may be more highly associated with hostility as compared to a waiting area that is clean, fresh-smelling, with a television, current magazines, newspapers, and various comfort supplies. This example is hypothetical but does have commonsense appeal.

Injury epidemiology, occupational psychology, and criminal justice offer interesting ways to view generalized society violence and more circumscribed occasions of violence, including those occurring in healthcare settings. An additional perspective described in nursing literature relates to violence as a response to oppression (Hedin, 1986; Hutchinson, Vickers, Jackson, & Wilkes, 2005; Roberts, 1983, 2000). Horizontal WPV or bullying is a significant concern in nursing; although it is not a phenomenon unique to the nursing profession (Hutchinson, Vickers, Jackson, & Wilkes, 2006). It has been suggested that bullying requires examination beyond the confines of oppressed group behavior theory to include broader environmental and organizational perspectives (Hutchinson et al., 2006; Hutchinson, Wilkes, Vickers, & Jackson, 2008).

Setting the Stage for Understanding Hospital Violence

"WPV is one of the most complex and dangerous occupational hazards facing nurses working in today's healthcare environment" (McPhaul & Lipscomb, 2004, p. 1). This danger reflects the risk of violent behavior victimization within society at large but may also be related to hesitancy and uncertainty within the healthcare system. Hospitals are concerned with patient satisfaction and recognize that healthcare consumers feel a sense of entitlement in terms of the quality of service.

Patient satisfaction is an important outcome measure used by most acute care facilities. It may be challenging to underscore the importance of treating staff with respect and using nonviolent methods of communication while simultaneously emphasizing the institution's friendliness, approachability, and interest in meeting individual "customer" needs. In addition, the culture of health care is to promote empathy and understanding, creating an environment in which there may be acceptance of unacceptable behavior (Rew & Ferns, 2005).

The United Kingdom (UK) is experiencing similar challenges and has responded with the National Health Service (NHS) Zero Tolerance Campaign (Rew & Ferns, 2005). In the UK, healthcare workers are four times more likely to experience WPV than the general public. Estimates suggest that healthcare workers are approximately 26 times more likely to be seriously injured than members of the general public (Rew & Ferns, 2005). The Zero Tolerance Campaign focuses on reinforcing to the public that violence against NHS healthcare workers is unacceptable while assuring staff that violent and intimidating behavior will not be tolerated. WPV continues to be a significant concern across the NHS with a persistently low level of reporting. Some fear that care providers, including physicians, may perceive WPV as inevitable (BBC News, 2008).

Each violent behavior depicted in the various typologies has the potential to occur in the hospital setting. Employees may behave in a violent fashion toward coworkers, supervisors, or patients. There may be lateral violence between nurses. Physicians and nurses may engage in verbal or physical assaults. Violence related to criminal behaviors associated with narcotics, robbery, or assault may occur. In addition, there is always the possibility of violence emanating from the patient or individuals connected to the patient.

Types of Violence in Healthcare Settings

Healthcare settings are at risk for a variety of violent behaviors. Violence may be manifested as verbal abuse, sexual harassment, racial harassment, bullying, property damage, threats, murder, and physical assault. In 2000, almost half of all nonfatal injuries from violent acts against workers occurred in the healthcare sector. These injuries include assault, bruises, lacerations, broken bones, and head injuries (McPhaul & Lipscomb, 2004).

The Bureau of Labor Statistics (BLS) does not collect data on verbal threats or assaults; it only reports on injuries severe enough to require time away from work. A direct result of inadequate or absent data collection specific to occasions of violence is the lack of clear descriptive statistics concerning the frequency of verbal and physical violence (Clements et al., 2005) and an accurate understanding of the measure of injuries resulting from violence (Love & Morrison, 2003).

Lateral or horizontal violence frequently occurs in healthcare agencies. Lateral violence is a form of bullying, nurse to nurse, and is usually directed toward nursing staff perceived as less powerful. Hutchinson et al. (2008) define bullying as referring to a variety of hidden behaviors that are difficult to substantiate. "Perpetrators aim to harm their target through a relentless barrage of behaviours that may escalate over time and include being harassed, tormented, ignored, sabotaged, put down, insulted, ganged-up on, humiliated, and daily work life made difficult" (p. 21). Bullying is tolerated because many nurses experienced it as a rite of passage and regard it as normal. Newly licensed nurses are one such group vulnerable to lateral violence during their early practice (Goldberg, 2006; Griffin, 2004). This type of violence may be considered an undesirable form of hazing as graduate nurses are initiated into the ranks of professional nurses.

When students or new nurses are victims of bullying behaviors, they may view such interactions as the norm in nursing and perpetuate the violent behaviors as they, in turn, progress to work with new nurses or students (Longo & Sherman, 2007). As with other types of violence, if institutions do not proactively protect staff through zero-tolerance policies, lateral violence goes unrecognized and unpunished, allowing it to perpetuate.

Violent verbal outbursts, aggressiveness, inappropriate criticisms, and publicly humiliating tirades are not atypical behaviors in healthcare organizations. Verbal abuse is common in the operating suite (Buback, 2004) and is largely unprovoked and unexpected when directed at a nurse from a surgeon. Nonphysical violence is normative in healthcare settings, and those employees who experience nonverbal violence are more than seven times more likely to experience physical violence (Lanza et al., 2006).

Upward vertical bullying occurs when staff members antagonize and continually challenge people in legitimate positions of authority (Goldberg, 2006), including new nurse managers or CNSs. It is also not uncommon for nurses to bully new residents or medical students or for physicians to abuse nurses with such regularity and aggressiveness that nurses are fearful to telephone or page with legitimate patient care concerns. Pharmacists also experience bullying and abuse, particularly from prescribers of all types, including physicians (Institute for Safe Medication Practices, 2004a).

Risk Factors for Violent Behaviors

Nurses and other healthcare providers work directly and intimately with unpredictable or explosive people thereby increasing exposure to violence risk. Patients may demonstrate unpredictability as a result of their medical condition such as brain injury (Pryor, 2005), psychiatric illness (Nachreiner et al., 2007), or dementia. Some exhibit explosiveness due to alcohol or drug use. Nursing work often requires one-on-one time with patients and family members. There are times when being alone increases vulnerability to violence, particularly when patients or family are impulsive, angry, and frustrated (Table 7-1).

Table 7-1 EXAMPLES OF OPPORTUNITIES FOR NURSE ASSAULT

1. Transporting a patient to a department for a necessary test during off-business hours with an on-call employee opening the department.
2. Traveling in an elevator confined with a confused, combative, or angry patient.
3. Transporting a deceased patient to the morgue, if the morgue is in a low-travel area.
4. Providing patient care in a room with doors closed and equipment or furniture blocking easy exit.
5. Sharing information with angry family members regarding a highly stressful patient care event.
6. Traveling to and from the parking facilities, particularly if it is later or earlier than the common shift end and start times.
7. Picking up medications or supplies during off-peak hours in distant, poorly monitored areas of the building.

Family members and visitors may present to healthcare facilities in angry or impaired states. Too few staff and staff members working alone either during direct-care interventions or simply as a result of a decreased personnel pool compound the risk for violence (McPhaul & Lipscomb, 2004). Long wait times, anxiety, and miscommunications or lack of communications can also trigger violence. These risks for violence relate to type II, customer/client violence (McPhaul & Lipscomb, 2004), personality conflicts, or any of the three types of violence described by Capozzoli and McVey (1996).

Other risk factors for victimization do not directly relate to patient care but are connected to types of healthcare-related enterprises or characteristics of individual nurses. Nursing educators are experiencing an increasing number of assaults by angry and violent students, particularly perpetrated by students who are failing or performing poorly (Love & Morrison, 2003). These violent episodes have the potential to spill into clinical education settings. In addition to setting, there is data suggesting that nurses with a history of victimization are more vulnerable to WPV (Anderson, 2002a, 2002b), and risk of violence varies by nurse license type (Nachreiner et al., 2007).

Larger societal influences directly affect the risk for violence in healthcare settings. Stress, substance abuse, economic pressures, and life's uncertainties contribute to the likelihood of violence. In the United States, over 50,000 people are murdered or commit suicide annually. Domestic violence is commonplace, manifested by high rates of spousal, child, and elder abuse. Individuals living in a violent home learn that violence is a normal coping mechanism. Over time, achieving a feeling of normalcy by behaving violently becomes a positive reinforcement (Capozzoli & McVey, 1996). Individuals who are accustomed to using violence to solve problems and who use anger as an early response to stress pose particular problems in hospitals when confronted with uncertainty, delays, confusion, grief, and perceived power inequities.

There were 14,920,000 people employed in healthcare and social assistance professions in 2006 with a projected increase of 4,034,000 by 2016 (BLS, 2007). This is a staggering number of citizens employed in settings providing medical care, health care and social services, and social services only. As hospitals struggle to provide care within an environment of fiscal shortages and resource competition, there are times when workforce reductions occur. Layoff and termination are highly stressful events and may trigger violent outbursts. Hospitals are not immune from personnel problems that may or may not be related to downsizing. Suspensions and other forms of disciplinary actions may also lead to violence.

In summary, many factors contribute to WPV and place nurses at risk. Typical interactions with patients, family, and visitors are potentially dangerous depending on the context of the interaction, the stress levels of the individuals involved, and the personal attributes and behavior patterns of each. Nursing is a "people business" and, as such, is risky. This risk is compounded by inadequate or nonexistent policies regarding WPV. Assaults, particularly verbal, occur between healthcare workers of all types, including physicians, nurses, ancillary staff, and multidisciplinary team members. An apathetic response to WPV in hospital settings contributes to the acceptability of lateral and vertical violence.

Hospitals are microcosms of society and are socialized to violence. Larger economic forces on local, regional, and national levels, reimbursement challenges, and resource shortages create circumstances addressed through labor downsizing, layoffs, and terminations. These few examples suggest that WPV is a multifaceted event with the potential to increase in frequency and scope. CNSs need to have a basic understanding of the risk for WPV to intervene in effective, efficient, and meaningful ways.

The Challenges of Establishing Violence Reporting Systems

Violent behaviors include assaults, domestic violence, stalking, threats, harassment in any form, and physical and emotional abuse (FBI, 2004). Cyberthreats, or threats via the Internet, are also considered prohibited threats or stand-alone criminal conduct (Turner & Gelles, 2003). The definitions of these behaviors are fairly well established and, in some instances, rather simple.

However, although violent behavior is recognized, its actual reporting rates are very low. Rationales for the low rates vary. Explanations offered specific to NHS staff include nurses' belief that they are "too busy" to take time out for reporting and also nurses' belief that some violent situations are not worth reporting, including unintentional aggression manifested by confused or disoriented patients and verbal abuse from elderly or pain-ridden patients (Ferns & Chojnacka, 2005).

The empathetic and caring nature of nursing care may also countermand a responsibility to report violence of any type. When patients react poorly to a diagnosis, for example, and lash out at the nurse, this behavior tends to be legitimized as a stress response. The threats of irate family members or verbal assaults of patient visitors are often rationalized as being a reaction to anxiety or an inappropriate response to a legitimate problem; for example, a lengthy wait in the holding area of the emergency department or an unanswered call bell.

Contributing to the inclination to not report may be that when nurses recognize systems problems but feel unable to correct them, they are more likely to excuse inexcusable behaviors. Reporting such behaviors and getting the patient, family, or visitor "in trouble" may seem an injustice. Ferns and Chojnacka (2005) suggested that nurses need to begin putting themselves first rather than patients to change the status quo perspective that violence is part of the job.

Another explanation may be that nurses are socialized to expect violence from physicians, managers, or those in roles perceived as powerful (Ferns & Chojnacka, 2005). When violent events occur, the nursing work must continue. Patients require care and attention, services need to be provided, and schedules must be followed. As a result, it may be that nurses are accustomed to carrying on regardless of violent exchanges, whether physical, emotional, or psychological assaults. There is little time to step back and step out from work and actually contemplate the impact of the event. An interesting aspect of this socialization is that nurses who experience occupational burnout are more likely to abuse other nurses (Rowe & Sherlock, 2005), and nurses who regularly experience verbal abuse may be more likely to experience burnout, thus perpetuating the cycle of violence.

Addressing the underreporting of violent incidences is a critical concern that must be corrected as an early step in violence prevention. Available data are incomplete, and the effectiveness of interventions cannot be fully researched without an accurate representation of the baseline characteristics and frequencies of violent events. A first step to collecting data is to develop consistent operational definitions of injuries and violent events that can be monitored using institutional and, eventually, national databases.

The Lingering Effects of Violence

Victims of violent behaviors have diverse responses to the events. Victims may internalize their feelings regarding verbal assault events or minimize the event (Antai-Otong, 2001) with initial reactions including anger, humiliation, shock, or surprise (Buback, 2004). Acute stress reactions are likely to follow traumatic encounters involving actual or threatened death, physical harm, or other threats to the physicality of self or others (Antai-Otong, 2001). Victims of lateral violence, particularly newly licensed nurses, often react to the violence by seeking other employment, particularly within the first 6 months (Griffin, 2004).

Needham, Abderhalden, Halfens, Fischer, and Dassen (2005) explored the nonsomatic effects of patient aggression on nurses by conducting a literature review spanning publications printed from 1983 to 2003. The initial retrieval produced 3009 publications with a final remaining number of 25 articles addressing nonsomatic effects of violence with empirical data and description. The literature revealed that nurses experienced anxiety or fear. A minority experienced post-traumatic stress disorder (PTSD) or some symptoms of PTSD. There were a variety of cognitive effects including victims feeling disrespected, unappreciated, violated, humiliated, compromised, or robbed of rights. Some shared feelings of guilt and shame, whereas others became more callous toward patients and were doubtful of their personal security and competency. The researchers call for research-based interventions to prevent patient aggression and to assist nurses' coping mechanisms when confronted with violence from patients (Needham et al., 2005).

A specific form of violence that may trigger nonsomatic effects in nurses is verbal abuse. Rowe and Sherlock (2005) investigated stress and verbal abuse in nursing using survey methodology. Respondents (N = 213) completed an adapted survey that incorporated the Verbal Abuse Scale and the Verbal Abuse Survey.

The sample included RNs and LPNs employed at a Philadelphia teaching hospital with level I trauma designation. The response rate was 69%. Interestingly, the respondents had been verbally abused by a diverse group of people including patients (79%), other nurses (75%), attending physicians (74%), patients' family members (68%), resident doctors (37%), interns (24%), and others (19%). The most frequent source of verbal abuse reported by these nurse respondents was nurses (27%) followed by patients' families, doctors, patients, residents, others, and interns. Staff nurses were the most frequent nursing source of abuse, responsible for 80% of the events, followed by nurse managers at 20%. Although most of the respondents were able to handle the anger, judging, criticizing, and condescension that were most often encountered as the abusing tactic, many did report response patterns of silence, passivity, calling out sick after the encounter, and having negative feelings about the workplace and the job (Rowe & Sherlock, 2005).

Not all violent events are nonphysical. Homicides, although uncommon, do occur. The 2004 Bureau of Labor Statistics report of fatal occupational injuries by occupation and selected event or exposure counts eight fatalities in healthcare support occupations, consisting of nursing, psychiatric, and home health aides (2005a).

The average cost of a workplace violent incident in terms of lost work time and legal expenses is approximately $250,000 excluding medical fees (Love & Morrison, 2003). The dollar amount suggests that there are both physical and psychoemotional effects associated with WPV. The expense of violence is high, not only in terms of human suffering but also in economic costs.

It may be that the effects of violence on nurses are made more profound by its apparent acceptability. Love & Morrison (2003) noted that there are very few states in which assaulting a nurse while on the job is considered a felonious act. They commented that in California, assaulting a lifeguard, bus driver, animal regulations officer, umpire, referee, juror, or emergency medical technician is a felony, but it is not felonious to assault a physician or nurse working in a healthcare setting. This inequity persists despite attempts to change the law because of the strong lobbying efforts of opponents. It is also important to remember that employees who witness violence are also victims (Capozzoli & McVey, 1996) and may experience the emotional shock, trauma, loss, and depression felt by those directly traumatized.

Strategies for Violence Reduction

Understanding the basics of WPV encourages an appreciation of its multifaceted nature and justifies the need to establish reporting mechanisms, national databases, policy changes, institutional programming, and multidisciplinary task forces. The CNS is uniquely suited to participate in these activities and is challenged to accept responsibility for influencing staff, patients, and systems to recognize WPV as a problem. The CNS is obliged to intervene with strategies that are reasonable and realistic. CNSs should research the impact of these interventions to establish an evidence base for policies and procedures.

There are resources available to CNSs and other healthcare leaders interested in effecting change in the phenomenon of violent workplaces. Formal study of threat assessment and WPV curtailment did not begin until the late 1980s with more obvious efforts in the 1990s. As a result, this field of study is relatively new, particularly as it relates to healthcare systems.

Establishing a Policy of Nonviolence

It is probably wise to begin with suggestions related to policy environment specific to WPV. Policy is not generally emphasized as a vehicle for change within programs of nursing education. Policy shapes what nurses do (Malone, 2005), and although not all nurses can be policy experts, it is important for nurses, including CNSs, to understand that policy environment provides the context and boundaries in which nursing is practiced. Malone offers a working framework for assessing the policy environment. This framework is useful for evaluating the policy environment specific to WPV and the deficiencies and strengths of such an environment.

Malone (2005) asserted that policy is a process rather than a static point and puts forth four distinctive policy characteristics that CNSs should keep in mind:

1. A policy is always general.
2. A policy establishes a norm of behavior. Policies formalize decision making about what course of action is good or better than alternative actions.
3. Policy has scale and is intended to apply to different levels of a social organization.
4. There is always someone who makes policy decisions. The CNS must figure out who this individual is within the healthcare system as part of assessing the policy environment of the system.

Ten questions drive the policy environment assessment (Malone, 2005). The questions provide a useful organizing framework for the CNS assessing the policy environment specific to WPV. Each question should be considered carefully to identify gaps and opportunities and to develop an appropriate plan for WPV reduction that encompasses policy change rather than simply rule approval, a less-substantive change. Policy requires "ongoing implementation activities, monitoring, and evaluation" (Malone, 2005, p. 137). The questions have been addressed based on the generic state of affairs at most institutions and the issues identified previously in the chapter. The policy framework questions should be applied to the CNS's practice setting. Answers may vary depending on the institution under consideration.

What Is the Problem?

The problem of note is the occurrence of violent behaviors in hospitals and other healthcare settings directed toward all types of care providers, including nurses. These behaviors can be categorized and include verbal and physical assaults, threats, and occasions of lateral or horizontal violence. To provide a more accurate definition of the "what" of this problem, it is necessary to define violence and to determine how to apply this definition when it is related to patient illness. Is violent behavior, when part of a medical condition, a policy problem or a medical management problem? One example is aggressive behaviors manifested by elderly patients with dementia and consisting of hitting, scratching, pinching, or screaming at nurses. These behaviors are violent and undesirable. They may be reflective of inadequate medical management or ineffective nursing interventions.

Using the FBI model (2004), it may be reasonable to view all violent behaviors as unacceptable and reportable. In the example of the elderly patient with dementia, the behaviors would be reported, but management of the situation would rely on medical and nursing interventions. This situation is different than a violent threat of harm from an emergency department visitor toward a nurse. Both behaviors would be reportable, although the interventions triggered by each would be markedly different.

The problem includes the lack of national and institutional reporting mechanisms to allow for benchmarking, intervention studies, and trending. An additional problem may be hospitals' current emphasis on patient satisfaction and service. The emphasis on servicing patient and family needs may promote a sense of entitlement that encourages the belief of patients, visitors, and families that they may act in ways that are usually unacceptable but are forgiven in the hospital setting due to the stressful effects of illness, anxiety, and pain. This perspective minimizes the value of staff and negates the importance of civility and respect in all forms of human interaction. It also encourages staff to avoid reporting violent incidences.

One additional problem is that while many healthcare professionals report experiences as victims of violence (Anderson, 2006; Hutton & Gates, 2008; Lanza et al., 2006; Nachreiner et al., 2007; Trossman, 2006; Winstanley & Whittington, 2002) there is little published addressing the various ways that nurses negatively influence violent encounters. Negative staff interactions characterized by hostile or aggressive responses to patient, family, or visitor encounters do contribute to an escalation of anger and negative inpatient cultures (Duxbury & Whittington, 2005). Violence-enhancing reactions may relate to personal tendencies to address emotionally heightened encounters with aggression (Anderson, 2002a).

Nurses experiencing burnout may be more vulnerable to aggression (Winstanley & Whittington, 2002), and nurses with unresolved issues of childhood abuses may have an increased susceptibility to violence, particularly during their early years of professional practice (Anderson, 2002a). CNSs need to consider that nurses involved in perpetrating violence, including lateral WPV, may be disinclined to identify themselves as abusers and may require opportunities for candid dialogue and introspection following occasions of nonphysical or physical violence.

Where Is the Process?

The process of garnering attention for policy issues related to WPV is not simple and is in its infancy. It is preferable to draw attention to this issue within an institution before a dramatically violent event unfolds. Violence should be addressed proactively rather than reactively.

The insidious nature of lateral or horizontal violence and incivility in the workplace has far-reaching implications in terms of human and economic costs. The NHS campaign of the UK offers ideas for CNSs employed in the U.S. healthcare system. As mentioned, a major thrust of the NHS Zero Tolerance Zone Campaign is educating the public that violence against NHS staff is unacceptable. The American public may require similar reminders.

Nurses need to be reminded that their safety is important, and the Federal Occupational Safety and Health Act (OSHA) requires employers to take steps to ensure a safe and healthful workplace for employees (Capozzoli & McVey, 1996). Consistent with OSHA's stance, the American Nurses Association (ANA) released its Bill of Rights for Registered Nurses asserting that nurses have the right to work in an environment that is safe for themselves and their patients (Wiseman, 2001). The American Association of Critical-Care Nurses (AACN) (2004) has a Zero Tolerance for Abuse public policy that recognizes the relationship between abusive work environments and nurse turnover.

CNSs must keep in mind that politics do affect policy. Effecting political change requires coalition-building activities and activism. Establishing WPV as a political priority means that CNSs need to galvanize rank-and-file nurses to apply pressure on government officials and the public remembering that there are many worthwhile political issues demanding resources and recognition. It may be a struggle to move the issue of WPV into the forefront of policy making.

How Many Are Affected?

When a problem affects only a few people, it is difficult to get the problem addressed through policies. In the case of WPV, many healthcare workers are affected. There is a need to mobilize this large number of nurses and other healthcare providers to give weight to the significance of the problem. WPV is an international concern. The International Council of Nurses (ICN) prioritized violence in 2001 by partnering with the World Health Organization, the International Labour Organization, and Public Services International to develop an effective worldwide antiviolence campaign (International Council of Nurses [ICN], 2007). Case studies specific to WPV in the healthcare sector across a variety of countries including South Africa (Steinman, 2003) and Brazil (Palácios et al., 2003), as well as ICN work related to workplace bullying (ICN, 2007) reveal the international scope of WPV.

What Possible Solutions Could Be Proposed?

Before committing to any single solution, it is important for the CNS to consider alternatives. The CNS should consider whether the preferred solutions to address WPV are politically palatable, practical, or achievable. It is important to select interventions that are acceptable to hospital staff (McPhaul & Lipscomb, 2004). For example, metal detectors in the emergency department (ED) may be the most desirable strategy for eliminating weapons threats but may present insurmountable manpower and budgetary challenges in small hospital facilities. Restricted access to the ED setting by reducing the number of entrances or locking the doors during low- or high-activity periods may be less expensive and actually solve the concurrent problem of too many people in crowded, tense circumstances waiting for access to inpatient areas.

A recent ED shooting event during which a police officer was slain by a criminal suspect illustrates that both suburban and urban care settings have risk for WPV and offers some real-world considerations for promoting safety in EDs. After the tragedy, medical center staff reevaluated hospital security and made improvements after consulting with law enforcement officials (Roman, 2007). Improvements included keeping criminal suspects separate from other ED patients, building a public safety room for the use of police officers taking suspects to the ED for testing, modifying entryways into the ED, bolting furniture to the floor in the sparsely furnished public safety room, and improving communication processes within the hospital. These interventions have led to effective improvements evaluated following a subsequent event of ED violence (Roman, 2007).

CNSs may want to explore using evidence-based tools for proactive identification of patients at risk for perpetrating violence. Kling et al. (2006) described the use of a violence risk assessment tool in an acute care hospital as a strategy for identifying potentially violent or aggressive patients. CNSs may find it useful to consider options for identifying patients that may have a propensity for violence so that staff can implement strategies designed to de-escalate aggression during care encounters.

What Are the Ethical Arguments Involved?

Distribution of resources (justice), privacy, nonmalificence (do not cause harm), autonomy, veracity, and fidelity are key ethical principles requiring consideration when examining strategies for reducing WPV. It is just to allocate scarce resources to protect nurses and patients from violence, although these security expenditures may be chosen over competing and worthy budgetary demands. Patient and employee privacy must be maintained and protected to ensure that rights are not compromised. Autonomy relates to independent decision making based on honest information. Hospitals may need to consider both publicly acknowledging rates of violence and installing programs designed to curtail or eliminate assaults or threats in any form. Fidelity refers to promises and keeping vows. Certainly healthcare facilities are obliged to provide a safe environment for workers and patients.

At What Level Is the Problem Most Effectively Addressed?

WPV must be addressed on a variety of levels including policy making at the federal level. Legislation should be passed that recognizes healthcare worker assault as a felony. Violence must be recognized as unacceptable, and the public needs to be informed that healthcare settings are not required to tolerate violent behaviors.

At the unit level, educational programs and staff training exercises may increase awareness of WPV and provide staff with the skills necessary to avoid escalating patient and family aggression, particularly since there is considerable evidence that some nurses may poorly handle aggressive encounters with patients (Duxbury & Whittington, 2005; McGill, 2006), visitors, and colleagues, and also contribute to episodes of horizontal WPV (Longo & Sherman, 2007).

Clinicians should be able to identify situations that trigger anger and diffuse these angry responses (Hollinworth et al., 2005; McGill, 2006). Hospitals may need to establish policies regarding lateral and vertical violence as well as policies and procedures concerning safety improvements in patient transport and security systems. Healthcare facilities may also need to consider broader programs that include institutional threat assessment (Turner & Gelles, 2003), signage, and flexible staffing levels to avoid nurses practicing in isolation without rapid access to emergency support. WPV policy change also requires legislative backing through employee protection statutes.

Who Is in a Position to Make Policy Decisions?

Within healthcare systems, it can be challenging to determine where the "buck stops" in terms of policy making. Identifying a persuasive and powerful administrative champion is critical for success. A zero tolerance for violence policy as a method of risk management is appealing for a number of reasons including institutional protection from lawsuits and negative publicity. The CNS should evaluate the healthcare facility's executive level to ascertain who might be in a position to either implement policy decisions or influence key individuals who are directly able to determine policy.

Healthcare system administrators will be compelled by the Joint Commission, formerly the Joint Commission on Accreditation of Healthcare Organizations (JCAHO), to address concerns related to security risks in Standard EC.2.10 of the 2008 Standards, Management of the Environment of Care (Joint Commission, 2008). This standard requires healthcare organizations to reduce and control environmental hazards and risks, prevent accidents and injuries, and maintain safe conditions. The standard expects that the institution consider the threat of workplace violence as part of its risk assessment. Standard EC.9.10 requires the organization to monitor conditions in the environment. These conditions include tracking injuries and security incidents and responding methodically (Joint Commission, 2008).

What Are the Obstacles to Policy Intervention?

Nurses are good problem solvers but often address issues indirectly rather than directly. Nurses' reluctance to report violent or threatening behaviors is an obstacle to developing and implementing effective nonviolence policies. Nurses may also be reluctant to confront patients, families, and visitors who may be dissatisfied with the suggestion that their behaviors need to be curtailed or modified.

What Resources Are Available?

CNSs need to consider informational, advocacy, and economic resources (Malone, 2005). Nurses are viewed in a positive way in terms of the public's perception of nurses' genuine desire to help. Nurses have high social capital but may need to more effectively use this social capital to the profession's advantage. Similar to the NHS, public campaigns by the media and public service messages may be useful in directing attention to WPV in healthcare settings. Nursing organizations at the international, national, regional, and local levels may be useful allies. The American Academy of Nursing (AAN) Expert Panel on Violence recommends that the ANA and other bargaining units representing nurses seek advisors so that they can adequately represent nursing violence-prevention interests and call for reliable measures to protect nurses (Love & Morrison, 2003).

Scholarly resources describing horizontal WPV including bullying and incivility are increasingly available through refereed publications. The development of a valid instrument for measuring workplace bullying provides a potential mechanism for better understanding the WPV experience (Hutchinson et al., 2008). Quantifying the bullying phenomenon may provide CNSs with the means to measure the effect of programs designed to reduce workplace bullying in nursing.

How Can the CNS Get Involved?

CNSs should consider learning advocacy skills and developing an understanding of the political process. Becoming well informed is essential. CNSs need to join lobbying efforts and initiate grassroots efforts to bring WPV topics to the forefront of public health discussion. CNSs must commit to nonviolence in the workplace and model this behavior for their professional counterparts.

Whether addressing horizontal violence with newly licensed graduates or verbal assaults from physician colleagues, effecting changes in violence reporting policies and procedures related to patients and families, or forming and participating in multidisciplinary security task forces, CNSs have the potential to positively influence the frequency and type of violent behaviors manifested in the work environment. Other strategies for eliminating healthcare violence include addressing personnel problems and establishing violence response teams.

Address Personnel Problems

Capozzoli and McVey (1996) offered suggestions for managing personnel problems with a focus on preventing WPV. These recommendations may be viewed as preemployment, employment, and postemployment strategies. CNSs may find themselves involved both peripherally and directly in these personnel events, depending on the type of employee and job responsibilities of the CNS.

Preemployment Strategies Background checks of job applicants should be conducted to the full extent allowed by the law. It is important to ascertain the credibility of the applicant's work history, degrees, military record, and licensing. Negligent hiring suits are becoming more common, and employers are losing because they have performed inadequate background checks (Capozzoli & McVey, 1996). It may be reasonable to include personality testing and drug screening with preemployment testing, but institutions must bear in mind that personality tests must be administered by skilled professionals, and the Americans with Disabilities Act protects people with recognized disabilities. In addition, the preemployment interview is an important screening activity. There are times when CNSs contribute to applicant interviews. Expertise in conducting interviews is an important CNS skill.

During Employment Strategies Employee performance problems must be addressed in a timely fashion using accurate documentation. The institution's disciplinary process should be used, and employees should be afforded the protection and dignity of due process, as outlined in employee handbooks. Managers should be trained in conflict resolution. CNSs may benefit from this training as well.

Postemployment Strategies When the progressive disciplinary process ends and the employee is terminated, Capozzoli and McVey (1996) warned that terminated employees cannot be expected to act rationally. All termination paperwork should be ready at the time of the final interview. Immediately following this meeting, the employee should gather personal effects and collect the last paycheck. It is important to collect keys, identification badges, and any other items to avoid creating a need for the employee to return to the work setting. Security services should be readily available.

From a broader perspective, healthcare facilities should anticipate occasions of violence. There should be a crisis management plan for violent events, and security procedures should be developed and disseminated. It may be helpful to have security drills to ensure that employees know where panic buttons, alarms, and security phones are located and to make certain that employees recognize red flag behaviors and respond appropriately.

Education Opportunities

WPV management requires educational programming at a variety of levels. Some educational challenges have been discussed. Identifying education programming needs using a circular model may assist the CNSs in planning education initiatives inclusive of all stakeholders (Figure 7-1). Establishing a conflict resolution process (Institute for Safe Medication Practices, 2004b) to nurture effective communication processes and facilitate healthy relationships is a wise investment and requires a commitment to education. ISMP recommends using vignettes and role-playing to strengthen employee communication skills. Organizations must also educate staff on how to recognize potentially violent situations and how to react during violent episodes, including occasions of extreme or lethal violence. As a WPV knowledge base builds, CNSs may have opportunities to attend conferences focused on WPV and violence-reduction strategies specific to healthcare settings.

Zero-Tolerance Policy

The FBI (2004) recognizes that zero tolerance has been criticized for overriding judgment and common sense. It recommends that employers should make clear that zero tolerance regarding WPV refers to the original sense of the phrase, absolutely no threatening or violent behavior is acceptable, and no violent incident will be ignored. This is a standard rather than a penalty. This differential is important because it recognizes that automatically generated penalties may be inappropriate and, ultimately, ineffective. Employees may be more reluctant to report violent behaviors of their counterparts if the perpetrator would be subject to automatic termination.

AACN (2004) has taken the position that a policy of zero tolerance for abuse is critical to reducing the incidence of abuse and intimidation in healthcare organizations. It recommends partnering a zero-tolerance policy and education programs for skill development. ISMP (2004a) concurs with the recommendation for zero tolerance for intimidating behaviors, regardless of the position held by the offender. Other organizations, including the Council on Surgical and Perioperative Safety (2007), have also committed to a policy of zero tolerance for both physical and nonphysical occasions of WPV.

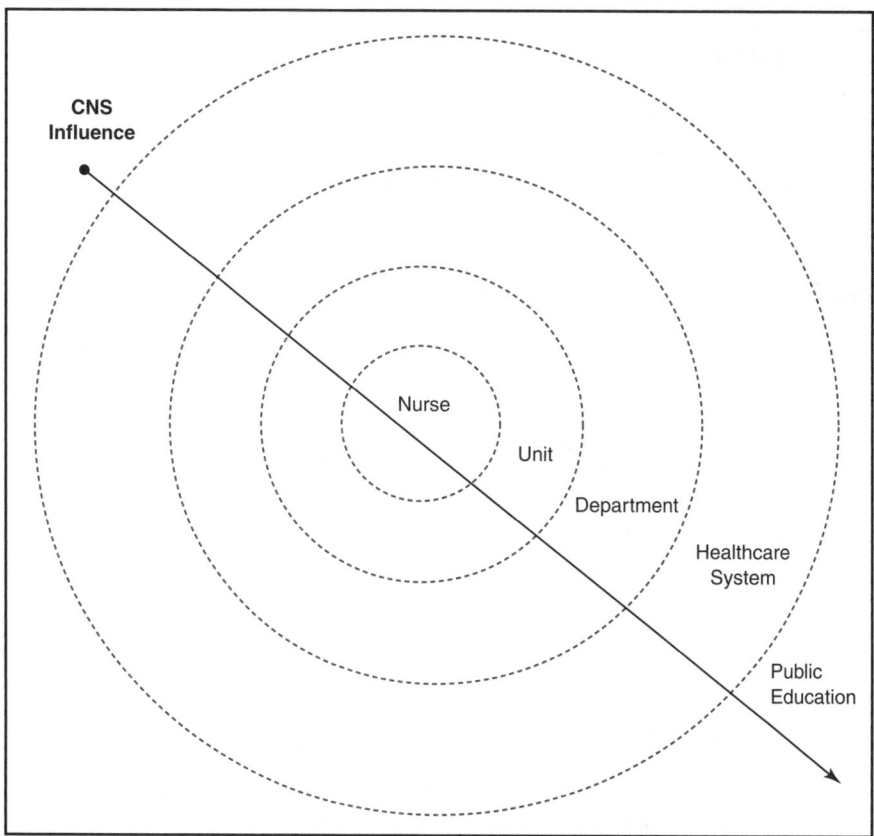

Figure 7-1   Stakeholders in CNS educational efforts addressing workplace violence.

Violence Response Team

CNSs need to think about the "what-ifs" surrounding potential WPV events. Hostage taking, gun violence, assault, and homicide are only a few of the more dramatic occasions of WPV. Of course, other types of violence are less physically destructive but still warrant consideration.

Critical incident stress debriefing is an intervention that provides immediate emotional support and education about normal stress reactions following an occasion of violence (Antai-Otong, 2001). The goal of critical incident stress debriefing is to promote a sense of psychological closure with regard to the concerning event. It is structured to assist the employee in making sense of the violence. Part of the challenge of working with nurses who have experienced violence at work is their tendency to dismiss the event as a normal occurrence in health care. This response, typical of psychiatric nurses and managers (Antai-Otong, 2001), is probably common for most nurses exposed to a wide range of patient and visitor behaviors, including emergency trauma, intensive care, and other high-acuity or long-term chronic settings.

Debriefing in some form should routinely occur within 24 to 72 hours after violent events in a safe, blame-free environment (Clements et al., 2005). Debriefing activities should be voluntary. CNSs should think about developing programs to assist nursing staff with the psychological, emotional, and physical responses to WPV. Programs need to be evaluated to determine effectiveness and modified accordingly.

Nursing Opportunities

A task force was created by the AAN, an arm of the American Nurses Association, to examine the issue of WPV and to put forth recommendations. The AAN Expert Panel on Violence Policy Recommendations on WPV was adopted in 2002 (Love & Morrison, 2003). This report provides richly descriptive data regarding WPV and offers policy recommendations. Many of the recommendations could involve CNSs, either directly as change agents and committee members or indirectly as voters and members of professional organizations. Policy recommendations include but are not limited to developing a national database, requiring healthcare organizations to adopt a zero-tolerance policy for violence and to create a plan for managing violent occurrences, requiring competency training initiatives of healthcare agencies and schools of nursing, and lobbying for stricter gun control laws (Love & Morrison, 2003).

Healthy Work Environments: Violence Free

The AACN Standards for Establishing and Sustaining Healthy Work Environments (2005) recognize that when work environments tolerate poor and ineffective relationships and fail to address these issues through policies and education programs, there is an increase in medical errors. Quality organizations develop and support relationship-building efforts. Violence, physical or verbal, is a manifestation of poor relationships and a direct contributor to unsafe patient care. It also contributes to sick work cultures that encourage nurse turnover and patient care staffing inadequacies. Abusive behaviors encourage intimidation, and when healthcare workers are intimidated, they are unlikely to freely communicate about care issues that could harm patients (Triola, 2006).

AACN (2005) has developed six standards for establishing and sustaining healthy work environments (Table 7-2). AACN recommends using the standards as a starting point for reflection and dialogue about individual work environments. The standards are interdependent, and each is necessary individually for the collective standards to facilitate optimal patient outcomes in an environment of clinical excellence (Figure 7-2).

The six standards (AACN, 2005) broadly address the work environment. When examined within the narrower scope of WPV, the six standards remain meaningful and important. Environments that nurture and expect collegial communication, col-

Table 7-2	STANDARDS FOR ESTABLISHING AND SUSTAINING HEALTHY WORK ENVIRONMENTS

The standards for establishing and sustaining healthy work environments are as follows.

Skilled Communication

Nurses must be as proficient in communication skills as they are in clinical skills.

True Collaboration

Nurses must be relentless in pursuing and fostering true collaboration.

Effective Decision Making

Nurses must be valued and committed partners in making policy, directing and evaluating clinical care, and leading organizational operations.

Appropriate Staffing

Staffing must ensure the effective match between patient needs and nurse competencies.

Meaningful Recognition

Nurses must be recognized and must recognize others for the value each brings to the work of the organization.

Authentic Leadership

Nurse leaders must fully embrace the imperative of a healthy work environment, authentically live it, and engage others in its achievement.

Source: © 2005, American Association of Critical-Care Nurses. Reprinted with permission.

laboration, and shared decision making while providing adequate staffing, recognition, and authentic leadership are environments that do not tolerate violence and bullying.

Conclusion

CNSs have a critical role to play in ensuring that healthcare environments are healthy for both patients and employees. An environment is healthy when verbal and physical abuse of any kind is not tolerated, regardless of the social stature of the offender or the nature of the relationship in question. Incidences of WPV are increasingly frequent. The more typical violent behaviors may be limited to social bullying or terroristic e-mail threats; however, these types of assaults have a significant cost in terms of nurse turnover rates and medical errors.

In addition, hospitals and other types of healthcare agencies are historically open systems. Visitors enter at will with cursory security checks. Rarely is identification

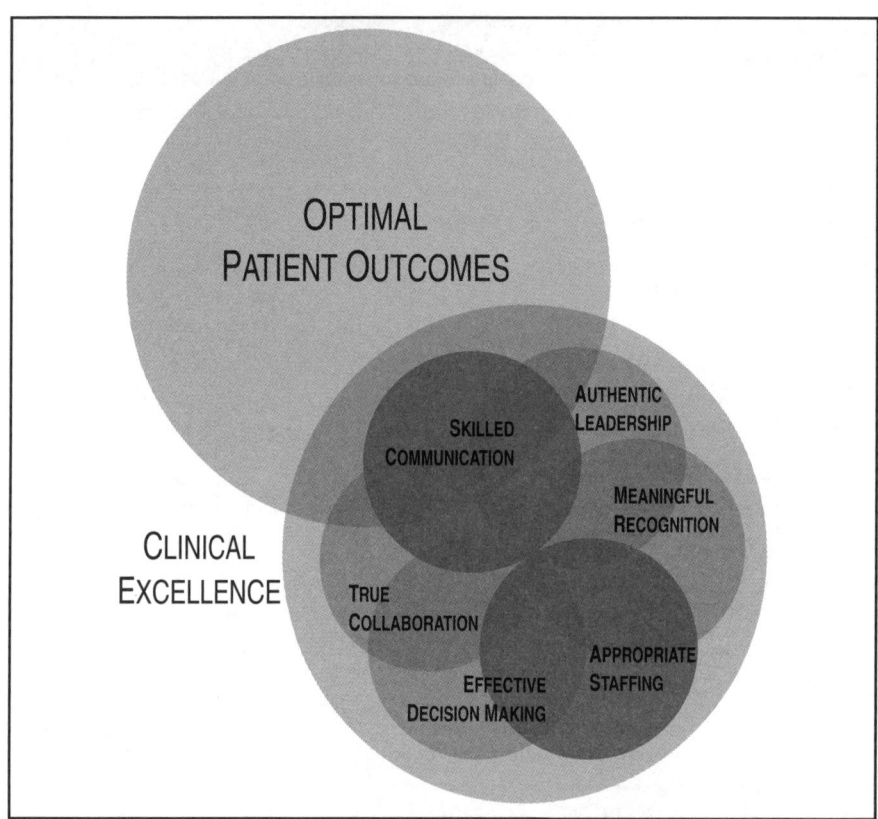

Figure 7-2 Interdependence of healthy work environment, clinical excellence, and optimal patient outcomes.

Source: © 2005, American Association of Critical-Care Nurses. Reprinted with permission.

required, particularly during daylight hours. Opportunities for extreme violence, including hostage taking, physical assault, or homicide, are significant. Although national terrorism events have evoked significant changes in some aspects of society, healthcare organizations have not yet attended to these issues in substantive ways. CNSs are in an ideal position to initiate dialogues about WPV and to participate in multidisciplinary activities aimed at reducing the potential for violence and responding to actual violence with effective action that minimizes the likelihood of harm.

References

American Association of Critical-Care Nurses (AACN). (2004). *AACN public policy position statement: Zero tolerance for abuse.* Retrieved July 7, 2006, from http://www.aacn.org/ AACN/pubpolcy.nsf/Files/ZeroPosStmt/$file/Zero%20 Tolerance%20for%20Abuse%

American Association of Critical-Care Nurses (AACN). (2005). *AACN standards for establishing and sustaining healthy work environments. A journey to excellence.* Retrieved July 7, 2006, from http://www.aacn.org/aacn/pubpolcy.nsf/Files/HWEStandards/$file/ HWEStandards.pdf

Anderson, C. (2002a). WPV: Are some nurses more vulnerable? *Issues in Mental Health Nursing, 23*(35), 351–366.

Anderson, C. (2002b). Future victim? *Nursing Management, 33*(3), 26–32.

Anderson, C. (2006). Training efforts to reduce reports of WPV in a community health care facility. *Journal of Professional Nursing, 22*(5), 289–295.

Antai-Otong, D. (2001). Critical incident stress debriefing: A health promotion model for WPV. *Perspectives in Psychiatric Care, 37*(4), 125–132, 139. Retrieved November 11, 2005, from CINAHL—Database of Nursing and Allied Health Literature.

BBC News. (2008). Doctors not reporting assaults. *BBC News.* Retrieved June 6, 2008, from http://news.bbc.co.uk/go/pr/fr/-/2/hi/health/7178777.stm

Buback, D. (2004). Home study program: Assertiveness training to prevent verbal abuse in the OR. *AORN Journal, 79*(1), 148–164.

Bureau of Labor Statistics (BLS). (2005). Table 1. *Fatal occupational injuries by occupation and event or exposure. All United States 2004.* Retrieved July 14, 2006, from http:// www.bls.gov/iif/oshwc/cfoi/cftb0200.pdf

Bureau of Labor Statistics (BLS). (2006a). Fatality rates by industry, occupation, and selected demographic characteristics, 2006. In *Census of fatal occupational injuries.* Retrieved June 1, 2008, from http://www.bls.gov/iif/oshwc/cfoi/CFOI_Rates_2006.pdf

Bureau of Labor Statistics (BLS). (2006b). *Fatal occupational injuries resulting from transportation incidents and homicides, all United States, 2006.* Retrieved June 1, 2006, from http://www.bls.gov/iif/oshwc/cfoi/cftb0215.pdf

Bureau of Labor Statistics (BLS). (2007). *Economic news release. Table 1: Employment by major industry sector 1996, 2006, and projected 2016.* Retrieved April 18, 2009, from http://www.bls.gov/news.release/ecopro.t01.htm

Bureau of Labor Statistics (BLS). (2008a). *Census of fatal occupational injuries charts, 1992–2006* (revised). Retrieved June 1, 2008, from http://www.bls.gov/iif/oshwc/ cfoi/cfch0005.pdf

Bureau of Labor Statistics (BLS). (2008b). Fatal injury events, by gender of worker, 2006. In *Census of fatal occupational injuries charts, 1992–2006* (revised). Retrieved June 1, 2008, from http://www.bls.gov/iif/oshwc/cfoi/cfch0005.pdf

Capozzoli, T. K., & McVey, R. S. (1996). *Managing violence in the workplace.* Delray Beach, FL: St. Lucie Press.

Clements, P. T., DeRanieri, J. T., Clark, K., Manno, M. S., & Kuhn, D. W. (2005). WPV and corporate policy for health care settings. *Nursing Economics, 23*(3), 119–124. Retrieved December 13, 2005, from CINAHL Database of Nursing and Allied Health Literature.

Council on Surgical and Perioperative Safety. (2007). *Statement on violence in the workplace.* Retrieved June 8, 2008, from http://www.cspsteam.org/education/education8.html

Denenberg, R. V., & Braverman, M. (1999). *The violence-prone workplace*. Ithaca, NY: Cornell University Press.

Duxbury, J., & Whittington, R. (2005). Causes and management of patient aggression and violence: Staff and patient perspectives. *Journal of Advanced Nursing, 50*(5), 469–478.

Federal Bureau of Investigation (FBI). (2004). *WPV issues in response*. Retrieved December 14, 2005, from http://www.fbi.gov/publications/violence.pdf

Ferns, T., & Chojnacka, I. (2005). Reporting incidents of violence and aggression towards NHS staff. *Nursing Standard, 19*(38), 51–56. Retrieved December 11, 2005, from CINAHL—Database of Nursing and Allied Health Literature.

Goldberg, E. (2006). Fight social bullying. *Men in Nursing, 1*(3), 45–49.

Griffin, M. (2004). Teaching cognitive rehearsal as a shield for lateral violence: An intervention for newly licensed nurses. *Journal of Continuing Education in Nursing, 35*(6), 257–263.

Hayes, L. J., O'Brien-Pallas, L., Duffield, C., Shamian, J., Buchan, J., Hughes, F., et al. (2006). Nurse turnover: A literature review. *International Journal of Nursing Studies, 43*, 237–263.

Hedin, B. (1986). A case study of oppressed group behaviour in nurses. *Image: Journal of Nursing Scholarship, 18*, 53–57.

Hollinworth, H., Clark, C., Harland, R., Johnson, L., & Partington, G. (2005). Understanding the arousal of anger: A patient-centred approach. *Nursing Standard, 19*(37), 41–47. Retrieved December 28, 2005, from CINAHL—Database of Nursing and Allied Health Literature.

Hutchinson, M., Vickers, M., Jackson, D., & Wilkes, L. (2005). "I'm gonna do what I wanna do." Organizational change as a legitimized vehicle for bullies. *Health Care Management Review, 30*(4), 331–336.

Hutchinson, M., Vickers, M., Jackson, D., & Wilkes, L. (2006). Workplace bullying in nursing: Towards a more critical organizational perspective. *Nursing Inquiry, 13*(2), 118–126.

Hutchinson, M., Wilkes, L., Vickers, M., & Jackson, D. (2008). The development and validation of a bullying inventory for the nursing workplace. *Nurse Researcher, 15*(2), 19–29.

Hutton, S., & Gates, D. (2008). Workplace incivility and productivity losses among direct care staff. *AAOHN Journal, 56*(4), 168–175.

Institute for Safe Medication Practices (ISMP). (2004a, March 11). *Intimidation: Practitioners speak up about this unresolved problem (Part I)*. ISMP Safety Alert. Retrieved July 1, 2009, from http://www.ismp.org/Newsletters/acutecare/articles/20040311.asp?ptr=y

Institute for Safe Medication Practices (ISMP). (2004b, March 25). *Intimidation: Mapping a plan for cultural change in healthcare (Part II)*. ISMP Safety Alert. Retrieved July 1, 2009, from http://www.ismp.org/Newsletters/acutecare/articles/20040325.asp?ptr=y

International Council of Nurses (ICN). (2007). *Workplace bullying in the healthcare sector*. Retrieved June 7, 2008, from http://www.icn.ch/matters_bullying.htm

Joint Commission. (2008). *History tracking report: 2009 to 2008 requirements.* Retrieved April 18, 2009, from http://www.jointcommission.org/NR/rdonlyres/11F3B7A3-77D0-48DA-B715-3D97124D8563/0/OME_EC_09_to_08.pdf

Kelling, G. L., & Wilson, J. Q. (1982, March). Broken windows: The police and neighborhood safety. *Atlantic Monthly, 249*(3), 29–38.

Kling, R., Corbière, M., Milord, R., Morrison, J., Craib, K., Yassi, A., et al. (2006). Use of a violence risk assessment tool in an acute care hospital. Effectiveness in identifying violent patients. *AAOHN Journal, 54*(11), 481–487.

Lanza, M. L., Zeiss, R. A., & Rierdan, J. (2006). Non-physical violence: A risk factor for physical violence in health care settings. *AAOHN Journal, 54*(9), 397–402.

Longo, J., & Sherman, R. (2007). Leveling horizontal violence. *Nursing Management, 38*(3), 34–37, 50–51.

Love, C. C., Morrison, E., for the AAN Expert Panel on Violence. (2003). American Academy of Nursing Expert Panel on Violence Policy recommendations on WPV (adopted 2002). *Issues in Mental Health Nursing, 24*, 599–604.

Malone, R. (2005). Assessing the policy environment. *Policy, Politics, and Nursing Practice, 6*(2), 135–143.

McGill, A. (2006). Evidence-based strategies to decrease psychiatric patient assaults. *Nursing Management, 37*(11), 41–44.

McPhaul, K., & Lipscomb, J. (2004). WPV in healthcare: Recognized but not regulated. *Online Journal of Issues in Nursing, 9*(3). Retrieved December 28, 2005, from http://www.nursingworld.org/ojin/topic25/tpc25_6.htm

Nachreiner, N., Hansen, H., Akiko, O., Gerberich, S., Ryan, A., McGovern, P., et al. (2007). Difference in work-related violence by nurse license type. *Journal of Professional Nursing, 23*(5), 290–300.

National Institute for Occupational Safety and Health (NIOSH). (1996). *Violence in the workplace. Purpose and scope.* Retrieved July 11, 2006, from http://www.cec.gov/nisoh/violpurp.html

National Institute for Occupational Safety and Health (NIOSH). (2002a). *The changing organization of work and the safety and health of working people* (NIOSH Publication No. 2002-116). Retrieved April 10, 2009, from http://www.cdc.gov/niosh/docs/2002-116

National Institute for Occupational Safety and Health (NIOSH). (2002b). *Violence: Occupational hazards in hospitals* (NIOSH Publication No. 2002-101). Retrieved April 10, 2009, from http://www.cdc.gov/niosh/docs/2002-101

National Institute for Occupational Safety and Health (NIOSH). (2006). *WPV prevention strategies and research needs* (NIOSH Publication No. 2006-144). Retrieved June 1, 2008, from http://www.cdc.gov/niosh/docs/2006-144/pdfs/2006-144.pdf

National Occupational Research Agenda. (1999). Background. In *An agenda for the 21st century.* Retrieved July 11, 2006, from http://www.cdc.gov/niosh/nora9904.html

Needham, I., Abderhalden, C., Halfens, R., Fischer, J. E., & Dassen, T. (2005). Non-somatic effects of patient aggression on nurses: A systematic review. *Journal of Advanced Nursing, 49*(3), 283–296.

Palácios, M., Loureiro dos Santos, M., Barros do Val, M., Medina, M. I., de Abreu, M., Soares Cardoso, L., et al. (2003). *Joint programme on workplace violence in the health sector.* Retrieved June 7, 2008, from http://www.icn.ch/SewWorkplace/WPV_HS_Brazil.pdf

Peter, E. H., Macfarlane, A. V., & O'Brien-Pallas, L. L. (2004). Analysis of the moral habitability of the nursing work environment. *Journal of Advanced Nursing, 47*(4), 356–367.

Pryor, J. (2005). What cues do nurses use to predict aggression in people with acquired brain injury? *Journal of Neuroscience Nursing, 37*(2), 117–121.

Rew, M., & Ferns, T. (2005). A balanced approach to dealing with violence and aggression at work. *British Journal of Nursing, 14*(4), 227–232.

Rippon, T. J. (2000). Aggression exposure and mental health among nurses. *Australian E-Journal for the Advancement of Mental Health, 1*(2). Retrieved April 10, 2009, from www.auseinet.com/journal/vol1iss2/Lam.pdf

Roberts, S. (1983). Oppressed group behavior: Implications for nursing. *Advances in Nursing Science, 5*(4), 21–30.

Roberts, S. (2000). Development of a positive professional identity. Liberating oneself from the oppressor within. *Advances in Nursing Science, 22*(4), 71–82.

Roman, L. (2007). Aftermath of a shooting. Tightened security in our ED. *RN, 70*(12), 39–42.

Rowe, M. M., & Sherlock, H. (2005). Stress and verbal abuse in nursing: Do burned out nurses eat their young? *Journal of Nursing Management, 13*, 242–248.

Runyan, C. W. (1998). Using the Haddon matrix: Introducing the third dimension. *Injury Prevention.* Retrieved July 11, 2006, from http://ip.bmjjournals.com/cgi/content/full/4/4/302#otherarticles

Steinman, S. (2003). *WPV in the health sector. Country case study: South Africa.* Retrieved June 7, 2008, from http://www.icn.ch/SewWorkplace/WPV_HS_SouthAfrica.pdf

Triola, N. (2006). Dialogue and discourse. Are we having the right conversations? *Critical Care Nurse, 26*(1), 60–66.

Trossman, S. (2006). Nurses want to put an end to workplace violence. *The American Nurse, 38*(2), 1, 6–7.

Turner, M. G., & Gelles, M. G. (2003). *Threat assessment. A risk management approach.* Binghamton, NY: Haworth Press.

University of Iowa Injury Prevention Research Center (IPRC). (2001). *WPV: A report to the nation.* Retrieved March 18, 2006, from http://www.publichealth.uiowa.edu/IPRC/NATION.PDF

Way, M., & MacNeil, M. (2006). Organizational characteristics and their effect on health. *Nursing Economics, 24*(2), 67–76. Retrieved July 5, 2006, from CINAHL—Database of Nursing and Allied Health Literature.

Winstanley, S., & Whittington, R. (2002). Anxiety, burnout and coping styles in general hospital staff exposed to workplace aggression: A cyclical model of burnout and vulnerability to aggression. *Work & Stress, 16*(4), 302–315.

Wiseman, R. (2001). *Issues update. The ANA develops Bill of Rights for Registered Nurses.* Retrieved July 13, 2006, from http://nursingworld.org/ajn/2001/nov/ajn_iu11.htm

Supplemental Resources

Publications

National Institute for Occupational Safety and Health. (2002). *Violence. Occupational hazards in hospitals* (Publication No. 2002-101). Retrieved July 14, 2006, from http://www.cdc.gov/niosh/2002-101.html

National Institute for Occupational Safety and Health. (n.d.). *NIOSH safety and health topic: Traumatic occupational injuries.* Retrieved July 14, 2006, from http://www.cdc.gov/niosh/injury/traumaviolence.html

United States Department of Labor Occupational Safety and Health Administration. (n.d.). *WPV: Hazard Awareness.* Retrieved July 14, 2006, from http://www.osha.gov/SLTC/workplaceviolence/recognition.html

Video Resources (Formats: Real Media Streaming Videos, and Downloadable Flash Video)

National Institute for Occupational Safety and Health. (2004). *Program #1. Violence on the job* (Publication No. 2004-100d). Retrieved July 14, 2006, from http://www.cdc.gov/niosh/docs/video/violence.html

National Institute for Occupational Safety and Health. (2004). *Program #2. Violence on the job case study* (Publication No. 2004-100d). Retrieved July 14, 2006, from http://www.cdc.gov/niosh/docs/video/violence.html

National Institute for Occupational Safety and Health. (2006). *WPV prevention strategies and research needs* (NIOSH Publication No. 2006-144). Retrieved June 1, 2008, from http://www.cdc.gov/niosh/docs/2006-144/pdfs/2006-144.pdf

CHAPTER EIGHT

Influencing Outcomes: Improving Quality at the Point of Care

Patti Rager Zuzelo, EdD, MSN, RN, ACNS-BC

The CNS role is under scrutiny within and outside the profession as new regulatory models are proposed, budgets are scrutinized, Magnet requirements are considered, and new nursing roles are created. The clinical nurse leader (CNL) role, an advanced generalist role originally conceived as an opportunity for people with college degrees interested in changing careers and entering nursing with a master's degree in nursing, presents challenges to CNSs as the delineation between CNL and CNS job responsibilities and skill sets appears murky, overlapping, and poorly articulated in real-world practice environments. In states without CNS title protection, nurse practitioners (NPs) and other RNs with or without graduate degrees in nursing view CNS opportunities as appropriate career options, while administrators, confronted with shortages of CNS applicants and confused by the unique skills each APRN role offers, hire an assortment of nurses into CNS positions. It is noteworthy that there has been some progress in CNS title protection as Pennsylvania has recently passed House Bill 1254, amending the Professional Nursing Law and providing for the definition of CNS (Pennsylvania General Assembly, 2009).

Another area of recent concern is the elimination of CNS positions as cost-savings measures during the current national economic downswing. Job insecurities perhaps contribute to lower than needed CNS program university enrollment figures that vary by region and contribute to subsequent CNS program closures. The proposed requirement by the American Association of Colleges of Nursing (AACN) (2004) of a doctorate in nursing practice (DNP) as the minimum level of entry into advanced nursing practice may further challenge the attractiveness of the CNS role for those nurses interested in graduate studies but not at the doctoral level. These identified challenges, coupled with the Centers for Medicare and Medicaid Services (CMS) lengthened list of noncovered hospital-acquired conditions (HACs) (Infectious Diseases Society of America, 2008) provide the context for considering the question, "What differences in care processes and outcomes are directly attributable to CNS efforts?" CNSs need to collect, analyze, and share outcome data supporting the premise that CNSs, prepared as such, make unique contributions to positive patient outcomes.

The increasing focus on improving outcomes and reaping cost benefits presents opportunities for motivated and savvy CNSs to make the case that CNS efforts are vitally important for quality nursing care. The CNS is the only advanced practice nursing role focused squarely on advancing *nursing* practice; therefore, this "super nurse" must tease out the outcomes that are unique to nursing and demonstrate how CNS efforts improve these measures. This effort is particularly important given the possibilities afforded by anticipated reforms in the U.S. healthcare system. CNSs must keep in mind that the *worth* of the CNS role becomes evident in CNS-influenced outcomes. Although CNSs recognize that they make a difference in healthcare quality, policy makers, administrators, and the public must be convinced. This chapter introduces some important ideas about outcomes, discusses trends, describes resources and tools, identifies challenges, and offers suggestions. The next chapter will offer the Patient Safety CNS role as an exemplar of an outcome-driven opportunity.

What Is an Outcome?

An outcome is the end result of particular healthcare practices and interventions. The paramount need for outcomes research was made obvious in the early 1980s when studies confirmed that surgical procedures and medical practices varied in frequency and type based upon geography rather than disease rates. In addition, there was no established way to compare the results of differing treatment approaches (Agency for Healthcare Research and Quality [AHRQ], 2000). These early discussions focused on patient outcomes related to prescribed medical therapies and interventions and stimulated outcomes discussions related to nursing practice as well as other types of clinical services.

Kleinpell and Gawlinski (2005) define outcomes as a "measure of healthcare quality, and often, effectiveness is measured by the outcomes that are produced" (p. 43). Nursing-sensitive outcomes are influenced by nurses' care practices. Nursing-sensitive patient outcomes (NSPOs) are best understood as "patient outcomes that are amenable to nursing intervention" (Given & Sherwood, 2005, p. 773).

Nurses do not influence all patient outcomes, but many outcomes are responsive to nursing interventions. Outcomes that are influenced by nurses in collaboration with other healthcare providers are important, but these particular outcomes, while affected by nurses, do not reflect nursing's *unique* contributions to healthcare structures and processes. Identifying the unique contributions of nurses, including those directly attributable to CNS influence, is key to the future of CNS practice. Nurses recognizing and marketing the differences that they make in patient outcomes, including mortality, morbidity, and length of stay, is critical to improving the healthcare system.

If CNSs are able to discern which end results of patient care are directly affected by nursing interventions, then CNSs are able to determine better ways to intervene, and thus contribute to improving patient outcomes. This linkage between nursing care and NSPOs provides justification for the current emphasis on evidence-based nursing (EBN). While there is ambiguity in the definition of EBN and continued discussion as to what EBN should and should not be, the synergy is clear between outcomes and evidence.

Evidence in all its forms, qualitative and quantitative, should inform nursing interventions (Zuzelo, 2006) and should assist in the measurement of nurses' affect on outcomes as well as on improvements in the structures and processes of healthcare systems. NSPOs should be evaluated and future interventions should be revised or maintained depending upon the outcomes. Quality of care is determined by outcomes (Figure 8-1). Measuring CNSs influence on outcomes and quality of care is important to marketing advanced nursing practice, justifying the fixed costs associated with competitive CNS compensation, and securing the full-time equivalents necessary for hiring CNSs.

Outcomes Measures: Key Players and Driving Forces

Each CNS must become well informed about the National Database of Nursing Quality Indicators (NDNQI), a program of the National Center for Nursing Quality within the American Nurses Association. NDNQI is a national database that collects data at the nursing unit level. Indicators are regularly added and new projects are developed and implemented regularly. The database is dynamic and offers a variety of reports that enable institutions to compare their outcomes to those of other similar institutions across the country (American Nurses Association [ANA], 2002).

The best way to appreciate the importance of NDNQI is to understand its history (ANA, 2009a). The American Association of Nursing (ANA) launched the Safety

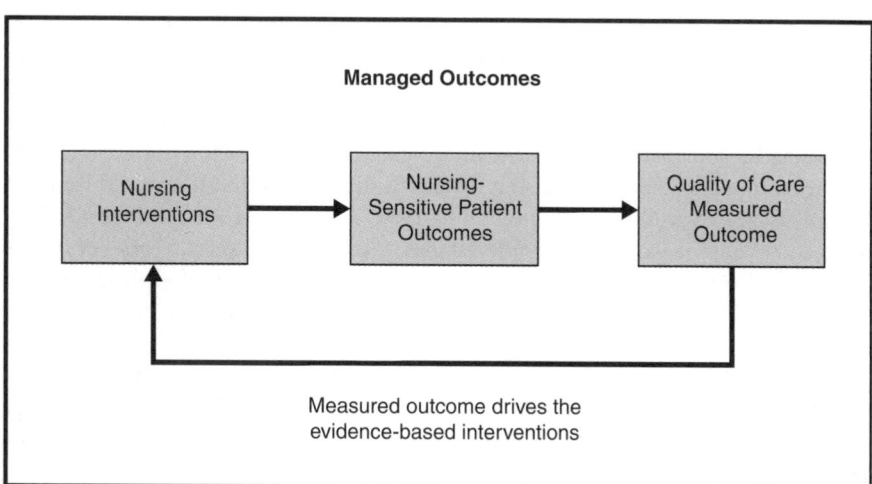

Figure 8-1 EBP, outcomes management, and quality.

and Quality Initiative in 1994 for the purpose of investigating and describing the empirical linkages between nursing care and patient outcomes. This project was early in the outcomes measurement movement and served to guide and support discussions about the connection between nurse staffing patterns and nurse preparation to patient care outcomes. Other organizations had called for outcomes measurement as early as the 1970s, including the Joint Commission, the Visiting Nursing Association (VNA) of Omaha, and the National League for Nursing (NLN). The ANA's initiative was the first report card–style report specific to acute care hospital nursing.

The outcome of the Safety and Quality Initiative was a report entitled, *The Nursing Care Report Card for Acute Care* (ANA, 1995). This report card identified 21 measures of hospital performance with a conceptual or quantifiable link to nursing services in acute care. The report card also established 10 nursing quality indicators that had a direct relationship to nursing services within acute care settings. Each indicator was operationally defined in careful terms to promote consistency in data collection and analysis. It is worthwhile for CNSs to go back to this original ANA report and review the complexity and detail of the measures used to establish reliable and valid indicators.

One of the most reliable predictors of outcome indicators was the percentage of RNs of the total staff (Moore, Lynn, McMillen, & Evans, 1999). Staff mix and the numbers of available RNs continues to be an important indicator with a direct effect on patient mortality in the hospital setting (Aiken, Clarke, Sloane, Sochalski, & Silber, 2002). Moore et al. caution that findings of the ANA report card, as well as summative evaluations compiled by other outcomes studies, should be considered within the framework of several contextual concerns.

First, there is no clear agreement about the indicators that should be included in a report card. Second, the availability, reliability, and validity of these indicators have not always been demonstrated. Third, once indicators have been consensually selected, there is no consensus about how long it will take to have valid and reliable measures for the indicators. Fourth, many databases contain compromised data from which report cards are generated; and, fifth, report card data may be meaningful to one stakeholder group to the exclusion of others that are important (Moore et al., 1999). Despite these concerns, the ANA report card was an important and significant beginning to formalized, nursing specific outcomes measurement.

The National Database of Nursing Quality Indicators (NDNQI) evolved from the *Nursing Care Report Card for Acute Care*. In 1997, ANA issued a request for development and maintenance of the national database. For the next 3 years, a series of ANA-funded pilot studies established the selected indicators and developed operational definitions and data collection methodologies for each indicator. In 1998, NDNQI began accepting data from participating hospitals and providing fee-based reports (ANA, 2009a). There are 10 nursing-sensitive quality indicators, and each has a recommended definition. ANA (2002) recommends that all hospitals collect and report on these 10 indicators to make clear the difference that RNs make in the provision of safe, high-quality patient care.

Many CNSs are employed in acute care institutions that are interested in pursuing Magnet status through the American Nurses Credentialing Center (ANCC). To seek accreditation, institutions are required to participate in NDNQI. Magnet certification achievement recognizes and celebrates exceptional nursing departments. NDNQI reports provide one view of quality evaluation that is nursing specific. The reports offer an opportunity for benchmarking or comparing within and between participating nursing departments. There are three requirements for joining the database: (1) a completed NDNQI Database Agreement; (2) designation of an institutional liaison between NDNQI and the facility with documentation on the NDNQI Site Coordinator Contact Information form; and (3) fee payment (ANA, 2009b).

Measuring outcomes is important but should not be performed independent of outcomes management. Unless measurement is conducted and results are managed as components of quality improvement, problems arise related to data collection activities that are not valued as meaningful and meaning making. This potential problem is similar to the issues that arise when research studies are conducted but findings are not used to inform and improve practice. CNSs should measure outcomes that are important to their particular institution or type of clinical practice and then manage these outcomes to improve quality using available evidence.

When the CNS considers Magnet accreditation processes, NDNQI and its historical roots in ANA's Nursing Care Report Card for Acute Care, and outcomes mandates from public and private foundations, organizations, and accreditors, linkages between quality improvement, evidence-based practice, and outcomes become evident and fairly simple to explain to nursing colleagues who may not have an understanding of the connecting relationships (Figure 8-2).

Leaders and Partners in Outcomes Measurement and Management

There are a number of organizations focusing efforts on improving healthcare outcomes and quality, in addition to ANA's efforts. Some organizations have a multidisciplinary focus while others predominately serve a particular stakeholder group. Overall, there are many stakeholders with significant vested interest in the outcomes measurement and management movement (Figure 8-3).

Corporations and smaller businesses have vital interest in outcomes measures as a data source to facilitate decision making about which plans and services provide employees with the best care (as measured by outcomes) in the most cost-effective manner (a fiscal outcome). For example, the Leapfrog Group is a voluntary program focused on using the purchasing power of employers to alert the U.S. health industry that big leaps in healthcare safety, quality, and customer value will be acknowledged and rewarded (2008a). This program intends to reduce preventable medical mistakes and improve the quality and affordability of health care, encourage public reporting of healthcare quality and outcomes, and reward doctors and hospitals for improving health care (Leapfrog Group, 2008b).

Another stakeholder group, healthcare consumers, has increasing access to outcomes-driven data that can be used to make informed decisions as to where to seek

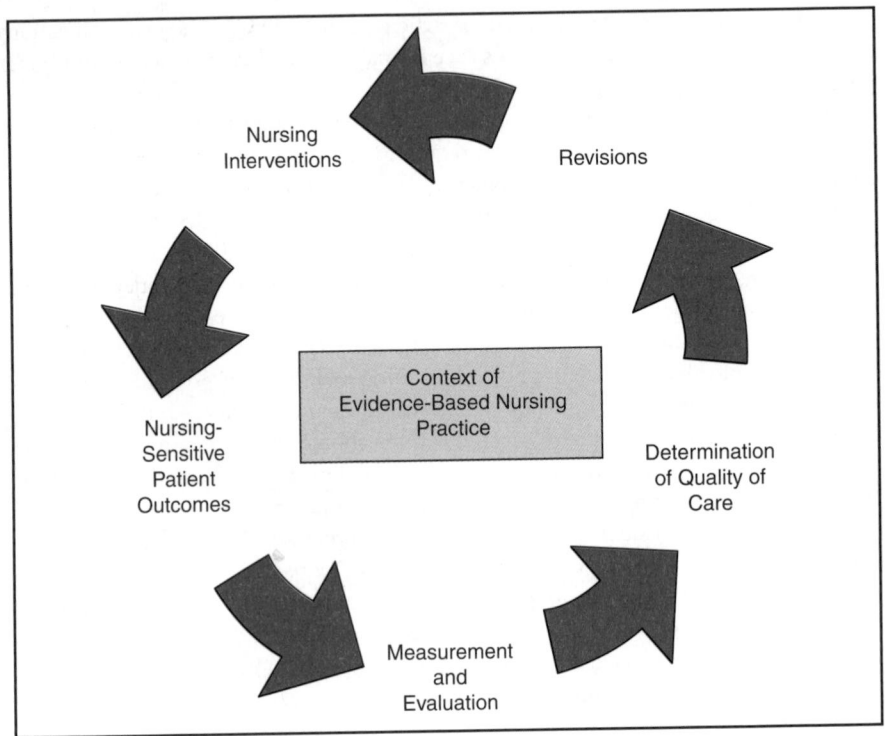

Nursing
Interventions

Revisions

Context of
Evidence-Based Nursing
Practice

Nursing-
Sensitive
Patient
Outcomes

Determination
of Quality of
Care

Measurement
and
Evaluation

Figure 8-2   Nursing-sensitive quality loop.

general or specialty care services. The Joint Commission Quality Check and Quality Reports provides consumers with access to information about how well a hospital performs against National Quality Improvement Goals (Joint Commission, 2009). As an example, potential "customers" can ascertain the percentage of patients with a suspected cardiac event who receive aspirin therapy upon arrival to local emergency departments (ED) and make informed decisions as to which provides better care, based upon this criterion. The Quality Reports and Quality Check build upon the data submitted to the Joint Commission database, ORYX, from healthcare organizations.

Another resource for helping consumers and employers choose between competing health maintenance organization (HMO) plans is the Health Plan Employer Data and Information Set (HEDIS). HEDIS is a program of the National Committee for Quality Assurance (NCQA) that facilitates decision making based upon value and cost of service. HEDIS consists of standardized performance measures that are related to many significant public health issues. HEDIS also includes a standardized survey of consumers' experiences related to service, access, and claims (National Committee for Quality Assurance [NCQA], 2006)

Other stakeholders in healthcare outcomes include practitioners and the public. Practitioners are affected by outcomes-driven data in a variety of ways. They need to

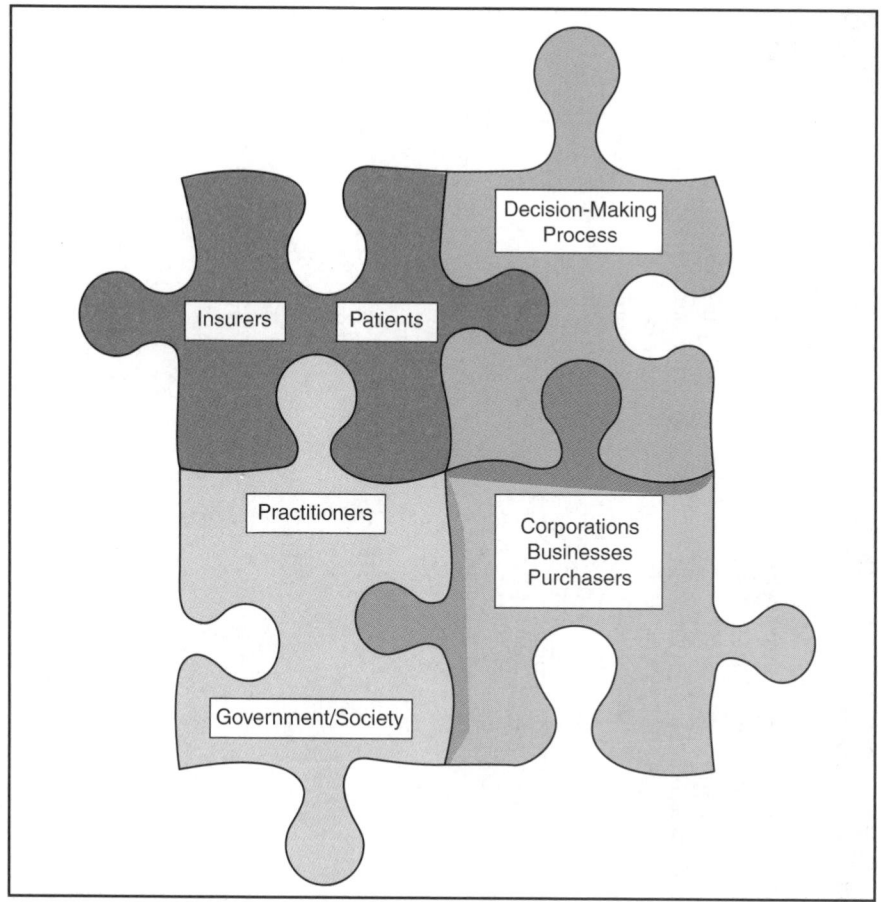

Figure 8-3   Healthcare outcomes stakeholders.

compile and submit this data, and these data collection processes require time and effort. Practitioners' records are available for public review: specifically, malpractice cases and complaints through the National Practitioner Data Bank-Healthcare Integrity and Protection Data Bank (n.d.); and indirectly, through publicly available outcomes data related to the practitioners' employing institution. Society is certainly affected by outcomes as morbidity and mortality influence public health, and gross domestic product expenditures relate to quality of life, including taxation and opportunity costs.

Some of the more established organizations and foundations are directly partnered with nursing while others do not have a formal relationship but do provide a variety of supports, in the form of electronic resources, conferences, database information, benchmarking, public education initiatives, or printed materials. CNSs need to become familiar with some of the critical contributors to the outcomes movement (Table 8-1).

Table 8-1 SELECT PARTNERS IN OUTCOMES MEASUREMENT, MANAGEMENT, AND QUALITY OF HEALTHCARE

Organization	General Description	Web Site	CNS Resources
Medical Outcomes Trust (MOT)	The Medical Outcomes Trust is a not-for-profit organization dedicated to improving health and health care by promoting the science of outcomes measurement (2006).	http://www.outcomes-trust.org	Medical Outcomes Trust provides access information for high-quality instruments that measure health outcomes that may be of interest to CNSs. Contact information is provided for access to and use of instruments.
Institute for Healthcare Improvement (IHI)	Non-for-profit organization dedicated to improving the quality of health care and accelerating the measurable and continual progress of healthcare systems throughout the world (IHI, n.d. 1).	http://ihi.org/ihi	CNSs may access program reports, white papers, improvement stories, and success headlines via the Web site. Many IHI initiatives have reports that may be helpful to CNSs including Transforming Care at the Bedside, and the Safer Patients Initiative. The reports are content validated by experts.
			The white papers may also be useful as they provide findings and tools related to breakthrough improvements or issues.
			The IHI Open School (http://www.ihi.org/IHI/Programs/IHIOpenSchool/?TabId=4) provides free, online courses that come with prepared quiz opportunities.

Table 8-1 (continued)

Organization	General Description	Web Site	CNS Resources
Hospital Quality Alliance (HQA)	This alliance includes the Centers for Medicare and Medicaid Services (CMS), American Hospital Association (AHA), and the Association of American Medical Colleges. Other organizations support the alliance, including the American Nurses Association. The program's goal is to identify standardized, user-friendly hospital quality measures that could be used by all healthcare stakeholders to improve the ability of consumers to make informed healthcare decisions (HQA, 2009).	http://www.cms.hhs.gov/HospitalQuality Inits/33_Hospital QualityAlliance.asp	CNSs may find the HQA tool, Hospital Compare, useful for patient, nursing student, and community teaching. This tool shares honest and user-friendly information about the quality of delivered care in hospitals as measured by Care Quality Measures for select medical conditions.
National Quality Forum (NQF)	NQF's mission is to improve American healthcare through endorsement of consensus-based national standards for measurement and public reporting of healthcare performance data that provide meaningful information about whether care is safe, timely, beneficial, patient-centered, equitable and efficient (NQF, 2008).	http://www.qualityforum.org	CNSs should be familiar with NQF's consensus reports and activities, including consensus reports pertaining to cancer, safe care practices, mammography, and others.

(continues)

Table 8-1 (continued)

Organization	General Description	Web Site	CNS Resources
National Patient Safety Foundation*	Mission: Improve the Safety of Patients We accomplish this through our efforts to: Identify and create a core body of knowledge; Identify pathways to apply the knowledge; Develop and enhance the culture of receptivity to patient safety; Raise public awareness and foster communications about patient safety; and Improve the status of the foundation and its ability to meet its goals. NPSF can make a long-term, measurable difference by serving as a central voice, and NPSF will lead the transition from a culture of blame to a culture of safety.	http://www.npsf.org	NPSF offers a variety of excellent and comprehensive resources via its Web site. This foundation sponsors education and research activities and publishes the *Journal of Patient Safety*. There are a variety of brochures available for download that are useful resources for professionals and patients/families (Figure 8-12). The videotape offerings are excellent opportunities to enliven staff meetings and discussions. There is a free 30-day review period for DVDs and CDs, and purchase prices are competitive.

Table 8-1 (continued)

Organization	General Description	Web Site	CNS Resources
Institute for Safe Medication Practices (ISMP)	This not-for-profit organization is a leader in medication use safety and medication error prevention. It is a long-standing organization with over 30 years experience. ISMP's mission is "to advance patient safety worldwide by empowering the healthcare community, including consumers, to prevent medication errors" (ISMP, 2009).	www.ismp.org	This organization is an outstanding resource for CNSs. The Web site offers medication safety tools, product information, error-reporting programs, and a variety of other cutting-edge resources. There are also FDA safety alerts and medication safety videotapes and DVDs that may be very useful for influencing patient safety outcomes. ISMP offers many newsletters including several practice specific editions of *ISMP Safety Alert: Nurse Advise-ERR*, *Community Ambulatory Care* edition, and the *Acute Care* edition. ISMP also publishes *Safe Medicine*, a consumer health education newsletter.

Source: *Reprinted with permission of the NPSF. © 2006 National Patient Safety Foundation. All rights reserved.

Most outcomes-focused organizations offer a variety of materials that are useful to CNSs evaluating clinically based patient care operations and looking for opportunities to positively influence patient outcomes. Many times CNSs are directed to investigate and solve specific clinical issues. These directives may be driven by complaints, benchmarking analyses that reveal room for improvement, new programs, or other types of critical incidents. Other times, CNSs identify the problems and opportunities that are apparent to them because of their expertise and experiences.

CNSs should investigate available resources for practice improvements before planning interventions. It is not uncommon for practitioners to brainstorm and problem solve without first reviewing the tools that are already established as valid, reliable, and accessible. Many organizations have readily available, relevant, free materials that are very user-friendly and well organized (Figure 8-4). There are excellent Web-based resources that offer tools and models designed to support efforts aimed at improving healthcare quality (Skinner, 2007).

For example, central line infection is a significant clinical concern across a variety of care settings but particularly in high-acuity nursing practice. Preventing central line infections was one of the six outcomes initiatives of the Institute for Healthcare Improvement (IHI) established as part of the early *100,000 Lives Campaign* and continuing as a priority in the *5 Million Lives Campaign* (Institute for Healthcare Improvement [IHI], 2008) (Table 8-2). A review of IHI's Web site (www.ihi.org) reveals a central line care bundle (Table 8-3), a group of evidence-based interventions that when used concurrently results in better outcomes than when followed individually. *A Getting Started Kit: Prevent Central Line Infections How-To Guide* (IHI, 2008) is available as a free download. This kit is an evidence-based booklet with clear instructions, defined outcomes, and supporting data for bundled interventions that promote teamwork and reduce infection rates. A CNS interested in improving the central line infection rate of a particular service or across an institution would be wise to begin by reviewing the IHI resources, available for public use, before attempting to develop a policy, procedure, or program based upon a literature review.

IHI supports the end-stage renal disease networks in their efforts to increase placement of arteriovenous (AV) fistula placement and use for U.S. dialysis patients. The Fistula First National Vascular Access Improvement Initiative is endorsed by IHI. As a result, IHI has valuable resources available for CNSs practicing in nephrology settings that provide care to patients requiring hemodialysis services. Resources posted on IHI may be used by the CNS to influence ingrained end-stage renal disease intervention habits and move the standard of care to best practice (IHI, n.d. 2)

Establishing an Outcomes Project of Interest

CNSs may have difficulty selecting a project that pertains to an outcome of interest. There are many competing demands for CNS attention, and prioritizing these demands can be frustrating. At times, CNSs may feel pulled in multiple directions and may be tackling multiple outcomes simultaneously thereby contributing to CNS burnout. CNSs often have some sort of responsibility, directly or indirectly, for

Tools

Diabetes

The Institute for Healthcare Improvement and Improving Chronic Illness Care, a national program of the Robert Wood Johnson Foundation, have both developed and adapted tools to help organizations accelerate their work to improve the care for patients with chronic conditions. In addition, many organizations have developed tools in the course of their improvement efforts—successful flowcharts, forms, instructions and guidelines for implementing key changes—and are making them available on IHI.org for others to use or adapt in their own organizations. We invite you to submit tools you have found useful!

The tools below are grouped according to the key areas of the Chronic Care Model where changes must be made to improve care for people with chronic conditions.

(→ Submit a Tool)

Delivery System Design Tools

Organization of Health Care Tools

Self-Management Tools

Self-Management/Consumer Involvement

Tools Icon Key

 PDF (Downloadable)   PowerPoint (Downloadable)

(Downloadable)   Word (Downloadable)   Access

 Excel (Downloadable)   Interactive Tool (Online)

Delivery System Design Tools

  Health Disparities Collaboratives Training Manual for Chronic Conditions

This step-by-step manual was developed to help healthcare organizations improve chronic care for their patients with diabetes, asthma, depression, and other chronic diseases; developed by the Institute for Healthcare Improvement (Boston, MA).

Rated by Users: ☆☆☆☆☆   (→ Rate This)

  Continuing Care Clinic Handbook

The Continuing Care Clinic Handbook is a step-by-step guide to establishing more efficient patient visits using periodic half-day visits to your clinic to meet multiple patient needs; developed by Improving Chronic Illness Care (Seattle, WA).

(continues)

Figure 8-4 Example of a Web-based resource from the Institute for Healthcare Improvement.

Rated by Users: ☆☆☆☆☆   (→ **Rate This**)

Organization of Healthcare Tools

  Quality Compass 2003 Benchmarks

Touchpoint Health Plan (Appleton, WI) uses this benchmarking tool to compare its results for preventive care, diabetes, asthma, depression, and more with other organizations in its network and with national averages.

Rated by Users: ☆☆☆☆☆   (→ **Rate This**)

  Chronic Care Model Audiovisual Presentation

A 57-minute presentation walking through the Chronic Care Model as presented by Dr. Ed Wagner, Director of the Improving Chronic Illness Care national program; developed by Improving Chronic Illness Care (Seattle, WA)

Rated by Users: ☆☆☆☆   (→ **Rate This**)

  Assessment of Chronic Illness Care Survey

A simple, comprehensive survey tool to assess your organization's current levels of care with respect to the six components of the Chronic Care Model (community resources, health organization, self-management support, delivery system design, decision support, and clinical information systems); developed by Improving Chronic Illness Care (Seattle, WA)

Rated by Users: ☆☆☆☆☆   (→ **Rate This**)

Self-Management Tools

  My Shared Care Plan

A self-management support tool used for long-term planned care; developed by Whatcom County Pursuing Perfection Project (Bellingham, WA)

Rated by Users: ☆☆☆☆   (→ **Rate This**)

  Self-Management Support: Patient Planning Worksheet

The Patient Planning Worksheet is a form to help people with chronic illnesses develop a personal plan to learn a new behavior, such as starting a program to increase their physical activity; developed by Improving Chronic Illness Care (Seattle, WA)

Rated by Users: ☆☆☆   (→ **Rate This**)

  Stoplight (Red-Yellow-Green) Tools for Patients with Diabetes

"Stoplight" tools assist patients with monitoring and managing their chronic condition by dividing various signs and symptoms into "green," "yellow," and "red" management zones; developed by Improving Chronic Illness Care (Seattle, WA)

Rated by Users: ☆☆☆☆☆   (→ **Rate This**)

Figure 8-4   Continued.

Self-Management/Consumer Involvement

 Group Visit Starter Kit

The Group Visit Starter Kit provides you with step-by-step instructions on how to begin running group visits with your patients; developed by Improving Chronic Illness Care (Seattle, WA)

Rated by Users: ☆☆☆☆☆   (→ Rate This)

Figure 8-4   Continued.

Table 8-2   *5 Million Lives Campaign* **INTRODUCTION AND RECOMMENDED INTERVENTIONS**

The Campaign

Do No Harm. It is a fundamental principle for healthcare providers: *primum non nocere*—first, do no harm. It is our duty, our responsibility. Patients ask and assume that the health care that intends to help them should, at the very least, not injure them.

Despite the extraordinary hard work and best intentions of caregivers, thousands of patients are harmed in U.S. hospitals every day. Hospital-acquired infections, adverse drug events, surgical errors, pressure sores, and other complications are commonplace.

Based on data collected over several years from multiple partner institutions, IHI estimates that nearly 15 million instances of medical harm occur in the United States each year—*a rate of over 40,000 per day.* This is a burden larger than most patients and professionals, and even some healthcare researchers, realize. It is time to declare this toll unacceptable; time to end it. You can help.

Proven Interventions

The *5 Million Lives Campaign* challenges U.S. hospitals to adopt 12 changes in care that save lives and reduce patient injuries:

The six interventions from the 100,000 Lives Campaign

* **Deploy rapid response teams** ... at the first sign of patient decline.
* **Deliver reliable, evidence-based care for acute myocardial infarction** ... to prevent deaths from heart attack.
* **Prevent adverse drug events (ADEs)** ... by implementing medication reconciliation.

(continues)

Table 8-2   (continued)

- **Prevent central line infections** ... by implementing a series of interdependent, scientifically grounded steps.
- **Prevent surgical site infections** ... by reliably delivering the correct perioperative antibiotics at the proper time.
- **Prevent ventilator-associated pneumonia** ... by implementing a series of interdependent, scientifically grounded steps.

New interventions targeted at harm

- **Prevent harm from high-alert medications** ... starting with a focus on anticoagulants, sedatives, narcotics, and insulin.
- **Reduce surgical complications** ... by reliably implementing all of the changes in care recommended by SCIP, the Surgical Care Improvement Project (www.medqic.org/scip).
- **Prevent pressure ulcers** ... by reliably using science-based guidelines for their prevention.
- **Reduce methicillin-resistant *Staphylococcus aureus* (MRSA) infection** ... by reliably implementing scientifically proven infection control practices.
- **Deliver reliable, evidence-based care for congestive heart failure** ... to avoid readmissions.
- **Get boards on board** ... by defining and spreading the best-known leveraged processes for hospital boards of directors, so that they can become far more effective in accelerating organizational progress toward safe care.

Source: Reprinted from www.IHI.org with permission of the Institute for Healthcare Improvement (IHI), © 2009.

engaging staff in meaningful work designed to enhance the quality of patient care services. Working on outcomes projects with staff and colleagues is an ideal way for CNSs to influence the work environment and patient care. Actually selecting the outcome of interest may be one of the most difficult stages of project development.

Searching for "Gaps"

There are a number of ways to identify a pertinent outcome measure that may be amenable to nursing practice changes and that will positively affect the quality of care delivery. It is important to solicit input from the nursing staff members if their participation is needed for project success, including data collection and implementing practice changes. CNSs should consider available outcomes measurement data including benchmarking results from NDNQI, the Joint Commission, or the Reporting Hospital Quality Data for Annual Payment Update initiative. The National Patient

Table 8-3	IHI MATERIALS AVAILABLE FOR PREVENTING CENTRAL LINE–ASSOCIATED BLOODSTREAM INFECTION

1. One-page summary available for download
2. Updated How-To Guide
3. Updated Annotated Bibliography
4. PowerPoint presentation with Facilitator Notes
5. Recording of recent Central Line Infections Office Hours Call
6. Opportunity to join a Central Line-Associated Bloodstream Infection Web Discussion
7. Frequently Asked Questions about Central Line Infections
8. Prevent Central Line Infections: A Fact Sheet for Patients and Families
9. Prevent Central Line Infections: A Fact Sheet for Patients and Families—Spanish Translation
10. Central Line Insertion Checklist
11. Hand Hygiene Getting Started Kit
12. Improvement Stories
13. Resources

Source: Reprinted from www.IHI.org with permission of the Institute for Healthcare Improvement (IHI), © 2009.

Safety goals, updated and revised annually, are also a good source of project ideas and quality improvement activities.

There may be opportunities for outcomes improvement revealed through careful review of patient, physician, or staff complaints. Nurses often recognize systems problems that negatively affect outcomes, and these staff worries may provide insight into possible topics for project development. Incident reports offer opportunities for measuring and managing significant outcomes including but not limited to falls, medication errors, needlestick injuries, workplace violence, communication processes, transfusion errors, or compromised patient safety. Many times, staff has ideas for projects but need encouragement and support before they will attempt to address the issue in an organized, formal process (Figure 8-5).

Caldwell (2006) offers a strategy, Manager Quality Waste Walk, as an opportunity for managers to improve service and reduce cost in the healthcare setting. His strategy involves managers physically making rounds on the units of interest and observing for occasions of wastefulness that, if removed, would benefit the institution. This may be a useful exercise for CNSs who are interested in involving staff in projects that improve efficiencies by eliminating waste and that may serve as catalyst projects for encouraging staff on a trajectory of process improvement projects. These sorts of

OFFICE OF THE ASSOCIATE DIRECTOR OF
NURSING FOR RESEARCH
PATTI ZUZELO, EDD, APRN, BC, CNS
ASSOCIATE PROFESSOR, LASALLE UNIVERSITY
SCHOOL OF NURSING & HEALTH SCIENCES

WANTED: UNIT-BASED PROJECTS

Have a great idea for a unit-based project? Thinking about a better way of doing things?

Interested in arranging for a unit-based workshop on literature searches? Willing to take responsibility for gathering your colleagues and setting up a date and time?

I am looking for RNs interested in developing and initiating unit-based projects related to clinical practice. Leadership and enthusiasm are must-haves. " Technical skills and research expertise are not required.

Talk with your colleagues. Consider developing a simple project. Think about the possibilities of presenting your work at a local, regional, or national conference as either a poster or a paper presentation. I'll help you throughout the process.

If you have an idea and are willing to take charge of a project, please contact me! I'd be happy to sit down with you over a cup of coffee and chat! The coffee is on me.

Figure 8-5 Soliciting input.

activities are concrete, practical, have real-world benefits, and may facilitate staff engagement in quality improvement initiatives.

Project Identification

Once gaps in a system of care provision have been identified, it is often productive to elicit staff input via group discussion. Staff meetings, informal chats, and electronic discussions are good methods for soliciting input and garnering ideas. It may be useful to collectively develop a list of outcomes that staff believes may be better managed. This list should be prioritized and reduced to a reasonable number of projects. The CNS should facilitate the prioritization process by using some type of sensible procedure including casting votes, assigning numeric values to projects and rank ordering based upon collective scores, Q-sort methodology, or Delphi technique to reduce the number of projects and to include only the most valued. The decision-making group may also find that the priorities are clearly evident after discussion.

CNSs may want to consider competitions or contests to elicit quality improvement ideas or evidence-based practice projects from staff. One example of this type of competition is the *Unearthing the Evidence* contest sponsored by Albert Einstein Healthcare Network's Department of Nursing (Figure 8-6). This contest has its origins in a research utilization competition that had been known as the Sacred Cow competition. The Sacred Cow competition encouraged nurses to submit fully developed research projects proposing simple but elegant research questions that had relevance to nursing practice within the organization. The selected project was funded with a small grants award. The winning nurse, usually a novice first-time researcher, was required to present the study findings during a subsequent nursing grand round.

The "Unearthing the Evidence" Contest

Identify a nursing or medical practice that is used on a fairly regular basis BUT that should be changed based upon published evidence.

Example: Saline lavage with suctioning is not supported in the literature for adult patients requiring airway suctioning. The evidence is clear. NO SALINE! And yet . . . the practice continues in some institutions on some units or by some nurses . . . .

Submit a description of the current practice and offer a recommendation for change. Include copies of references

Entries will be judged on:

1. Commonness of the nursing or medical practice. Think about the things that we do every day in practice . . . are they really grounded in evidence? Are there alternative strategies we should be using? How do nurses accomplish these interventions in other countries?

2. Relevance to direct patient care

3. Quality of literature support

4. Realism of practice change suggestion (including fiscal reality)

Prize: $100 American Express Gift Certificate

Recognition in upcoming E^3 Newsletter

Admiration of nursing colleagues

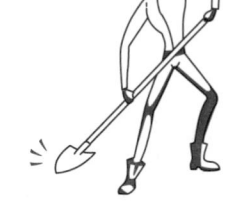

Submissioin Due Date: Entries may be e-mailed as attachments to zuzelop@einstein.edu or dropped off in my mailbox on 2nd floor Levy Building, Nursing Administration.

Figure 8-6   *Unearthing the Evidence* competition announcement.

After a number of years of dwindling submissions, the competition was stopped. The *Unearthing the Evidence* competition was created to encourage nurses to consider nursing and medical practices and offer suggestions for improvement based upon available evidence. The required format was narrative but also succinct with less of an academic structure. The first competition was a success with two well-crafted submissions and a number of electronic inquiries of interest.

The first winning submission addressed bladder catheterization practices and offered recommendations for change based upon a compelling need to reduce urinary tract infections (Exemplar 8-1). This project stimulated interest and was well received. Some recommendations were implemented by nursing in consultation with the physicians. A second project, Frequency of Vital Signs, explored the required frequency of postoperative vital signs for patients transferred from the postanesthesia care unit. The subsequent year, the winning project explored the frequency and type of saline lock use on a telemetry care unit in an effort to preliminarily explore the possibility of changing unit policy (Exemplar 8-2). This particular project also was the catalyst for a staff nurse to begin his journey as a beginning researcher and author.

Involving nurses in the identification of outcomes projects can accomplish several goals. Active involvement in project selection facilitates staff engagement, and this engagement improves participation. Outcomes projects provide opportunities to teach staff about outcomes management, measurement, and resources. For staff who have been practicing for more than 10 years and who have not been involved in formal

Clinical Project Exemplar

Unearthing the Evidence Competition **Submission**

Carolyn Jacobson, MSN, RN, CCRN
Albert Einstein Healthcare Network

Problem

The statistics are alarming: 5 million patients have urinary catheters inserted each year, and more than a million acquire catheter-related urinary tract infections (CAUTIs). CAUTI, the most common nosocomial infection in ICUs, leads to longer hospital stays and increased healthcare costs and precipitates the use of antibiotics at a time when resistance issues are a major healthcare concern. Despite research findings demonstrating the hazards and risks associated with the use of urinary catheters, they are routinely used, often unnecessarily. Research estimates that up to 25% of hospital patients have Foley catheters. The surgical/trauma unit urinary catheter use rate exceeds this benchmark figure. Patient acuity and severity of illness in the surgical/trauma unit frequently warrants urinary catheter placement to monitor output, but there are situations where its use is not justified, and nurses are in an empowered position to affect change in practice.

Evidence

Saint, Lipsky, and Goold (2002) cited a study where initial insertion was unjustifiable in 21% of hospitalized patients with a urinary catheter and that continued use was unwarranted for almost half the days the patient was catheterized. Other investigators (Maki & Tambyah, 2001) cited CAUTIs as the most common nosocomial infection in hospitals and identified risk factors for CAUTIs with prolonged catheterization >6 days as the most important, modifiable risk factor with a near universal infection rate by catheterization day 30. Tew, Pomfret, and King (2005) suggested that urinary catheterization is sometimes essential but also believe that catheters are forgotten once inserted. Research findings reveal that urinary catheters are the second most common cause of bacteremia (Tew et al., 2005). Saint and Lipsky (1999) conducted an extensive review of the literature published from 1966 to 1998 and concluded that catheter-related bacteriuria is associated with increased morbidity and mortality. Recommendations were offered, including catheterization avoidance and, if initiated, termination as soon as clinically possible. They also suggested use of silver-coated catheters as a means to reduce the risk of UTI.

Recommendations

1. Eliminate clinically unnecessary urinary catheterizations.
2. Prevent UTIs when catheter is warranted and inserted by following standardized protocols for catheter care.
3. Educate nurses and physicians to the potential hazards and risks associated with the urinary catheter.
4. Remove urinary catheters as soon as possible, preferably by the day 6 modifiable risk factor.
5. Explore possibility of pilot research study using silver-coated catheters.
6. Establish and monitor outcomes measures.

Proposed Plan

1. Collaborate with trauma and emergency departments to evaluate the Standard Trauma Admission Order Set inclusive of "insert Foley" checkbox, substituting "assess patients for Foley catheter need."
2. Revisit urinary catheter policy and procedure for possible changes based on research findings.
3. Develop unit-based competency and poster. Collaborate with clinical educators for possible hospital-wide education program.
4. Label urinary catheters with insertion date and initiate a nurse-generated reminder or an automatic computer "stop order" requiring catheter removal or reorder on day 6.
5. Create a quality assurance indicator that tracks the labeling and dating of urinary catheters.
6. Collaborate with infection disease control department for feasibility of conducting a pilot study using the silver-alloy urinary tract catheter.
7. Utilize currently collected data to evaluate the effectiveness of proposed interventions.

References

Maki, D. G., & Tambyah, P. A. (2001). Engineering out the risk of infection with urinary catheters. *Emerging infectious diseases*, *7*(2). Retrieved March 7, 2006, from http://www.cdc.gov/ncidod/eid/vol7no2/maki.htm

Saint, S., & Lipsky, B. A. (1999). Preventing catheter-related bacteriuria: Should we? Can we? How? *Archives of Internal Medicine*, *159*(8), 800–808.

Saint, S., Lipsky, B. A., & Goold, S. D. (2002). Indwelling urinary catheters: A one-point restraint? *Annals of Internal Medicine*, *137*(2), 125–127.

Tew, L., Pomfret, I., & King, D. (2005). Infection risks associated with urinary catheters. *Nursing Standard*, *20*(7), 55–61.

Exemplar 8-2

Clinical Project Exemplar

Unearthing the Evidence Competition Submission: Describing Saline Lock Usage on a Telemetry Unit

Steven Szablewski, BSN, RN, PCCN
Albert Einstein Healthcare Network

Scope of Problem

It is estimated that 200 million saline locks (SLs) are used in U.S. hospitals each year. SLs have been routinely inserted in patients admitted to the telemetry unit based on the premise that these patients are at risk for life-threatening dysrhythmias requiring emergent intravenous (IV) drug administration. Research suggests that SLs are associated with risk because of the potential for infection, phlebitis, and patient discomfort. There is limited research exploring SL usage patterns, and the actual need for SLs is not substantiated; rather, SLs may be inserted because of tradition and history. Although SLs are commonly prescribed for patients admitted to telemetry units, a comprehensive literature review did not reveal a standard of care for SL usage in the telemetry care setting.

Unit-Based Problem

Two serious SL phlebitis events with associated sepsis elevated nurses' concerns specific to the risk of adverse events associated with SLs. Nurses noted that all patients had SLs inserted and maintained for the duration of the telemetry unit admission but observed that the SLs were rarely required for emergency therapies. SLs were most frequently used for intravenous diuretic dosing or antibiotic therapy. Nurses believed that these medications could have been reasonably delayed by the few minutes required for establishing intravenous access.

Evidence

A recent, national audit completed by members of the Royal College of Nursing IV Therapy Forum revealed that the majority of SLs in their sample (N = 625) were accessed at a rate of 75.5% (n = 472) within a 24-hour period while 23.2% (n = 145) of SLs were not accessed (Bravery et al., 2006). In contrast, a prospective study on SL use rates of emergent patient admissions (N = 86) in the United Kingdom calculated SL use at 51% (n = 44) with 49% (n = 42) of SLs never being used (Abbas, Klass de Vries, Shaw, & Abbas, 2007). While IV therapy has become the preferred route for its reliable delivery of medications, guidelines have recommended that every patient should have a documented, therapeutic and/or diagnostic purpose for SL insertion (Infusion Nurses Society, 2006; Weinstein, 2007). There have not been research studies exploring the relationships between SL usage rates, telemetry patient diagnosis, and medication classifications delivered via saline locks.

Recommendations

1. Design and conduct a research study describing rates and patterns of SL use categorized by high-frequency telemetry unit admitting diagnoses to assess the need for continuous SL access.
2. Ensure the timely removal of SLs inserted with questionable aseptic technique or those associated with patient discomfort, and/or signs and symptoms of SL-related complications.
3. Educate staff nurses on the risks associated with indwelling SLs and evidence-based guidelines regarding rotation and removal of SLs.
4. Institute standardized procedure for SL insertion and maintenance with utilization of SL insertion kit.

Proposed Plan

1. Collect data to explore SL usage patterns in the telemetry care unit.
2. Utilize research findings to develop a nursing decision tree regarding insertion and maintenance of SLs within certain telemetry patient diagnosis groups.
3. Collaborate with department of internal medicine and cardiology to set up protocol for removing clinically unwarranted SLs in telemetry patients at low risk for requiring emergent IV interventions.
4. Develop interdisciplinary charting record for daily assessment of SL access.

5. Educate staff regarding proper SL insertion techniques and risks associated with indwelling SLs.

References

Bravery, K., Dougherty, L., Gabriel, J., Kayley, J., Malster, M., & Scales, K. (2006). Audit of peripheral venous cannulae by members of an IV therapy forum. *British Journal of Nursing, 15,* 1244–1249.

Abbas, S. Z., Klass de Vries, T., Shaw, S., & Abbas, S. Q. (2007). Use and complications of peripheral vascular catheters: A prospective study. *British Journal of Nursing, 16,* 648–652.

Infusion Nurses Society. (2006). Infusion nursing standards of practice. *Journal of Infusion Nursing, 29,* S1–S92.

Weinstein, S. M. (2007). *Plumer's principles & practice of intravenous therapy* (8th ed.). Philadelphia: Lippincott, Williams & Wilkins.

academic programs, an outcomes project may be the first exposure to the outcomes movement. CNSs should keep in mind that an outcomes project does not have to be complex; rather, simple and elegant construction is ideal for a first-time venture.

Developing the Outcomes Project

As mentioned, CNSs may become involved in outcomes management through interest in improving a clinical outcome or through assignation by the chief nurse executive or other administrator. For example, if urinary tract infection (UTIs) rates increase within the surgical service line, the CNS may be asked to participate in a multidisciplinary ad hoc committee exploring strategies for reducing nosocomial UTI rates, or the CNS may initiate a nursing project to explore evidence-based practice changes that may improve this outcome measure. The current emphasis on outcomes management and measures fits nicely with the evidence-based practice (EBP) movement as the interventions that may be used to improve outcomes should be consistent with or based upon current EBP recommendations. The aggressive actions of the Centers For Medicare & Medicaid Services (CMS) (2008) to ensure safe, high-quality care by designating select hospital-acquired conditions (HAC) as nonreimbursed are also triggering the need for outcome management and quality improvement efforts (Table 8-4).

It is worth noting that there is much administrative consternation about HACs and benchmarked NDNQI data. The worrisome HACs and the important indicators collected through the NDNQI program offer CNSs meaningful opportunities to "show their stuff." Both data sets provide CNSs with opportunities to quantify their influence. CNSs should design useful continuous quality improvement projects using established methodology and established data sets to change processes that affect patients at the point of care. Seize the opportunities offered by HACs and nurse-sensitive indicators!

As CNSs construct a project, including the data collection plan, they need to consider the validity, reliability, and feasibility associated with the instruments that will be used in outcomes measurement (Duffy & Korniewicz, 2002). It is often better to

Table 8-4   HOSPITAL ACQUIRED CONDITIONS (HACs)

HAC categories:

1. Foreign object retained after surgery
2. Air embolism
3. Blood incompatibility
4. Stage III and IV pressure ulcers
5. Falls and trauma
   a. Fractures
   b. Dislocations
   c. Intracranial injuries
   d. Crushing injuries
   e. Burns
   f. Electric shock
6. Manifestations of poor glycemic control
   a. Diabetic ketoacidosis
   b. Nonketotic hyperosmolar coma
   c. Hypoglycemic coma
   d. Secondary diabetes with ketoacidosis
   e. Secondary diabetes with hyperosmolarity
7. Catheter-associated urinary tract infection (UTI)
8. Vascular catheter-associated infection
9. Surgical site infection following:
   a. Coronary artery bypass graft (CABG)—Mediastinitis
   b. Bariatric surgery
      i. Laparoscopic gastric bypass
      ii. Gastroenterostomy
      iii. Laparoscopic gastric restrictive surgery
   c. Orthopedic procedures
      i. Spine
      ii. Neck
      iii. Shoulder
      iv. Elbow
10. Deep vein thrombosis (DVT)/pulmonary embolism (PE)
    a. Total knee replacement
    b. Hip replacement

Source: Centers for Medicare and Medicaid Services, 2008.

use a preexisting instrument or a portion of an instrument rather than creating a new one. Creating a valid and reliable instrument requires careful processes that often involve quantitative methodologies, expert input, and pilot testing.

The Medical Outcomes Trust is an excellent resource for accessing instruments that measure health outcomes (Table 8-5). If no instrument is available that examines the outcome or process of interest and constructing a tool is the only option, CNSs should make certain to establish some type of content validity and ascertain the reliability of the tool. Choosing to use a tool that does not have established validity and reliability undermines the believability and worth of the entire outcomes project.

Table 8-5	SELECT INSTRUMENTS APPROVED BY THE SCIENTIFIC ADVISORY COMMITTEE OF MEDICAL OUTCOMES TRUST
Instrument	**Description**
SF-12 Health Survey	Multipurpose short-form generic measure of health status. Shorter, valid alternative to the SF-36.
SF-36 Health Survey	Measures health status and outcomes from the patient's point of view. Constructed to use in surveys, evaluations, and clinical practice and research. Measures eight health concepts.
Adult Asthma Quality of Life Questionnaire (AQLQ)	Disease-specific instrument with 32 items for adults with asthma.
Pediatric Asthma Quality of Life Questionnaires (PAQLQ)	Measures impact of children's asthma on their primary caregiver's quality of life.
Migraine Specific Quality of Life (MSQOL)	Twenty-five-item instrument designed to measure long-term effects of migraine and migraine treatment on quality of life.
Seattle Angina Questionnaire (SAQ)	Measures functional status of coronary artery patients.
Urinary Incontinence-Specific Quality of Life Instrument (I-QOL)	Self-report instrument that assesses three domains of quality of life specific to urinary incontinence.
Basis-32	Assesses outcomes of mental health treatment for populations experiencing inpatient psychiatric hospital care for a variety of disorders.
Child Health Questionnaire (CHQ)	Assesses a child's physical, emotional, and social well-being from the perspective of a parent or guardian or, at times, the child directly.

Once the CNS has determined the most appropriate instrument to use for data collection, it is important to keep in mind that data collection activities do have associated expenses related to personnel, data storage, and printing, purchasing, or other types of costs. The budgetary impact of data collection and outcomes tracking should be considered before beginning the project (Duffy & Korniewicz, 2002). In addition, data collection requires proactive planning. CNSs need to determine who will collect the data and what processes will be followed. Ensuring a consistent, reliable process of data collection, particularly if there is more than one data collector, is essential.

Duffy and Korniewicz (2002) note that data are worthless if clinicians believe the data is inaccurate. To protect data integrity, they offer a few suggestions including the use of a flowchart to graphically depict the data collection process, verifying that data entry processes have integrity, considering data analysis prior to actual data collection, and reporting on the data in a regular and timely fashion. Data reporting may include quarterly reports for staff review, updates during staff meetings, signage, or electronic messages.

Improving Quality by Systematically Examining and Managing Outcomes

Quality improvement (QI) is an important component of CNS practice. It is critical for CNSs to become adept at utilizing a systems approach to QI activities in order to test the effects of changes in practice on outcomes. There are typically a number of possible ways to influence outcomes, and discerning whether the selected interventions have yielded maximum positive effects given the committed resources is an important question.

Another important consideration in QI activities is the accessibility of organized data. There is a great amount of data that is collected in healthcare institutions, but it is often in disarray. Usually data collection activities are sporadic and inconsistently reported and discussed (Perkins, Connerney, & Hastings, 2000). Establishing organized systems of data collection, storage, and retrieval processes is important to QI initiatives.

IHI (2006) notes that there are differences between research and QI measurements (Table 8-6). CNSs are familiar with the research process and have experience with traditional measurement concerns through graduate research studies or clinical research projects. A key difference between research and QI measurements is that measurement for improvement occurs frequently and is often performed rapidly in small batches so as to accelerate the implementation of desirable changes.

The CNS needs to be able to compare the costs to benefits of practice changes, and this analysis requires a systematic, scientific approach. There are a number of approaches to QI that may be useful to CNSs, including plan-do-study-act (PDSA), Six Sigma, rapid cycle improvement, positive deviance, failure mode and effects analysis (FMEA), root cause analysis (RCA), and flowcharting. A brief overview of each technique or process may be useful to stimulate further exploration.

Table 8-6	CONTRASTING MEASUREMENT FOR IMPROVEMENT TO MEASUREMENT FOR RESEARCH	
	Measurement for Research	Measurement for Learning and Process Improvement
Purpose	To discover new knowledge	To bring new knowledge into daily practice
Tests	One large "blind" test	Many sequential, observable tests
Biases	Control for as many biases as possible	Stabilize the biases from test to test
Data	Gather as much data as possible, "just in case"	Gather "just enough" data to learn and complete another cycle
Duration	Can take long periods of time to obtain results	"Small tests of significant changes" accelerates the rate of improvement

Source: Reprinted from www.IHI.org with permission of the Institute for Healthcare Improvement (IHI), © 2006.

PDCA or Plan-Do-Check-Act

PDCA is the fundamental process of Total Quality Management (TQM) developed by W. Edwards Deming in the 1950s. PDCA is also referred to as PDSA, the Deming Cycle, Shewhart Cycle, or the Deming Wheel (American Society for Quality, n.d.). Regardless of its title, the process consists of four steps: plan, do, study (check), and act (Table 8-7). These steps should be viewed as circular and continuous. PDSA quality

Table 8-7	PDCA PROCEDURE
Procedure	
Plan.	Recognize an opportunity and plan a change.
Do.	Test the change. Carry out a small-scale study.
Study.	Review the test, analyze the results, and identify what you've learned.
Act.	Take action based on what you learned in the study step: If the change did not work, go through the cycle again with a different plan. If you were successful, incorporate what you learned from the test into wider changes. Use what you learned to plan new improvements, beginning the cycle again.

Source: Reprinted with permission from ASQ Quality Press. © 2005 American Society for Quality.

improvement uses the scientific method to implement and test the effects of changes on the performance of the healthcare system (Speroff, James, Nelson, Headrick, & Brommels, 2004; Williams & Fallone, 2008). When used in TQM or continuous quality improvement (CQI) projects, PDCA is user-friendly and may be useful when working with multidisciplinary groups or staff nurses unfamiliar with CQI processes.

PDCA may be used to accomplish a number of goals. It was originally designed as a model for CQI and is successfully used for such activities in the private and public sector and in all types of ventures, including health care (Williams & Fallone, 2008). PDCA is also a useful tool in root cause analyses and when developing a new or improved design of a care delivery process. There are a number of Web-based, print, and program resources to help the CNS become expert with this quality tool.

FOCUS-PDCA Quality Improvement Model

FOCUS is an acronym for *find, organize, clarify, understand,* and *select* (Bader, Palmer, Stalcup, & Shaver, 2003). FOCUS is frequently added as a forerunner to the PDCA cycle (Figure 8-7). FOCUS facilitates the discovery process and problem identification required for PDCA to begin. The CNS begins by finding a process requiring improvement. As mentioned previously, this process may be discovered by the CNS using a variety of methodologies, or it may be assigned to the CNS as part of a department or institution initiative.

Once a problem is found, the second step is to organize in order to improve the current state of the process. The CNS may elect to form a multidisciplinary committee, nursing committee, or may determine that the best organizational structure is to use an existing standing committee. Brainstorming with colleagues may offer insights that the CNS would not have considered.

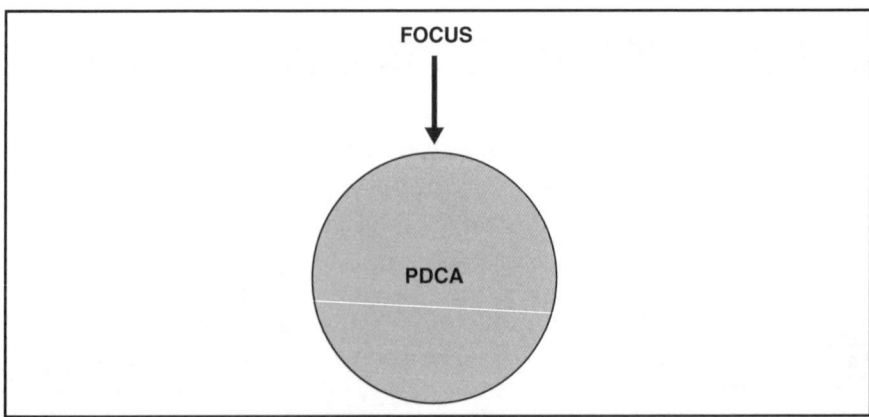

Figure 8-7 FOCUS-PDCA cycle for continuous improvement.

It is imperative to establish a team that will be responsive, enthusiastic, and expert. Identifying the appropriate team members is also critical. The CNS needs to make certain that key players are represented and that the individuals who know the way that the current process "really works" are essential for quality improvement. This may also be a good opportunity to establish ownership of the project not only in terms of budgetary responsibility but also specific to authorship and presentation rights, should the activity result in a scholarly outcome. The CNS should determine whether secretarial, technical, or fiscal supports are in place.

Clarification follows organization. This stage is concerned with accurately describing the process and identifying the details that may contribute to opportunities for improvement. Organizing activities may include searching the literature, examining available evidence, scrutinizing benchmarked data, flowcharting or diagramming current processes, or exploring the problem of interest using some type of descriptive data collection method including focus groups, interviews, or surveys, among others.

Organizing activities are important as they provide the fodder for developing a clear understanding of the current processes and identifying the gaps and shortcomings. Chart audits and medical records reports may also provide useful information, depending upon the process requiring improvement. There are times when systems are needlessly complex and processes are onerous. Flowcharting or diagramming the process of interest in a step-by-step, detailed fashion are helpful exercises.

Understanding or uncovering the sources of variation or the problems in the process is the fourth step. The CNS may discover that some of the problems cannot be solved. For example, if a group is working on improving patient wait times in a small but busy emergency department and a key problem area is a lack of physical space, there may not be a realistic way to correct this problem until a new waiting room is constructed. However, there may be other opportunities in the process of entering the ED to obtaining a examination bed in the ED that could be addressed and that could contribute to reducing waiting room time.

The CNS should think about variable measurement during this step. An important aspect of outcomes management and CQI is outcomes measurement. The CNS needs to consider the ways that variables and processes are measured and make certain that these measurements are useful and practical. Remember that data will need to be collected, compiled, and analyzed. It makes sense to establish a data collection plan early. If possible, take advantage of data collection processes that are already in play.

Once the process has been selected, dissected, and understood, PDCA activities begin. In general, PDCA should focus on particular aspects of the selected process. Complex processes should not be tackled all at once. Rather, the CNS should start the process by selecting exactly what portion of the process will be examined. The selection criteria should include the feasibility of changing the selected process.

At this point, the CNS plans the improvement. The working group needs to decide whether the identified changes will be made in a pilot program or initiated on a large scale. This decision depends upon the recommended change and the process.

For example, if the recommended change is dramatic and the consequences are not entirely understood, or if there is little in the literature or experientially that describes the potential impact of the change, a pilot study may be the wisest course. If the change is based upon research and is consistent with the recommendations of leading authorities, it may be acceptable to proceed on a larger scale. The CNS needs to remember that a data collection plan should be in place prior to implementing changes.

The next step is to "do" or implement the recommendation. Part of the challenge of "doing" is to make certain that the recommended changes are being done correctly and consistently. The CNS should be auditing processes, talking with people involved in the implementation, and maintaining careful data collection that follows the developed data collection plan.

After implementing the changes and collecting data, the CNS "checks" for improvement, deterioration, or no change from the status quo. In the event of little or no positive change, the group needs to analyze how the intervention was implemented and whether the processes rather than the recommendation were deficient. Brainstorming and interviewing are effective strategies for collecting this information. Remember that there is a possibility that the change was not conducted as planned and that unaccounted intervening influences had a negative effect on the outcomes. Theory-driven evaluation strategies and considerations are necessary to avoid discarding appropriate changes to the system based upon faulty data (Chen, 1994).

The final stage is "act," but the CNS needs to keep in mind that PDCA is a circular model when used for quality improvement (American Society for Quality, n.d.) (Figure 8-8). At this point, the CNS and colleagues need to decide whether to adjust, abandon, or adopt the change. If data reveals that the change has positively affected the system, the group will need to devise strategies for establishing this change as fixed.

The final activities should include updating policies and procedures and informing key personnel of the changes. The CNS may also want to give thought to potential ways to continuously improve the process. The group may also want to apply PDCA to other areas of the process in order to further affect quality measures.

FOCUS-PDCA and PDCA are popular methods for quality improvement endeavors. CNSs will find this method useful and user-friendly as it provides a context for planned change based upon careful analysis. Changing systems and processes takes time and FOCUS-PDCA is a careful, deliberate strategy. Certainly there are aspects of patient care that can be swiftly and effectively changed without engaging in PDCA; however, it is very useful for correcting and improving processes based upon clear understanding that has arisen from careful, informed analysis.

The Six Sigma Revolution: A Measure of Quality Striving for Perfection

Six Sigma is a disciplined, data-driven approach and method for eliminating defects in any process (iSixSigma, 2009), including health care. It is an improvement process

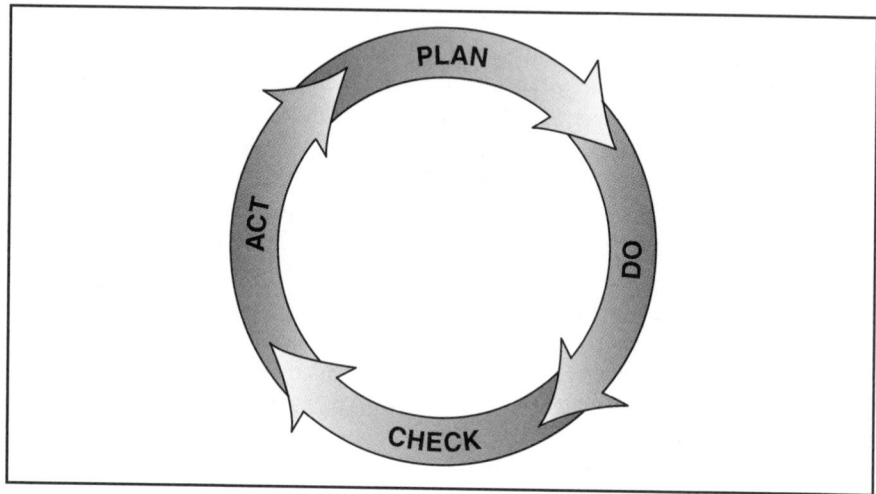

Figure 8-8   The plan-do-check-act cycle is a four-step model for carrying out change. Just as a cycle has no end, the PDCA cycle should be repeated again and again for continuous improvement.

Source: Reprinted with permission from ASQ Quality Press. © 2005 American Society for Quality.

that is committed to excellence. Six Sigma originated in Motorola in the mid-1980s, and soon other industries, including General Electric, Allied Signal, Sony, Motorola, and Polaroid, became users as well (Chowdhury, 2001).

Six Sigma focuses on eliminating defects by reducing variability. Sigma is the Greek letter used to describe variability as standard deviation (Figure 8-9). The "six" standard deviation refers to the sixth standard deviation or a 99.9996% success rate (Chowdhury, 2001), or not more than 3.4 defects per million opportunities (iSixSigma, 2009). As the name implies, Six Sigma relies heavily on the quantitative analysis of data.

Six Sigma methodology is appealing to the healthcare industry because of its emphasis on variation or error reduction. Hospitals and healthcare systems continue to display variability in outcomes that contribute to patient dissatisfaction and inefficiencies in processes and outputs (Woodward, 2005). Perioperative services are using Six Sigma to

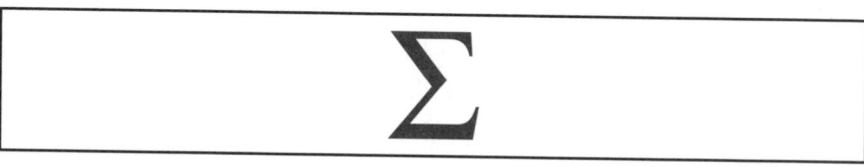

Figure 8-9   Greek capital letter sigma.

improve operating room turnover time (Adams, Warner, Hubbard, & Goulding, 2004) and reduce surgical case delays (Anonymous, 2004), while other hospitals are using Six Sigma to reduce the incidence of ventilator-associated pneumonia (VAP) (Simmons-Trant, Cenek, Hockenbury, & Litwille, 2004), reduce the mean time from emergency department arrival to cardiac catheterization laboratory (Porter, 2005), and improve quality and patient safety (Nimtz-Rush & Thompson, 2008).

There are critics of Six Sigma concerned about how a quality improvement process with its roots in manufacturing can be applied to the healthcare industry. However, Six Sigma demands identification of specification limits that define acceptable performance. Healthcare systems are not always inclined to evaluate performance within tight, prescriptive constraints despite the fact that continuous improvement requires accurate measurements. Lazarus (2003) asserts that Six Sigma is adaptable to the development of best clinical practices and that the language of Six Sigma will benefit healthcare consumers.

Improving an existing process using Six Sigma methodology follows a five-step analysis: (1) define the opportunity, (2) measure to establish baseline performance; (3) analyze data and critical elements; (4) improve the new process; and (5) control the new process (DMAIC) (Adams et al., 2004). DMAIC (pronounced *duh-may-ick*) (iSixSigma, 2003) uses statistical analysis to find the most defective part of the process under scrutiny and applies rigorous control procedures to maintain improvement (Lazarus, 2003). A second key methodology in Six Sigma is DMADV, representing: define, measure, analyze, design, and verify. DMADV is used to create new product or process designs (iSixSigma, 2009).

Six Sigma creates new positions within the organization. These positions have names taken from the martial arts. A black belt is a team leader. This position is full time and is responsible for the DMAIC processes. Green belts are trained in Six Sigma and can run initiatives, but they continue to have their full-time position responsibilities within the organization. Change agents are facilitators who move a group through the change process using change acceleration process and work-out tools.

Change acceleration process identifies change barriers and works through them. Work-out is a process that brings approximately 10 to 12 key people together for 4 to 8 hours to concentrate on reaching the best decision for improvement or change (Adams et al., 2004). The basic working premise of Six Sigma is $Q \times A = E$ (Chowdhury, 2001). This formula denotes that the effectiveness of the results (E) is equal to the quality of the solution (Q) times the acceptance of the idea (A).

There is a substantial amount of training involved in Six Sigma, and it is not a trivial commitment. As an example, Adams et al. (2004) describe the education commitment within their institution after having committed to using Six Sigma as 7 days for executive leadership training, 4 days for managers, 35 days for green belts, 7 days for change agents, and 21 days for team planning and training. When these days are distributed across a significant number of employees, the start-up costs are high.

Six Sigma is an increasingly popular methodology for quality improvement. Healthcare institutions are looking for opportunities to reduce care process outcomes variances more than those provided in traditional quality improvement models. The published results of Six Sigma are impressive and suggest that CNSs should at least be comfortable with the basic underlying premises of this method as their exposures to Six Sigma may increase.

LEAN Thinking

LEAN is a process improvement strategy designed to eliminate unnecessary steps and redundancies that are not critical to quality for the user. Within the healthcare enterprise, this user, or customer, may be the nurse, physician, patient, or other key stakeholder that is the direct beneficiary of the particular service. It is common to find LEAN combined with Six Sigma methodology. For example, LEAN Six Sigma (LSS) may offer benefits to the purchasing departments of healthcare systems; although, the tools and methodologies associated with LSS may have applicability to any number of healthcare processes (Barlow, 2008). LEAN is meant to eliminate waste, identified as waste in inventory, overproduction, waiting, transportation, defects, excess motion or walking, and processing. Underutilizing employee skills is also considered a waste (Blecker-Shelly & Mortensen, 2008).

Rapid Cycle Improvement Model (RCIM)

The rapid cycle improvement model builds on organizations' desires to accelerate the change process in order to make rapid improvements in outcomes. The model is also referred to as rapid cycle tests (RCTs) of change (Pape et al., 2005) or rapid cycle change (RCC) methodology (Bisaillon, Kelloway, LeBlanc, Pageau, & Woloshyn, 2005). RCC is based on the premise that traditional methods of quality improvement are too slow, fail to engage people, and inadequately utilize current evidence (Bisaillon et al., 2005).

This accelerated improvement method asserts that if an organization wants to make rapid gains in quality, it must be able to answer three questions: (1) What does the organization want to accomplish? (2) How will change be recognized as an improvement and how will it be measured? and (3) What changes can be made that will result in an improvement? (Martin, 2003).

RCTs of change processes are often used in conjunction with DMAIC steps. The basic process is to follow the initial DMAIC steps and after analyzing the problem or gap, use RCTs to improve the system (Pape et al., 2005). RCTs may also be used in partnership with PDSA as a component of the "do" step. If results are positive, the improvements should be controlled and perpetuated. If results are not positive, or not positive enough, the action plan requires revision.

RCC can be used in a variety of clinical venues. It has been used successfully as a process for improving medication use systems by addressing nurses' distractions during medication administration (Pape et al., 2005). It has also been used to establish best practices in stroke care by incorporating small improvement changes, measuring results, and using the measured successes to facilitate further improvements in stroke care practices for both patients and care providers (Bisaillon et al., 2005).

RCIM has been an effective process for increasing the use of the American College of Cardiology's *Acute Myocardial Infarction Guidelines Applied in Practice* quality initiatives' evidence-based guidelines (Montoye et al., 2003) and has offered a strategy for decreasing the incidence of pneumothorax in a neonatal intensive care unit (Walker, Shoemaker, Riddle, Crane, & Clark, 2002). Martin (2003) utilized RCIM methods to improve the accuracy of patient identification at a pediatric hospital that was confronted with significant numbers of patients with similar or same last names creating opportunities for medical errors.

Walker et al. (2002) offer an excellent clinical example of affecting positive clinical changes using RCIM. After reviewing the published evidence on strategies for pneumothorax reduction in preterm infants, Walker et al. developed a policy to electively intubate all infants less than 28 weeks gestational age in the delivery room and administer a surfactant extract. A multidisciplinary team was formed and a rapid cycle for learning and improvement was instituted.

The target measurement of interest, pneumothorax, was established at an incidence reduction of 50%. The group devised a one-page data collection sheet. Other clinical plans of care were incorporated into the study and other endpoints were established. Study results revealed a decrease in the incidence of pneumothorax and an improvement in the time frame for pneumothorax diagnosis. There was also a reduction in study group mortality rates as compared to the control. Walker et al. (2002) assert that evidence-based practice changes can improve outcomes. RCIM methods, in partnership with evidence-based practice, were offered as strategies for improving select morbidity and mortality outcomes.

IHI (2006) offers tips for testing changes that should be considered when using RCTs. The suggestions include staying ahead of the tests based upon the possible findings that were identified in the study phase of PDSA efforts. Other recommendations include working with people who want to work on the project, picking changes that are simple and reasonable, scaling down the breadth of the tests whenever possible, and preparing to eliminate a change if it is not improving the measure of interest (IHI).

Positive Deviance Approach

Positive deviance (PD) describes uncommon, beneficial health behaviors that some people already practice. Positive deviant behavior is atypical and confers benefits to people who practice it as compared to the rest of the community (Marsh, Schroeder, Dearden, Sternin, & Sternin, 2004) without any difference in available resources (Bertels & Sternin, 2003). In the 1990s, the PD approach was used to influence the nutritional status of children. Since this time, it has been used to affect changes via a variety of projects including the eating strategies of low-income pregnant women (Fowles, Hendricks, & Walker, 2005), breastfeeding in rural Vietnam (Dearden et al., 2002), and female genital cutting (Centre for Development and Population Activities, 1999).

PD addresses problems that require behavioral or social change. The approach is consistent with Six Sigma because it provides a design that Six Sigma projects can amplify and replicate (Bertels & Sternin, 2003). For Six Sigma to be successful in reducing outcomes variability, Six Sigma projects must be replicable across entire organizations. Replication is challenging and yet, is crucial to benefiting fully from Six Sigma project efforts. The PD approach offers a way for Six Sigma organizations to spread successes.

PD comprises six steps: define, determine, discover, design, discern, and disseminate (Bertels & Sternin, 2003). The focus of PD is on behavior replication. Rather than targeting the acquisition of knowledge related to why people behave in the ways that they do, PD demonstrates that it is possible to find successful solutions before all the underlying causes are addressed. Marsh et al. (2004) identify six steps to the PD approach with the community as an active partner. The approach includes:

1. Developing case definitions
2. Locating four to six people who have managed to achieve an unanticipated good outcome despite their high level of risk
3. Interviewing and observing these deviants to uncover the atypical behaviors or enabling factors that might explain the positive outcome
4. Analyzing the findings to confirm that the behaviors really are atypical and are available to the people who would benefit by adopting the behaviors
5. Designing activities to change behaviors and to encourage the community to adopt the new behaviors
6. Monitoring performance and evaluate outcomes

Marsh et al. (2004) suggest that there are three important processes that occur in response to the PD approach. The first is the positive reaction of community members when they learn that they are doing something right rather than hearing only negative feedback. The second process involves information seeking and gathering to identify the positive behaviors that may be spread and the factors that encourage this spread. The third process is the actual behavior change.

Dearden et al. (2002) provide a good example of the PD process as it relates to exclusive breastfeeding in a rural Vietnam village. The goal of the project was to improve breastfeeding practices. Examination of Vietnamese breastfeeding practices revealed that women who return to work are confronted with barriers that hinder exclusive breastfeeding. Data were collected and women were grouped into (1) those who were not exclusively breastfeeding and had returned to work; (2) women who were exclusively breastfeeding and had returned to work; (3) women who were not exclusively breastfeeding and had not yet returned to work; and (4) women who were exclusively breastfeeding and had not yet returned to work.

The women in the second group were identified as the positive deviants. These women were working and yet were able to maintain exclusive breastfeeding while other women in similar circumstances were not exclusively breastfeeding. The researchers explored the differences between these groups of women and determined the facilitators and barriers to exclusive breastfeeding. Based upon these findings, the researchers offered suggestions for programmatic changes that might increase the incidence of exclusive breastfeeding. The focus of the researchers' activities was to identify the experiences of the positive deviances in an effort to promote this deviant or abnormal behavior within the community of interest.

Sternin (2002) defines positive deviance as "a departure, difference, or deviation from the norm resulting in a positive outcome" (p. 1). Sternin sees this deviance as proof that there are viable solutions to today's complex problems that can be utilized before addressing all the factors underlying the problem. In other words, the PD approach offers hope. Sternin offers this assertion within the context of childhood malnutrition and points out that these children need immediate help if they are to survive and thrive. These children do not have time to wait for problem analysis; rather, they need immediate solutions. PD offers these solutions. Sternin states:

> A critical component of the definition of "positive deviants" is that PD individuals have exactly the same resource base as their non-positive deviant neighbors. Hence, whatever they are doing, whatever resources they are using to achieve their successful outcomes, are by definition, accessible to their neighbors. By identifying the special beliefs and practices of the positive deviants and then making them accessible to the community, a *demonstrably successful* strategy is provided which can be acted upon *today*. (p. 2)

Sternin (2002) comments that if a project's objective is social or behavioral change and if there are some individuals exhibiting the behavior within the community, then PD is a useful tool. The advantage of PD is the sustainability that occurs because the resources required for change already exist within the community. In other words, external resources are not required. Positive deviants are successful with the resources that are available to them illustrating that the fundamental structure of PD is the belief that there is "wisdom and untapped resources" within the community of interest (Sternin, 2002, p. 6).

PD offers opportunities to improve outcomes and to sustain these changes within the healthcare system just as it offers opportunities within communities. Handwashing behaviors, best practice implementation, infection control practices, and nursing documentation are examples of healthcare concerns that fundamentally rely on behavior and social changes. If there are units within a hospital or nurses employed on a particular unit whose practices are associated with uncommon but positive outcomes, these individuals may be identified as positive deviants.

There are several examples illustrating the potential impact of PD on problem solving in health care. A recently awarded Pioneer Grant by the Robert Wood Johnson Foundation (2008) for a project targeting methicillin-resistant *Staphylococcus aureus* infections in hospitals by implementing the PD approach illustrates the importance of and interest in the PD approach for quality improvement projects within the healthcare system.

Cusano (2006) describes using the PD approach to improving medication use processes for patients at time of discharge and transfer. This medication reconciliation project included identification of positively deviant staff and practices related to those positively deviant patients who had no problems with their medical regimen after discharge. During the course of the study, the researchers identified that the uncommon but successful practices included following up discharge with a telephone call, using written instructions with specific information for complex regimens, providing instructions to caregivers, as well as other strategies. These practices were shared in small-group meetings with other professionals, and 6 months later the PD team found that patients were 66% more likely to use their medications without troubles (Cusano, 2006).

Of course, one of the challenges of successful endeavors is to figure out strategies for replicating the success across an entire organization. Difficulties duplicating successful results are the result of a lack in communication, transferability, processes and systems, and incentives (Bertels & Sternin, 2003). Six Sigma relies on the successful implementation and spread of changes that have been demonstrated as positive and useful via pilot studies or rapid change testing. If successes are not replicated, Six Sigma is ineffective as an improvement process. The PD approach may help to facilitate the spread of the improvements. Six Sigma pilots can be treated as positive deviants and then magnified. The potential connection between PD and Six Sigma may be useful to the CNS employed by an organization who is using either or both of these approaches to QI. A basic understanding of the two methodologies and their interconnectedness may be helpful as CNSs begin to learn and implement both processes.

Bertels and Sternin (2003) caution that benchmarking and PD have similar objectives but that there are profound differences between the two concepts. They point out that the PD approach recognizes successful and accessible behaviors as critical while benchmarking targets efficiency and effectiveness. PD attends to the context of a process, and benchmarking applies the principles and attributes of an effective process as enacted by a different entity.

Finally, benchmarking focuses on opportunities external to the organization that may be borrowed and applied; PD looks for successful ideas from within the organization. Bertels and Sternin (2003) appreciate the benefits of benchmarking as a helpful process when organizations are seeking to redesign or duplicate results but note that benchmarking is more applicable to situations that require unconventional ideas; for example, thinking that is "outside the box." Positive deviance works best when an organization is looking for results that can be nurtured and replicated.

In addition to using the PD approach to improving clinical outcomes, PD may also be useful to improve norms in the workplace, including healthcare organizations. Spreitzer and Sonenshein, as shared by DeGroat (2004), describe PD in workplace situations in which people conduct themselves honorably and with extreme excellence. They relate PD to positive organizational scholarship (POS), which focuses on workplace virtuosity and is consistent with the PD emphasis on positive behaviors.

CNSs may find the PD-POS connection useful as they attempt to positively influence problems in nursing work environments including laterally violent behaviors or poor end-of-shift reports. PD may provide a method for exploring the positive deviants who nurture young, inexperienced staff members or who provide excellent, timely, and succinct end-of-shift reports. PD may be a wiser and more effective approach than telling staff what it is that they are doing that is wrong and inappropriate. The PD approach offers an alternative means of influencing behavioral and social outcomes within healthcare organizations and in clinical practice.

Failure Mode and Effects Analysis (FMEA)

Failure mode and effects analysis (FMEA) is a proactive process focusing on predicting the negative outcomes of human, system, and machine failures (Senders, 2004). FMEA was created as an industrial tool and was developed by reliability engineers to evaluate complex processes in a systematic fashion, to identify the elements that may cause harm, and to prioritize remedial measures (Apkon, Leonard, Probst, DeLizio, & Vitale, 2004). FMEA is based on the idea that the amount of risk associated with a process, system, machine malfunction, or human behavior relates not only to the probability of a failure occurrence but also to the degree of severity of the failure and the ease with which failure might be noticed and addressed before causing harm. FMEA uses a variety of information sources to determine failure rates and then predicts the behavior of a system in the event of failure (Apkon et al.).

FMEA has been used in health care to improve the safety of intravenous drug infusions (Apkon et al., 2004) and to reduce vulnerabilities in healthcare systems before mistakes or near misses occur (DeRosier, Stahhandske, Bagian, & Nudell, 2002; Institute for Safe Medication Practices, 2001), as well as addressing other healthcare systems concerns. Although it has existed for a long time in engineering circles, there is relatively little published about FMEA in the healthcare literature (Senders, 2004). Root cause analysis (RCA) is much more common in health care simply because it is a reactive approach to understanding the intervening mechanisms associated with adverse incidents. RCA, as compared to FMEA, is a reactive approach that takes place after a negative event. Senders (2004) predicts that FMEA usage will increase in medicine particularly given The Joint Commission's requirement compelling organizations to select at least one high-risk process for annual proactive risk assessment.

The Department of Veterans Affairs (VA) National Center for Patient Safety (NCPS) has devised a hybrid risk analysis system that uses five steps to proactively evaluate a healthcare process. This hybrid model, Health Care Failure Mode and Effect Analysis (HFMEA), uses an interdisciplinary team, process flow diagramming, and a unique scoring matrix and decision tree to identify and scrutinize potential vulnerabilities (DeRosier et al., 2002). NCPS has a root cause analysis process in place that responds to actual events and near misses in order to improve patient safety.

NCPS recognized that the VA system also needed a prospective system to further their patient safety improvement agenda. NCPS reviewed the opportunities of the FMEA system but found that the definitions and scoring required revision so as to be more applicable to healthcare processes. Ultimately NCPS modified a system in use by the National Advisory Committee on Microbiological Criteria for Foods for the U.S. Department of Agriculture and, in combination with concepts used from

FMEA, Hazard Analysis and Critical Control Point (HACCP), and root cause analysis (RCA), developed HFMEA.

HFMEA is based upon five steps:

1. Define the high-risk or high-vulnerability area as the HFMEA topic.
2. Assemble the multidisciplinary team making certain to include a subject matter expert, advisor, and leader.
3. Create and confirm a process flow diagram to visually depict the steps of the process.
4. Analyze the possible or potential failure modes for each of the graphically identified subprocesses and determine the severity and probability of each potential failure using the Hazard Scoring Matrix.
5. Develop actions and outcome measures for each failure mode cause (DeRosier et al., 2002).

Similar to FMEA, HFMEA involves the use of a numeric severity rating scale. FMEA uses severity, probability, and hazard scores to rank items for action (Institute for Safe Medication Practices, 2005).

FMEA and RCA processes do improve healthcare outcomes, and may be particularly useful for improving patient safety systems. Senders (2004) labels *FMEA* and *RCA* acronyms as "mantras of modern risk management" (p. 249). It is obvious that simply because a potential error is identified and associated with quantified risk, this does not guarantee a cause–effect relationship between one specific error and one specific injury. However, as Senders points out, using FMEA and RCA methodologies may also serve as protective mechanisms against lawsuits by demonstrating that the organization was working diligently to prevent avoidable patient injuries.

CNSs need basic familiarity with FMEA and RCA processes and, in some instances, require a more thorough understanding in order to participate in these activities as a fully engaged member of a multidisciplinary committee. CNSs may be more familiar with RCAs, particularly CNSs employed in acute care settings, because of the linkage between RCAs and sentinel event reporting requirements through the Joint Commission (2007). The Joint Commission defines a sentinel event as an

> unexpected occurrence involving death or serious physical or psychological injury, or the risk thereof. Serious injury specifically includes loss of limb or function. The phrase, "or the risk thereof" includes any process variation for which a recurrence would carry a significant chance of a serious adverse outcome. Such events are called "sentinel" because they signal the need for immediate investigation and response. (2007, ¶ 2–3)

The Joint Commission requires an analysis of the root causes of sentinel events and an action plan. However, this is a retrospective review that may improve outcomes for future patients but does not work to prevent the event from occurring in the first place. FMEA may assist by providing a prospective analysis of risk thereby enhancing improved outcomes management and measurement. It is very likely that CNSs will play increasing roles in working with FMEA and RCA groups as healthcare professionals make environments safer for patients and for employees.

Flowcharts and Diagrams: Visual Tools for Successful Outcomes Improvements

The use of flowcharts and diagrams as pictorial representations of a process is a common practice in QI initiatives. To improve outcomes, CNSs must understand the processes leading to the outcome. Many people grasp material best when information is presented using a variety of modalities. Graphic representations of processes and group discussions that "fill in" gaps and ensure accuracy in the diagrammed steps are very important to multidisciplinary QI efforts. There is an array of helpful process tools including flowcharts, cause–effect or fishbone diagrams (also known as Ishikawa diagram), histograms, and Pareto diagrams (IHI, 2006).

In general, providing that the process under scrutiny is not too complicated, flowcharts can be user-friendly and efficient. It may also serve as a blueprint for the activities of a group. There are common symbols used in flowcharts. Microsoft Word has a flowchart option in its AutoShapes feature. Each shape is tagged with an identifier making it easy for the novice flowchart creator to depict simple processes (Figure 8-10). There are also flowchart software programs available for purchase.

Cause–effect diagrams or Ishikawa diagrams are useful to explore sources of variability within a process (Figure 8-11). This diagram appears as a fish bone skeleton. The name of the problem of interest is on the right side of the diagram at the end of the main "backbone" of the fish. The possible causes of the problem are pictorially represented as bones off the backbone.

In general, there should be enough substance to the problem that there are approximately three to six main categories of causative factors; otherwise, the fish bone diagram is superfluous. The main bones off the backbone may be further elaborated upon to give more bones to the skeleton. Generally, the practical depth of detail is four to five levels of bone fragments or else the chart becomes too cumbersome (Vanderbilt University, School of Engineering, n.d.)

Pareto diagrams depict the variables that contribute to a particular outcome or overall effect (Figure 8-12). The variables are arranged in the order of their contribution to the outcome of interest as a histogram or bar graph (IHI, 2006). Identifying the influences responsible for the greatest effects assists team members with making decisions as to which variables should be addressed in terms of costs and benefits. The contributions of the variables should be determined in a rigorous, objective fashion rather than through opinion gathering.

CNSs may find it useful to incorporate diagramming and flowcharting activities into group discussions, staff meetings, and multidisciplinary committee work. Visual aids are useful in establishing a common perspective and facilitate communication. There are times when problems become self-evident once details are diagrammed.

Standardizing the Language of Nursing

CNSs should be familiar with the progress made toward the electronic health record (EHR) specific to the use of standardized nursing languages. By 2010, all U.S. healthcare events will be electronically recorded, and healthcare organizations

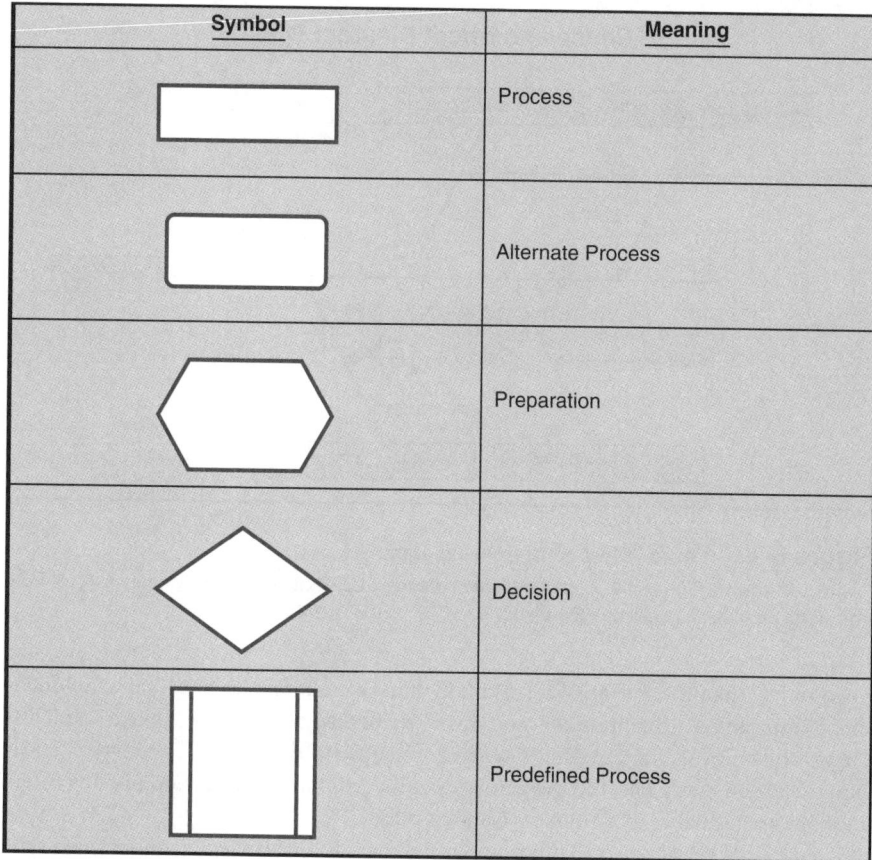

Symbol	Meaning
	Process
	Alternate Process
	Preparation
	Decision
	Predefined Process

Figure 8-10   Select flowchart symbols available on Microsoft Word in Microsoft Office XP Small Business.

will be required to submit data to data banks regarding these events (Lunney, 2006). Sharing data requires a common nursing language such as the nomenclature published by NANDA International, the Nursing Outcomes Classification (NOC), and the Nursing Interventions Classification (NIC). An EHR facilitates data aggregation that encourages knowledge development, including a better understanding of outcomes and quality (Lunney). To examine the quality of nursing care and its associated costs, outcomes and interventions must be connected in the clinical record to the relevant nursing diagnoses (Moorhead & Johnson, 2004).

Using the standardized languages of NANDA, NIC, and NOC (NNN) differs from using the customary nursing process. NNN compel data interpretation rather than data collection. Patient outcomes and nursing interventions are in a standardized

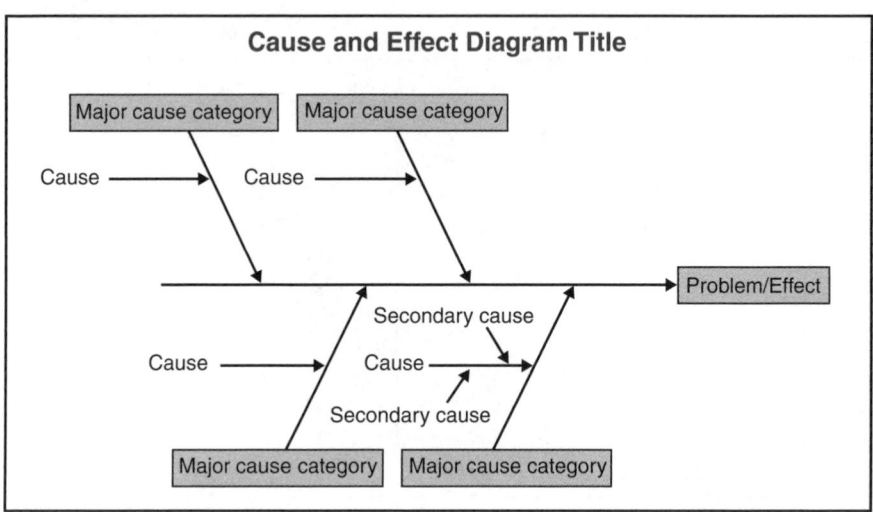

Figure 8-11 Cause–effect or fishbone diagram.
Source: Microsoft Office. (2009). Cause and effect diagram. U.S. Units. Retrieved January 6, 2009, from http://office.microsoft.com/enus/templates/TC010265451033.aspx

form rather than the narrative forms many nurses are familiar with. Narrative documentation can be difficult to interpret owing to inconsistencies, inadequacies, and different style forms that make drawing comparisons difficult. NNN in an EHR supports consistency because the names used for patient outcomes and nursing interventions are available to all nurses (Lunney, 2006).

Lunney (2006) suggests that both novice nurses and advanced beginners are capable of proficiently learning and using NNN. More experienced nurses may need encouragement to document and think differently than the status quo. As the EHR is implemented into the healthcare system, nurses will become more accountable for their diagnoses, outcomes, and interventions and the impact these processes will have on cost and quality. Educators will need to make certain that nursing curriculums include NNN so that nurses learn how to collect data, rule in or rule out diagnoses, and perform complex nursing interventions (Lunney).

Moorhead and Johnson (2004) note that NNN is built on expert opinion that requires validation. Clinical testing and examination of the linkages between outcomes and diagnosis are consistent with the outcomes chosen for that diagnosis in the clinical setting. Moorhead and Johnson identify several issues that need to be addressed to eliminate obstacles to evaluating linkages and conducting effectiveness studies. The posed concerns that require study include identifying what a diagnostic-specific outcome describes, determining the pertinent outcomes for each nursing diagnosis, establishing the information set that should be available for analysis beyond the linkages, and devising and creating clinical information storage systems.

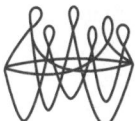

NATIONAL PATIENT SAFETY FOUNDATION® (NPSF)

What You Can Do to Make Healthcare Safer:

A Consumer Fact Sheet

If a medical error occurs, it is often a result of a series of small failures that are individually not big enough to cause an accident, but combined can result in an error. Patients can ensure a safer experience with the health care system by being involved and informed about their treatment. Improving patient safety requires continuous learning and constant communication between caregivers, organizations, and patients. Everyone has a role in patient safety, and everyone will benefit from its successes.

What can consumers do to make sure they have a safer experience with the health care system? NPSF suggests these steps to help make your health care experience safer:

Become a more informed health care consumer:
- Seek information about illnesses or conditions that affect you.
- Research options and possible treatment plans.
- Choose a doctor, clinic, pharmacy, and hospital experienced in the type of care you require.
- Ask questions of your doctor, nurse, pharmacist, or benefits plan coordinator.
- Seek more than one opinion.

Keep track of your history
- Write down your medical history including any medical conditions you have, illnesses, immunizations, allergies, hospitalizations, all medications and dietary supplements you're taking, and any reactions or sensitivities you've experienced.
- Write down the names and phone numbers of your doctors, clinics, and pharmacies for quick and easy reference.

Work with your doctor and other health care professionals as a team
- Share your health history with your care team.
- Share up-to-date information about your care with everyone who's treating you.
- Make sure you understand the care and treatment you'll be receiving. Ask questions if you're not clear on your care.
- Pay attention. If something doesn't seem right, call it to the attention of your doctor or health care professional.
- Discuss any concerns about your safety with your health care team.

Involve a family member or friend in your care
- If you're not able to observe or participate fully in your care, ask a family member or friend to assist. They can accompany you on appointments or stay with you, help you ask questions, understand care instructions and suggest your preferences.

Follow the treatment plan agreed upon by you and your doctor
- Be sure you receive all instructions verbally and in writing that you can read and understand. Ask questions about any instructions that are confusing or unclear.
- Take medications exactly as prescribed.
- Use home medical equipment and supplies only as instructed.
- Report anything unusual to your doctor.

National Patient Safety Foundation - 1120 MASS MoCA Way, North Adams, MA 01247
(413) 663-8000   www.npsf.org   @2003

Figure 8-12   Sample of NPSF patient teaching resource available for download.

CNSs with a particular interest in nursing language and development will find Nursing Language in Nursing Knowledge Systems (NLINKS) informative. This international organization has a mission to "advance the development, testing, and refinement of language and informatics in nursing knowledge systems" (Nursing Language in Nursing Knowledge Systems, n.d.). NLINKs was approved at the NANDA 2000 conference. NLINKs has a concept analysis center charged with providing Web-based written protocols, consultation, and resources for concept analysis that international nurses can use for language development that is meaningful and culturally relevant (Nursing Language in Nursing Knowledge Systems).

Another good source of information is the Web site of the University of Iowa College of Nursing's (n.d.) Center for Nursing Classification and Clinical Effectiveness. The center's home page offers information about NIC and NOC and has resources for purchase, translations, and reports available for review.

Conclusion

CNSs have a critical role to play in outcomes measurement and management. NACNS (2004) has developed a model for CNS practice that is based upon the belief that CNS practice is "consistently targeted toward achieving quality, cost-effective *outcomes* through patient/client care, by influencing the practice of other nurses and nursing personnel, and by influencing the healthcare organization to support nursing practice" (p. 18). The crux of CNS practice is influencing processes, organizations, and systems to achieve desired outcomes.

Urden (1999) identified outcome evaluation as an essential component for CNS practice. In this classic piece, Urden describes five types of outcomes: clinical, psychosocial, functional, fiscal, and satisfaction. It may be that safety is another outcome worthy of separate distinction. Certainly the current emphasis on patient safety, catapulted to the forefront of public attention with the published report *To Err Is Human* (Institute of Medicine, 1999), has become a critical quality indicator in health care.

CNSs need to recognize that there is a partnership between outcomes, quality improvement processes, and evidence-based practice. Outcomes measures provide indicators of quality that may be improved through the use of systematically applied evidence. In addition to using outcomes measures to demonstrate quality improvements within systems and processes, CNSs are challenged to demonstrate their impact on patients/families, nurses, and organizations by using outcomes measures that are sensitive to CNSs' unique contributions.

Selecting measurable and meaningful outcomes is not an easy task. It can be challenging to discern the "best" outcome measure out of the plethora of potential outcomes that exist related to a specific aspect of health care. Garnering input from multidisciplinary teams can be very helpful. CNSs should use the established resources that are available to them from the exceptional foundations and organizations that have made outcomes improvement their reveille call. Tools from expert safety and quality organizations including but not limited to the Institute for Safe Medication

Practices, NPSD, IHI, the Joint Commission, and the Agency for Healthcare Research and Quality, and benchmarking opportunities like NDNQI provide valid and reliable measures of quality. As CNSs use these tools to improve systems of care, they should also consider contributing to the concept analyses so important to nursing language so as to eventually facilitate the creation of powerful databases obtained through EHR data collection activities and research studies. Outcomes management and QI can be overwhelming to new CNSs, but starting with unit projects or small-scale department activities can be a good way to develop a repertoire of QI process tools.

References

Adams, R., Warner, P., Hubbard, B., & Goulding, T. (2004). Decreasing turnaround time between general surgery cases: A Six Sigma initiative. *Journal of Nursing Administration, 34*(3), 140–148.

Agency for Healthcare Research and Quality. (2000). *Outcomes Research.* Fact Sheet (AHRQ Publication No. 00-P011). Retrieved January 12, 2009, from http://www.ahrq.gov/clinic/outfact.htm

Aiken, L. H., Clarke, S. P., Sloane, D. M., Sochalski, J., & Silber, J. H. (2002). Hospital nurse staffing and patient mortality, nurse burnout, and job dissatisfaction. *Journal of the American Medical Association, 288,* 1987–1993.

American Association of Colleges of Nursing (AACN). (2004, October). *Position statement on the practice doctorate in nursing.* Retrieved January 7, 2009, from http://www.aacn.nche.edu/DNP/pdf/DNP.pdf

American Nurses Association (ANA). (1995). *The nursing care report card for acute care.* Washington, DC: Author.

American Nurses Association (ANA). (1999). Nursing-sensitive quality indicators for acute care settings and ANA's safety and quality initiative. Retrieved January 12, 2009, from http://www.nursingworld.org/MainMenuCategories/ThePracticeofProfessional Nursing/PatientSafetyQuality/NDNQI/Research/QIforAcuteCareSettings.aspx

American Nurses Association (ANA). (2002). *The National Database of Nursing Quality Indicators NDNQI. Frequently asked questions.* Retrieved January 7, 2009, from http://www.nursingquality.org/FAQPage.aspx#2

American Nurses Association (ANA). (2009a). *The national database. About the database.* Retrieved April 4, 2009, from http://www.nursingworld.org/MainMenuCategories/ ThePracticeofProfessionalNursing/PatientSafetyQuality/NDNQI/NDNQI_1.aspx

American Nurses Association (ANA). (2009b). How to join NDNQI. Retrieved January 12, 2009, from http://www.nursingworld.org/MainMenuCategories/ThePracticeof ProfessionalNursing/PatientSafetyQuality/NDNQI/NDNQI_1/HowtoJoin.aspx

American Society for Quality (n.d.). *Quality tools: Project planning and implementing tools.* Retrieved January 7, 2009, from http://www.asq.org/learn-about-quality/project-planning-tools/overview/pdca-cycle.html

Anonymous. (2004). Six Sigma gives leaders tools for improving processes in OR. *OR Manager, 20*, 6. Retrieved January 7, 2009, from CINAHL Database of Nursing and Allied Health Literature.

Apkon, M., Leonard, J., Probst, L., DeLizio, L., & Vitale, R. (2004). Design of a safer approach to intravenous drug infusions: Failure model effects analysis. *Quality and Safety in Health Care, 13*, 265–271.

Bader, M. K., Palmer, S., Stalcup, C., & Shaver, T. (2002). Using a FOCUS-PDCA quality improvement model for applying the severe traumatic brain injury guidelines to practice: Process and outcomes (Document number 4C). *On-Line Journal of Knowledge Synthesis for Nursing*. Retrieved January 7, 2009, from http://www.stti.org/articles/cc_doc4c.pdf

Barlow, R. D. (2008). Erasing the stigma of Six Sigma and LEAN principles. *Healthcare Purchasing News, 8*, 42–45. Retrieved February 1, 2009, from http://www.hpnonline.com/inside/2008-08/0808-PS-sixsigma.html

Bertels, T., & Sternin, J. (2003). Replicating results and managing knowledge. In T. Bertels (Ed.), *Rath & Strong's Six Sigma leadership handbook* (pp. 450–457). Hoboken, NJ: John Wiley & Sons.

Bisaillon, S., Kelloway, L., LeBlanc, K., Pageau, N., & Woloshyn, N. (2005). Best practices in stroke care. *Canadian Nurse, 101*(8), 25–29.

Blecker-Shelly, D., & Mortensen, J. (2008). An introduction to LEAN. *Continuing Education Topics and Issues*. Retrieved February 1, 2009, from http://findarticles.com/p/articles/mi_6944/is_3_10/ai_n31007007?tag=content;col1

Caldwell, C. (2006). *Healthcare Financial Management*. Retrieved February 1, 2009, from http://www.asq.org/perl/search-Google-Mini.pl?q=cache:y_flp4p9-dw:http://www.asq.org/pdf/articles/lean-ss-hfm.pdf+Caldwell+Healthcare+Financial+Management&site=my_collection&output=xml_no_dtd&client=my_collection&access=p&proxystylesheet=my_collection&oe=UTF-8

Centers for Medicare & Medicaid Services (CMS). (2008). *Hospital-acquired conditions*. Retrieved January 12, 2009, from http://www.cms.hhs.gov/HospitalAcqCond/06_Hospital-Acquired_Conditions.asp

Centre for Development and Population Activities. (1999). *Ending female genital cutting: A positive deviance approach in Egypt. Promoting Women in Development (PROWID) program*. Retrieved January 7, 2009, from http://www.positivedeviance.org/projects/egypfgc/egypfgc_rep2.pdf

Chen, H. (1994). *Theory-driven evaluations*. Newbury Park, CA: Sage.

Chowdhury, S. (2001). *The power of Six Sigma*. Chicago, IL: Dearborn Trade.

Cusano, A. J. (2006). *Use of the positive deviance approach to improve reconciliation of medications and patients medication management after hospital discharge: The experience of Waterbury Hospital (Connecticut)*. Retrieved January 7, 2009, from http://www.positivedeviance.org/projects/waterbury/waterbury_narrative_final.pdf

Dearden, K., Quan, L. N., Do, M., Marsh, D. R., Pachón, H., Schroeder, D. G., et al. (2002). Work outside the home is the primary barrier to exclusive breastfeeding in rural

Viet Nam: Insights from mothers who exclusively breastfed and worked. *Food and Nutrition Bulletin, 23*(4), 99–106.

DeGroat, B. (2004, April 7). Understanding the impact of positive deviance in work organizations. *Michigan in the News—Stephen M. Ross School of Business.* Retrieved January 7, 2009, from http://www.bus.umich.edu/NewsRoom/ArticleDisplay.asp?news_id=2925

DeRosier, J., Stalhandske, E., Bagian, J., & Nudell, T. (2002). Using health care failure mode and effect analysis: The VA National Center for Patient Safety's prospective risk analysis system. *Journal on Quality Improvement, 28*(3), 248–267.

Duffy, J. R., & Korniewicz, D. (2002). *Quality indicators: Outcomes measurement using the ANA Safety and Quality Indicators.* ANA Continuing Education. Retrieved January 7, 2009, from http://nursingworld.org/mods/archive/mod72/ceomfull.htm

Fowles, E. R., Hendricks, J. A., & Walker, L. O. (2005). Identifying healthy eating strategies in low-income pregnant women: Applying a positive deviance model. *Health Care for Women International, 26*(9), 807–820.

Given, B., & Sherwood, P. (2005). Nursing-sensitive patient outcomes: A white paper. *Oncology Nursing Forum, 32*(4), 773–784.

Hospital Quality Alliance (HQA). (2009). *Hospital Quality Alliance hospital quality initiatives.* Retrieved July 2, 2009, from http://www.cms.hhs.gov/HospitalQualityInits/33_HospitalQualityAlliance.asp

Infectious Diseases Society of America. (2008). Medicare adds only one new HAC to the list for non-payment in 2009. *ISDA News, 18*(8). Retrieved January 12, 2009, from http://news.idsociety.org/idsa/issues/2008-08-01/6.html

Institute for Healthcare Improvement (IHI). (2006). *Tips for testing changes.* Retrieved January 7, 2009, from http://www.ihi.org/IHI/Topics/Improvement/ImprovementMethods/HowToImprove/tipfortestingchanges.htm

Institute for Healthcare Improvement (IHI). (2008). 5 Million Lives Campaign. A Getting Started Kit: *Prevent Central Line Infections How-to Guide.* Retrieved January 12, 2009, from http://www.ihi.org/NR/rdonlyres/0AD706AA-0E76-457B-A4B0-78C31A5172D8/0/CentralLInesHowtoGuide.doc

Institute for Healthcare Improvement (IHI). (n.d. 1). *About us.* Retrieved July 2, 2009, from http://www.ihi.org/about

Institute for Healthcare Improvement (IHI). (n.d. 2). *End stage renal disease.* Retrieved January 12, 2009, from http://www.ihi.org/IHI/Topics/ESRD

Institute for Healthcare Improvement (IHI). (n.d. 3) *Implement the central line bundle.* Retrieved January 12, 2009, from http://www.ihi.org/IHI/Topics/CriticalCare/IntensiveCare/Changes/ImplementtheCentralLineBundle.htm

Institute for Healthcare Improvement (IHI). (n.d. 4). *Pareto diagram (IHI tool).* Retrieved January 7, 2009, from http://www.ihi.org/IHI/Topics/Improvement/ImprovementMethods/Tools/Pareto+Diagram.htm

Institute for Safe Medication Practices (ISMP). (2001). *Failure mode and effects analysis (FMEA): A tool to help guide error prevention efforts.* Retrieved January 7, 2009, from http://www.ismp.org/Tools/FMEA.asp

Institute for Safe Medication Practices (ISMP). (2005). *Example of a health care failure mode and effects analysis for IV patient controlled analgesia (PCA).* Retrieved January 7, 2009, from http://www.ismp.org/Tools/FMEAofPCA.pdf

Institute for Safe Medication Practices (ISMP). (2009). *ISMP mission and vision statement.* Retrieved July 2, 2009, from http://www.ismp.org/about/mission.asp

Institute of Medicine. (1999). *To err is human: Building a safer health system.* Washington, DC: National Academies Press.

iSixSigma. (2003). *Dictionary. DMAIC.* Retrieved January 7, 2009, from http://www.isixsigma.com/dictionary/DMAIC-57.htm

iSixSigma. (2009). *Six Sigma—What is Six Sigma?* Retrieved January 7, 2009, from http://www.isixsigma.com/sixsigma/six_sigma.asp

Joint Commission. (2007). *Sentinel events policy and procedure.* Retrieved January 7, 2009, from http://www.jointcommission.org/SentinelEvents/PolicyandProcedures/se_pp.htm

Joint Commission. (2009). *Quality check.* Accessed on January 7, 2009, from http://www.qualitycheck.org

Kleinpell, R., & Gawlinski, A. (2005). Assessing outcomes in advanced practice nursing practice: The use of quality indicators and evidence-based practice. *AACN Clinical Issues, 16*(1), 43–57.

Lazarus, I. (2003, January 1). Six Sigma. Raising the bar. *Managed Healthcare Executive.* Retrieved January 7, 2009, from http://www.managedhealthcareexecutive.com/mhe/article/articleDetail.jsp?id=43331

Leapfrog Group. (2008a). *About us.* Retrieved January 12, 2009, from http://www.leapfroggroup.org/about_us

Leapfrog Group. (2008b). *Home.* Retrieved on January 12, 2009, from http://www.leapfroggroup.org/home

Lunney, M. (2006). Helping nurses use NANDA, NOC, and NIC: Novice to expert. *Journal of Nursing Administration, 36*(3), 118–125.

Marsh, D. R., Schroeder, D. G., Dearden, K. A., Sternin, J., & Sternin, M. (2004). The power of positive deviance. *British Medical Journal, 329*, 1177–1179.

Martin, M. L. (2003). Rapid-cycle improvement in pediatric health care: A solution for patients with similar or same last names. *Journal for Specialists in Pediatric Nursing, 8*(4), 148–154. Retrieved January 9, 2009, from CINAHL Database of Nursing and Allied Health Literature.

Medical Outcomes Trust (MOT). (2006). *Goals and objectives.* Retrieved October 16, 2006, from http://www.outcomes-trust.org/about.htm

Medical Risk Management Associates. (2006). *FOCUS-PDCA model: A nine step process guide to quality improvement.* Retrieved January 7, 2009, from http://www.sentinel-event.com/focus/ppframe.htm

Montoye, C. K., Mehta, R. H., Baker, P. L., Orza, M., Elma, M. A., & Parrish, R. (2003). A rapid-cycle collaborative model to promote guidelines for acute myocardial infarction. *Joint Commission Journal on Quality and Safety, 29*(9), 468–478.

Moore, K., Lynn, M., McMillen, B., & Evans, S. (1999). Implementation of the ANA Report Card. *Journal of Nursing Administration, 29*(6), 46–54.

Moorehead, S., & Johnson, M. (2004). Diagnostic-specific outcomes and nursing effectiveness research. *International Journal of Nursing Terminologies and Classifications, 15*(2), 49–57. Retrieved January 8, 2009, from CINAHL Database of Nursing and Allied Health Literature.

National Association of Clinical Nurse Specialists 2004 Statement Revision Task Force. (2004). *Statement on clinical nurse specialist practice and education.* Harrisburg, PA: Author.

National Committee for Quality Assurance. (2006). *NCQA programs. HEDIS and quality measurement.* Retrieved January 7, 2009, from http://www.ncqa.org/tabid/59/Default. aspx

National Council of State Boards of Nursing. (2006). *Draft: Vision paper: The future regulation of advanced practice nursing.* Retrieved January 7, 2009, from http://www.nacns. org/02_17_06%20APRN%20Vision%20Paper.pdf

National Practitioner Data Bank-Healthcare Integrity and Protection Data Bank. (n.d.). NPDB-HIPDB home page. Retrieved January 7, 2009, from http://www.npdb-hipdb. com

National Quality Forum. (2008). *Mission.* Retrieved July 2, 2009, from http://www. qualityforum.org/about/mission.asp

Nimtz-Rusch, K., & Thompson, J. (2008). Nursing and Six Sigma: A perfect match for safety and quality improvement. *CHART, 105*(3), 10–13.

Nursing Language in Nursing Knowledge Systems. (n.d.). *Welcome to NLINKS.* Retrieved January 7, 2009, from http://www.nlinks.org/news_mainpage.phtml

Pape, T. M., Guerra, D. M., Muzquiz, M., Bryant, J. B., Ingram, M., Schranner, B., et al. (2005). Innovative approaches to reducing nurses' distractions during medication administration. *Journal of Continuing Education in Nursing, 36*(3), 108–116.

Pennsylvania General Assembly. (2009). *Bill information. Regular session 2007–2008. House Bill 1254.* Retrieved January 12, 2009, from http://www.legis.state.pa.us/cfdocs /billinfo/billinfo.cfm?syear=2007&sind=0&body=H&type=B&bn=1254

Perkins, S., Connerney, I., & Hastings, C. (2000). Outcomes management: From concepts to application. *AACN Clinical Issues, 11*(3), 339–350.

Porter, A. (2005 Fall-Winter). Six Sigma takes root at North Carolina Baptist Hospital. *Visions.* Retrieved January 7, 2009, from http://www1.wfubmc.edu/articles/Six+Sigma

QualityNet. (n.d.). *RHQDAPU program overview. Reporting hospital quality data for annual payment update.* Retrieved January 19, 2009, from http://www.qualitynet.org/dcs/ ContentServer?cid=1138115987129&pagename=QnetPublic%2FPage%2FQnet-Tier2&c=Page

Robert Wood Johnson Foundation. (2008). *Grants: Pioneer.* Retrieved January 12, 2009, from http://www.rwjf.org/portfolios/pioneer/grant.jsp?id=55726&iaid=140

Senders, J. W. (2004). FMEA and RCA: The mantras of modern risk management. *Quality and Safety in Healthcare.* Retrieved January 7, 2009, from http://qhc.bmjjournals. com/cgi/content/full/13/4/249

Simmons-Trant, D., Cenck, P., Counterman, J., Hockenbury, D., & Litwille, L. (2004). Reducing VAP with SixSigma. *Nursing Management, 35*(6), 41. Retrieved January 8, 2009, from CINAHL Database of Nursing and Allied Health Literature.

Skinner, B. (2007). Web alert: Tools and models for quality improvement in health care. *Quality in Primary Care, 15*, 373–377. Retrieved January 8, 2009, from CINAHL Database of Nursing and Allied Health Literature.

Speroff, T., James, B., Nelson, E., Headrick, L., & Brommels, M. (2004). Guidelines for appraisal and publication of PDSA Quality Improvement. *Quality Management in Health Care, 13*(1), 33–39.

Sternin, J. (2002). *Positive deviance: A new paradigm for addressing today's problems today.* Retrieved January 7, 2009, from http://www.i-p-k.ch/subsites/Report_LEAP/dateien/www_barbwaugh_com_articles_positive_deviance.pdf

Tague, N. R. (2004). *The quality toolbox* (2nd ed., pp. 390–392). Milwaukee, WI: ASQ Quality Press.

University of Iowa College of Nursing. (n.d.). *Center for nursing classification and clinical effectiveness.* Retrieved January 7, 2009, from http://www.nursing.uiowa.edu/excellence/nursing_knowledge/clinical_effectiveness/index.htm

Urden, L. (1999). Outcome evaluation: An essential component for CNS practice. *Clinical Nurse Specialist, 13*, 39–46.

Vanderbilt University School of Engineering (n.d.). *Ishikawa diagram.* Retrieved January 7, 2009, from http://mot.vuse.vanderbilt.edu/mt322/Ishikawa.htm

Walker, M. W., Shoemaker, M., Riddle, K., Crane, M. M., & Clark, R. (2002). Clinical process improvement: Reduction of pneumothorax and mortality in high-risk preterm infants. *Journal of Perinatology, 22*, 641–645.

Williams, H., & Fallone, S. (2008). CQI in the acute care setting: An opportunity to influence acute care practice. *Nephrology Nursing Journal, 35*(5), 515–517.

Woodward, T. (2005). Addressing variation in hospital quality: Is Six Sigma the answer? *Journal of Healthcare Management, 50*(4), 226.

Zuzelo, P. (2006). Evidence-based nursing and qualitative research: A partnership imperative for real-world practice. In P. Munhall (Ed.), *Nursing research: A qualitative perspective* (4th ed.). Sudbury, MA: Jones and Bartlett.

Patient Safety: Preventing Unintended Consequences and Reducing Errors

Patti Rager Zuzelo, EdD, RN, MSN, ACNS-BC*

The patient safety movement was galvanized by the Institute of Medicine (IOM) report, *To Err Is Human: Building a Safer Health System* (Kohn, Corrigan, & Donaldson, 2000). This report fundamentally changed how providers, policy makers, and the public view healthcare safety and focused national attention on the mistakes and errors occurring in a deficient system that permits 44,000 to 98,000 needless patient deaths each year due to medical error (Kohn et al., 2000). Although certainly one of the most highly recognized initiatives, the IOM report was not the first attempt to address healthcare safety concerns. White (2004) noted that the earliest safety and quality efforts can be traced to 1955, although this work was not specific to patient safety initiatives but rather to patient outcomes, complications, and strategies for establishing measures to monitor outcomes.

Approximately 40 years later, in the mid-1990s, interest in medical errors and patient safety peaked with the convening of the first Annenberg Conference on Patient Safety, the establishment of the National Patient Safety Foundation (NPSF), and President Clinton's formation of the Advisory Commission on Consumer Protection and Quality in the Health Care Industry. In 1996, the Joint Commission launched its Sentinel Event Policy for the voluntary reporting of sentinel events. By 2000, continued momentum in the patient safety and quality movement led the Agency for Health Care Policy and Research (AHCPR) to change its name to the Agency for Healthcare Research and Quality (AHRQ) and become a funding powerhouse for research focused on patient safety, error reduction, strategic planning specific to patient safety, and technology utilization in the interest of enhancing quality of care (White, 2004).

---

* Dr. Zuzelo would like to acknowledge the contributions of JoAnne Phillips, MSN, RN, CCRN, CCNS. Her first edition chapter, The Patient Safety CNS: A New Role for an Established Systems Expert, is incorporated into this revised chapter.

Within this same period of time, the Business Roundtable established the Leapfrog Group, an organization with the mission of triggering "giant leaps forward in the safety, quality, and affordability of health care by supporting informed healthcare decisions by those who use and pay for health care; and promoting high-value health care through incentives and rewards (Leapfrog Group, 2007).

CNSs have been involved in workplace safety initiatives throughout this trajectory and are uniquely positioned to serve as patient safety experts across a variety of care settings. As patient safety is indistinguishable from quality care (Aspden, Corrigan, Wolcott, & Erickson, 2004), the CNS's goal of delivering quality patient care is in concert with, and contributes to, creating and sustaining an environment of safety. This chapter introduces CNSs to current patient safety perspectives and opportunities while sharing suggestions for Web sites, tools, and resources that may be used to create and sustain a culture of safety through the integration of evidence-based practice with patient safety practices, as defined by the Agency for Health Research and Quality (AHRQ) (2001).

Human Error and Types of Error

Most practicing nurses are well aware of the high rates of errors and near misses that occur on a daily basis across the healthcare system. The number of actual errors and prevented errors is staggering. Appreciating the various types of errors and their triggers may assist CNSs in planning and implementing targeted strategies that minimize error likelihood and improve patient outcomes. Reason's work (1990) on human error provides interesting theoretical and practice perspectives on basic error mechanisms, types and consequences of errors, and techniques for assessing and reducing the risks of errors.

Human error theory (HET) (Reason, 1990) suggests that organization failures in complex systems cause accidents. Reason (1990) asserts that the term *error* denotes an intentional act. Other error types depend upon two kinds of failure—slips and lapses—and mistakes. Errors may be active or latent. Latent errors lie dormant for a long period of time until they align with enough other factors to breech the system's defenses.

The alignment of latent failures and a variety of triggering events is referred to as the dynamics of accident causation, or the Swiss cheese model of accident causation (Figure 9-1). The figure illustrates a trajectory of accident opportunity that penetrates several defensive systems and is the result of complex interactions between latent failures and triggering events. In this model, latent failures at the managerial levels combine with psychological precursors, and unsafe acts within a context of local triggering events lead to an accident opportunity. When these factors and influences align, accidents are more likely to occur, characterized by the holes of a Swiss cheese wedge aligning to allow for unimpeded passage through the cheese wedge. A few examples of organizational failures include lack of administrative commitment to safety, blurred safety responsibilities, and poor training (Wolf, 2007).

Reason (1990) points out that very few unsafe acts actually result in damage or injury, even in systems that are unprotected. Findings from a focus group study exploring the influence of technologies on registered nurses' work illustrate the many ways that nurses work around and bypass technology-related rules and routines in efforts

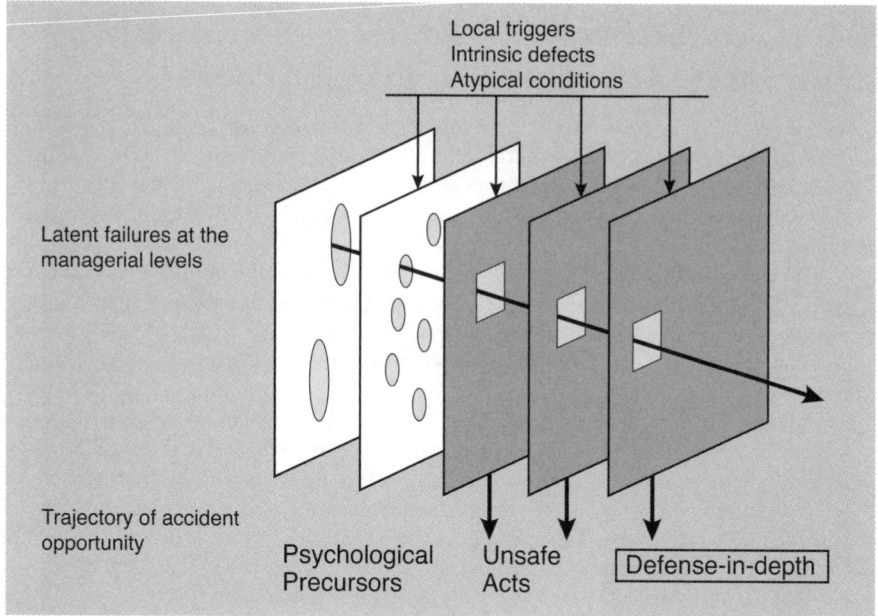

Local triggers
Intrinsic defects
Atypical conditions

Latent failures at the
managerial levels

Trajectory of accident
opportunity

Psychological
Precursors

Unsafe
Acts

Defense-in-depth

Figure 9-1   The dynamics of accident causation. The diagram shows a trajectory of accident opportunity penetrating several defensive sysems. This results from a complex interaction between latent failures and a variety of local triggering events. It is clear from this figure, however, that the chances of such a trajectory of opportunity finding loopholes in all of the defenses at any one time is very small.

Source: James Reason (1990). *Human error.* © Cambridge University Press, 1990. Reprinted with permission of Cambridge Univerity Press.

to meet patient care needs, save time, or minimize frustrations. Rarely do these system breeches lead to patient harm (Zuzelo, Gettis, Hansall, & Thomas, 2008). However, when mistakes do occur, they may be catastrophic.

Reason (1990) pessimistically observes that while engineered safety devices offer barriers against most single errors, human and mechanical, there are no guaranteed technological defenses against the accumulation of latent failures that provide opportunities for errors within organizations, including high-risk healthcare systems (see Exemplar 9-1). Reducing the likelihood of errors by minimizing latent failures, scrutinizing and improving systems, and rapidly evaluating the effectiveness of process changes are requisite activities to promote safety and certainly fall within the purview of CNS practice.

Accident causation theory is very relevant to CNS practice and is applicable to large healthcare organizations as well as to specific types of clinical care areas. As an example, critical care poses great risk for patients related to (1) increased patient acuity, (2) high frequency of invasive interventions, (3) high medication volume, (4) need for

Exemplar 9-1

The Unsafe Act: Case of the Infusion Pump

Tim Bradley, RN, is a new intensive care unit nurse with 1 year experience. One evening, Tim is presented with a newly admitted, critically ill patient requiring intravenous antibiotics, high-volume fluid resuscitation, and vasopressor and inotropic support therapy to treat progressive shock. The patient is deteriorating, and Tim is rapidly responding to each ailing system.

This particular shift, there had been a registered nurse sick call. This individual was not replaced. The remaining nurses were very busy providing care to unstable patients. As a result, Tim was independently handling his patient's care needs.

Tim's patient was prescribed dopamine 400 mg/250 ml @ 7 micrograms/kilogram/minute. The patient weighed 80 kilograms.

Unit policy required high-risk medication infusions via Smart Pump devices capable of identifying and preventing adverse drug events (ADE) when used as designed. Tim was familiar with the correct use of the Smart Pump infusion devices and had been correctly in-serviced; however, during his orientation, his preceptor had also encouraged Tim to bypass the pump technology. Tim's colleagues shared with him a variety of ways to avoid "dealing with the drug library and all those alerts!" The rationale was to "save time" by "bypassing" the information required when setting up the infusion device alerts.

Tim was in a hurry. His patient required many medications. Tim felt rushed and pressured. When he saw the dopamine infusion order, he decided to hang the medication without the use of the Guardrails alerts. His intent was to go back after hanging the remaining medications and set up the dopamine infusion as per policy.

Tim calculated the dopamine infusion rate. He set the infusion pump as per his calculation. Tim did not realize that he had mistakenly calculated an infusion rate of 70 micrograms/kilograms/minute. Within a short period of time, the patient exhibited tachycardia and ventricular irritability with increased blood pressure significantly above the desired mean arterial pressure. Scared that he had made an error, Tim immediately rechecked the dopamine dosage and quickly discovered his error. The patient did not suffer apparent untoward effects once the dose was corrected; however, certainly the ADE could have been fatal.

This exemplar provides an overview of an unsafe act that violated an established rule because the rule violation was perceived as a routine, common act. Nurses had violated this particular rule on many occasions but the preconditions of nurse inexperience, high acuity, and inadequate supports in combination with established workarounds or shortcuts contributed to the actual adverse drug event.

speedy decision-making processes and associated intervention, and (5) other factors, including patient characteristics. In one study, researchers found that critical care patients experienced 1.7 errors per day, 29% with the potential to cause significant harm or death (Pronovost, Thompson, Holzmueller, Lubomski, & Morlock, 2005). Across the United States, that data extrapolates to 85,000 errors every day, of which 24,650 are potentially life threatening. Nursing homes and ambulatory care settings are also not immune from error. In fact, because the number of outpatient visits each year far exceeds the number of inpatient visits, the opportunity for error in that setting is also considerable (Aspden et al., 2004).

The frequencies and costs of patient safety incidents (PSI) that occurred in the hospitalized Medicare population are staggering. From 2004 to 2006, patient safety incidents (PSIs) cost the Medicare program $8.8 billion and resulted in 238,337 potentially preventable deaths (HealthGrades, 2006). HealthGrades analyzed 41 million Medicare patient records and identified that those patients treated at top-performing hospitals had approximately a 43% lower chance of experiencing one or more medical errors than if treated at the poorest-performing hospitals.

While HealthGrades found that the overall death rate among Medicare beneficiaries that developed one or more patient safety incidents had decreased by almost 5% during the 2-year period, four indicators had increased when compared to a 2004 baseline. These indicators included postoperative respiratory failure, postoperative pulmonary embolism or deep vein thrombosis, postoperative sepsis, and postoperative abdominal wound separation/splitting. These key areas are included in the current focus of regulatory (e.g., Joint Commission and Centers for Medicare and Medicaid Services [CMS]) (CMS and Joint Commission, 2008) and recommending (e.g., Institute for Healthcare Improvement [IHI]) agencies.

Since the release of the IOM report (Kohn et al., 2000), there has been an abundant volume of published patient safety-focused literature. Multiple recommending and regulatory agencies offer guidelines and mandates. Many organizations provide evidence-based practice guidelines to assist clinicians in providing standardized evidence-based care.

The volume of materials and ever-changing safety standards and best practices may be overwhelming to CNSs, particularly those who are new to putting patient safety principles into practice. The CNS is absolutely pivotal in assessing the clinical environment for accident and error opportunities, collaborating with appropriate team members to proactively improve systems or to meaningfully react to occurrences, and rapidly evaluating the outcomes of systems changes. Actively engaging in this work requires a preliminary review of the definitions of terms commonly used in patient safety projects and publications (Table 9-1). The CNS concentrating on a patient safety role integrates all the skill and competencies described in role-based CNS conceptualizations (Hamric, 1989; Oncology Nursing Society, 2003) and influence-based models (American Association of Critical-Care Nurses [AACN], 2002; National Association of Clinical Nurse Specialists [NACNS], 2004).

Creating a Just Culture for Patient Safety

Culture is a shared set of beliefs and values about how people work individually and together as teams (Phillips, 2005). It delineates a shared set of values and beliefs that influences communication, social relations, and actions (Friersen, Farquhar, & Hughes, 2006). Achieving and sustaining a culture of safety requires an understanding of the values and beliefs within a particular organization. The safety culture of an organization is the product of individual and group values, attitudes, perceptions,

Table 9-1	DEFINITIONS OF KEY TERMS IN PATIENT SAFETY
Term	**Definition**
Error	Mistakes made in the process of care that result in, or have the potential to result in, harm to the patient.
Near miss	An act of commission or omission that could have harmed the patient, but did not do so as a result of chance (IOM).
Patient safety	The absence of the potential for, or occurrence of, healthcare-associated injury to patients. Created by avoiding medical errors as well as taking action to prevent medical errors from causing injury. Mistakes include failure of a planned action to be completed as intended or the use of a wrong plan to achieve an aim. These can be the result of an action that is taken (error of commission) or an action that is not taken (error of omission).
Incident	Unexpected or unanticipated events or circumstances not consistent with the routine care of a particular patient, which could have, or did, lead to an unintended or unnecessary harm to a person, or a complaint, loss, or damage.
Adverse event	An injury resulting from a medical intervention.

Source: Aspden et al., 2004; Pronovost et al., 2005.

competencies, and patterns of behavior that combine to determine the commitment to, and the style and proficiency of, an organization's health and safety management (AHRQ, 2001).

The notion of a "just culture" is relatively recent and denotes a culture where people can report mistakes, errors, accidents, or waste without negative repercussions (AHRQ, 2008a). In a just culture, individuals remain accountable for their actions but they are not held responsible for flawed systems that permit earnest, trained people to err. Sharing and disclosure are prominent features of a just culture because efficiencies and quality improvement processes depend on the frontline staff to drive improvements, and such drive requires a sense of safety. Staff must feel empowered to point out errors, defects, and systems failures that could cause patient harm (AHRQ, 2008a). A just culture is not an "anything goes" culture. In other words, individuals may be held personally accountable for intended actions that are unsafe and violate rules. But, in highly protected systems with established defense systems, such unsafe acts are more likely in a highly specific, often atypical, set of circumstances (Reason, 1990).

Organizations with a positive safety culture have characteristics in common. These organizations have leaders who support bidirectional communications founded on mutual trust, with the ability for all employees to speak up and raise concerns, as well as the willingness to listen when others have a concern. In addition, there are shared perceptions of the importance of safety, coupled with a systems approach to analysis of safety issues (Friersen et al., 2006; Helmreich, 2005). Patient safety permeates the culture, and there is an emphasis on continuous improvement (Friersen et al., 2006). Highly reliable organizations (HROs) tend to be exceptionally consistent and are particularly good at avoiding error (AHRQ, 2008b). HROs are characterized by several organizing concepts: (1) sensitivity to operations with staff maintaining an ongoing organizational awareness; (2) reluctance to simplify; (3) preoccupation with failure; (4) deference to expertise; and (5) resilience (AHRQ, 2008b).

Progress toward creating a culture of patient safety requires honest, routine error reporting. Errors and near misses are reported in organizations in which staff feels safe reporting errors. In organizations with a culture of patient safety, the emphasis is on *why* the error occurred, versus *who* made the error (see Figure 9-2). Leaders use errors to help staff evaluate processes and learn how to prevent a recurrence of an error, rather than to blame. Two strategies encouraged by the Joint Commission that can assist with error analysis are failure mode and effects analysis (FMEA) and root cause analysis strategies (RCA) (De Rosier & Stalhandske, 2006; Duwe, Fuchs, & Hansen-Flashen, 2005).

What strategies can the CNS use to assess the culture of safety within the practice environment? AHRQ has tools posted on its Web site that can be downloaded free of charge to facilitate assessment of the safety culture within a hospital or nursing home. The tools are designed to provide institutions with the opportunity to assess their patient safety cultures, track changes in safety over time, and evaluate the influence of patient safety interventions (AHRQ, 2008c).

Results of the AHRQ survey will assist the CNS and other members of the leadership team to assess the perception of patient safety within their organizations, whether errors are reported and discussed in an appropriate forum, and whether there is an atmosphere of continuous learning based on the principles of patient safety. Each healthcare institution can use the completed survey data to calculate their percentage of positive responses on each item. Those data can be submitted to AHRQ for entry into a national database. The AHRQ Hospital Survey on Patient Safety Culture allows comparisons between the submitting hospital and other similar hospitals. This report enables each hospital to compare itself to the benchmark hospitals (AHRQ, 2008c).

Safety culture assessments are useful tools for measuring organizational conditions that lead to adverse events and patient harm in hospitals. The assessment is the starting point from which action planning begins and patient safety changes evolve (Sora & Nieva, 2003). Reassessments serve as barometers to measure the success of improvement interventions. Once the cultural assessment is complete, the CNS can use the data to integrate evidence-based guidelines into everyday practice for patient care.

Creating a Safe Environment

Armed with the culture assessment findings, the CNS must continue to examine the practice environment with an eye on safety. Through assessment and analysis of the

ASSESS - ERR™

Medication System Worksheet

Patient MR# _____
(if error reached patient)

Incident # _____
✓ if no callback identified: _____

Date of error:_____   Date information obtained: _____   Patient age: _____

Drug(s) involved in error: _____

Non-formulary drug(s)?	❏ Yes ❏ No
Drug sample(s)?	❏ Yes ❏ No
Drug(s) packaged in unit dose/unit of use?	❏ Yes ❏ No
Drug(s) dispensed from pharmacy?	❏ Yes ❏ No
Error within 24 hours of admission, transfer, or after discharge?	❏ Yes ❏ No
Did the error reach the patient?	❏ Yes ❏ No

Source of IV solution: ❏ Manufacturer premixed solution   ❏ Pharmacy IV admixture   ❏ Nursing IV admixture

Brief description of the event: (what, when, and why)_____
_____
_____
_____

Possible causes	Y/N	Comments
Critical patient information missing? (age, weight, allergies, BS, lab values, pregnancy, patient identity, location, renal/liver impairment, diagnoses, etc.)		
Critical drug information missing? (outdated/absent references, inadequate computer screening, inaccessible pharmacist, uncontrolled drug formulary, etc.)		
Miscommunication of drug order? (illegible, ambiguous, incomplete, misheard, or misunderstood orders, intimidation/faulty interaction, etc.)		
Drug name, label, packaging problem? (look/sound-alike names, look-alike packaging, unclear/absent labeling, faulty drug identification, etc.)		
Drug stoage or delivery problem? (slow turn around time, inaccurate delivery, doses missing or expired, multiple concentrations, placed in wrong bin,etc.)		
Drug delivery device problem? (poor device design, misprogramming, free-flow, mixed up lines, IV administration of oral syringe contents, etc.)		
Environmental, staffing, or workflow problems? (lighting, noise, clutter, interruptions, staffing deficiencies, workload, inefficient workflow, employee safety, etc.)		
Lack of staff education? (competency validation, new or unfamiliar drugs/devices, orientation process, feedback about errors/prevention, etc.)		
Patient education problem? (lack of information,noncompliance, not encouraged to ask questions, lack of investigating patient inquiries, etc.)		
Lack of quality control or independent check systems? (equipment quality control checks, independent checks for high alert drugs/high risk patient population drugs etc.)		

Did the patient require any of the following actions after the error that you would not have done if the event had not occurred?
❏ Testing   ❏ Additional observation ❏ Gave antidote ❏ Care escalated (transferred, etc.) ❏ Additional LOS ❏ Other_____

Patient outcome: _____

@2006 Institute for Safe Medication Practices

Figure 9-2   Assess-ERR Medication Safety System Worksheet.
Source: © 2006, Institute for Safe Medication Practices. Reprinted with permission.

practice environment, the CNS begins to understand potential root causes of errors within that environment. The majority of medical errors do not occur as the result of one person's actions, but are the result of faulty systems, processes, and conditions that lead people to make mistakes or fail to prevent them (Phillips, 2005).

AHRQ has identified factors that contribute to errors: communication, inadequate flow of information, human problems, patient-related issues, organizational transfer of knowledge, staffing patterns and work flow, technical failures, and inadequate policies and procedures (AHRQ, 2003). Table 9-2 presents each of these factors with an example of how they apply to bedside practice.

When assessing the role each factor plays in contributing to errors within the practice environment, the CNS must also assess how staff has adapted its practice to work around systematic obstructions to completing work. Nurses have unparalleled skill at developing workarounds. In other words, what can the nurse do to solve the issue for the patient today?

Although this strategy does garner short-term success, it creates long-term problems. As a simple example, if a nurse does not have a patient's medications and solves this problem by borrowing medications from another patient, this exemplifies first-order problem solving (Tucker & Edmondson, 2002). The nurse has met the needs of the patient in the immediate period by securing the needed medications. But, of course, the medications are now no longer available for the patient for whom they were intended.

In examining this simple issue, numerous other issues arise: What about the patient whose medications were taken (his or her dose is now missing)? What if it is a slightly different dose? What will keep this situation from arising tomorrow? Bedside nurses' role supports first-order problem solving. Nurses at the point-of-care do not have the resources (mainly time) to do second-order problem solving (Tucker & Edmondson, 2002).

The role of the CNS in this scenario is critical. Second-order problem solving involves a system analysis of why the error occurred—what part of the system failed the nurse and the patient (Tucker & Edmondson, 2002). To have more than a temporary fix, the root cause of the problem must be uncovered. It is often easier to work around problems, especially when the staff nurses believe that they have reported this issue previously and no action has been taken. The CNS must partner with the staff nurse to investigate the concern and to craft a reasonable, efficient solution to the clinical problem. Partnering facilitates staff buy-in, because the nurses helped to broker the solution. The CNS must make it easier for staff to do the right thing while making it more difficult to do a workaround.

One essential support to sustaining a culture of safety is the creation of a healthy work environment (HWE). The attributes of a healthy work environment are symbiotic with a culture of patient safety. The American Association of Critical-Care Nurses' (AACN) Healthy Work Environment standards demonstrate a commitment to creating a positive work environment that facilitates safety (Barden, 2005). Each standard is clarified by essential (absolutely required, fundamental), standard (authoritative statement), and critical elements (structures, processes, programs, and behaviors required for a standard to be achieved).

The first healthy work environment standard is skilled communication; nurses must be as proficient in communication skills as they are in clinical skills. The concept of communication is complex, encompassing verbal, written, and nonverbal skills. In reviewing sentinel events, the Joint Commission has identified team communication

Table 9-2   FACTORS THAT CONTRIBUTE TO ERRORS

Factor	Description	Examples of Interventions for CNS
Communication	Verbal/nonverbal, written (e.g., in e-mail communication). Between any members of the team: nurse, physician, family, support staff, therapists. NPSG #2: "Improve the effectiveness of communication among caregivers" (Joint Commission, 2006).	1. Conduct briefings: Role-model efficient and effective bidirectional communication with all team members. When preparing to perform a procedure, review each step before beginning to prevent miscommunication. 2. Be assertive: Create an environment where any member of the team feels comfortable in voicing their concern. Utilize the SBAR strategy to communicate a message that is clear and concise. 3. Develop situational awareness: Place signs outside the patient's door, be sure all staff are aware of patients who are "at risk" for falls or other clinical issues. 4. Understand the difference between the novice and the expert in making decisions: Decisions are made based on past experience, and because the novice has little past experience, he or she may rely more on the CNS to support his or her decision-making process. 5. Conduct debriefings: After a significant clinical event, review with the staff the pre-event situation, the event, and the response to the event. Listen to the staff's perception of what happened. The CNS may be able to use the information to plan future education.

Table 9-2   (continued)

Factor	Description	Examples of Interventions for CNS
Communication (continued)		6. SBAR strategy: Develop a template for the use of the SBAR strategy, including a few key clinical characteristics. For example, if caring for a thoracic population, always include an assessment of breath sounds and pattern of breathing.
Inadequate flow of information	Members of the team may not have the information they need to appropriately care for the patient. NPSG #2, to "Improve the effectiveness of communication," includes a requirement for a standardized handoff of communications (Joint Commission, 2006).	1. Examine the handoff process within the practice environment; include nurses, physicians, pharmacists, etc. 2. Partner with other members of the team to create a handoff tool that would enable clear, concise communication.
Human problems	How standards of care, policies, and procedures are followed. Other factors that play a role: fatigue, stress, distractions, interruptions, and	1. CNS plays a key role in the design, development, implementation, and evaluation of policies. 2. Partner with the nurse manager and bedside nurses to establish the standards of care within the practice environment. 3. Evaluate the practice environment for factors that may influence care. 4. Develop a peer-review process to enable the staff to hold each other accountable for care delivered.

(continues)

Table 9-2 (continued)

Factor	Description	Examples of Interventions for CNS
Patient-related issues	multitasking. Incomplete assessment, which may include allergies, or duplicate or missing medications. NPSG #8 requires accurate and complete reconciliation of medications across the continuum of care. Patient identification, utilizing two unique identifiers (NPSG #1) (Joint Commission, 2006).	1. Monitor patient identification: As you make rounds on each patient, ask the patient if the staff have been checking his or her identification. 2. Ensure that there is a clear process if the identification is incorrect. 3. Partner with bedside nurses, pharmacists, physicians, and nursing leadership to establish a process for medication reconciliation.
Organizational transfer of knowledge	Formal transfer of knowledge occurs during orientation, education, and competency assessments. Informal.	1. In collaboration with other experts, design, develop, and evaluate clinical competencies as they relate to the care of a defined population. 2. Develop a tool for a brief orientation to your practice area for staff who are pulled, pool nurses, or agency staff. Include emergency equipment, supplies, medications, a short lesson on how to contact the physicians; anything that is important about your patient population.
Staffing patterns/workflow	Supplies: disjointed, missing, not easily available to the nurse. Assignments geographically undesirable.	1. Review work by Ebright and colleagues who have studied the flow of "nurse work" (Ebright, 2004). 2. Start with one simple project: What does a nurse need to perform safe, aseptic intra-

Table 9-2 (continued)		
Factor	**Description**	**Examples of Interventions for CNS**
Staffing patterns/ workflow (continued)		venous line care? If the care is done at the patient's bedside, the supplies should be at the bedside, not in the supply room.
		3. Discuss with the staff changes in where/how medications are prepared to decrease, and eventually eliminate interruptions/distractions when preparing medications.
Technical failures	Frequent interruptions/ distractions. Mechanical devices can malfunction.	1. Ensure that contact numbers for experts (in house or from the companies) are easily accessible, particularly for life-sustaining equipment; for example, ventricular assist devices.
		2. Plan and execute drills for all equipment that is low volume, high risk (continuous renal replacement machines, postcardiac arrest hypothermia devices).
Inadequate policies and procedures	Policies that are too long, too wordy, out of date, or not easily accessible will not be utilized.	1. Participate in policy review and revision, with an eye for practicality (e.g., if the policy is 28 pages single spaced, it is not likely to be used).
		2. Promote electronic availability of nursing policies and medication information (e.g., online policy manuals or medication manuals).

Source: AHRQ, 2003; Phillips, 2005.

as a top contributor to sentinel events (Joint Commission, 2006). Healthcare organizations are obligated to help staff develop excellent communication skills. Skilled communicators focus on finding solutions and desirable outcomes, advancing collaborative relationships, listening as intently as they speak, and demonstrating mutual respect (Barden, 2005). The CNS must role model expert communication techniques and offer constructive feedback to staff nurses as they develop their communication skill sets.

One strategy that has been effective in facilitating clear, direct communication among caregivers is the SBAR strategy. SBAR is an acronym for *situation, background, assessment,* and *recommendation* (Leonard, Graham, & Bonacum, 2004). SBAR is a situational briefing model characterized by appropriate assertion, critical language, and awareness and education. It is a vital model designed to address the different communication styles used and valued by nurses, physicians, and other clinicians (Table 9-3).

Table 9-3 SBAR	
30–60 Second Communication	
Situation	**What is happening with the patient?**
	Example:
	"Hello, Dr. Jones, this is Susan, I am calling from 2 West. I am taking care of Mr. Green in room 212, a patient of Dr. Johnson's who went to the OR today for a colectomy. He has been back from the PACU for 4 hours. I have just reassessed him."
Background	**What is the important clinical information?**
	"Over the past 4 hours, his BP has dropped from 120/78 to 90/58, his heart rate has increased from 70 to 100, his respiratory rate is 24, and his urine output was 80 mL/hour for the first 2 hours and has dropped to 30 mL each hour for the past 2 hours.
	He is receiving IV fluids, D5.45NS + 20 meq KCL at 125 mL/hour.
	His postop labs were unremarkable, his hemoglobin was 10.2.
	His estimated blood loss was 450 mL."
Assessment	**What do you think the problem is?**
	"I think he is dry."
Recommendation	**What do you think he needs? If you think the patient needs to be seen by the physician or nurse practitioner, do not be afraid to say so.**
	"I think he needs more fluid."

Source: Leonard et al., 2004; Phillips, 2005.

The CNS can assist staff with developing a template for communicating with physicians and other team members using the SBAR strategy and incorporating the consistent use of particular elements that relate to the specific patient population. For example, if caring for a neuroscience population, the assessment of the Glasgow Coma Score (GCS) would always be included in every communication. Additional strategies to improve communication include conducting briefings, being assertive, developing situational awareness, understanding the differences in expert and novice decision making, and conducting debriefings (Volker & Clark, 2004). Communication successes will develop over time and will occur only with practice, repetition, and constructive feedback to staff.

The second healthy work environment standard is true collaboration: Nurses must be relentless in pursuing and fostering true collaboration. True collaboration can build on the relationships fostered through skilled communication. It is a relationship grounded in respect and trust. Nurse–physician collaboration is one of the three strongest predictors of nurse empowerment. One of the critical elements of true collaboration is that "every team member contributes to the achievement of common goals by giving power and respect to each person's voice, integrating individual differences, resolving competing interests, and safeguarding the essential contribution each must make in order to achieve optimal outcomes" (Barden, 2005, p. 21). Authentic collaboration is revealed through relationships with other nurse leaders, physicians, and administrators.

The third standard is effective decision making: Nurses must be valued and committed partners in making policy, directing and evaluating clinical care, and leading organizational operations (Barden, 2005). Nurses have primary responsibility for patient safety, but only 8% of physicians recognize the nurse as part of the decision-making team (Cook, Hoas, Guttmannova, & Joyner, 2004). Effective decision making bridges the autonomy–accountability gap by empowering nurses to be the decision-making authority in the care of their patient.

The fourth healthy work environment standard addresses appropriate staffing: Staffing must ensure the effective match between patient needs and nurse competencies (Barden, 2005). Some CNSs may play a functional role in staffing by either being accountable to make sure enough staff is present or filling in when staffing is short. One clear role for the CNS in any staffing pattern is to collaborate with the nurse manager and staff nurses to look at the nurse work flow and the relationship to staffing. Are there staff members uninvolved in patient care for parts of the day that could have time schedules flexed? Are there times when the CNS must partner with the manager to assert that the staff has reached a critical workload point and cannot take any more patients? This standard builds on the first, second, and third standards, wherein all the skills can combine to provide excellent communication, collaboration, and decision making to solve complex staffing issues.

Meaningful recognition is the fifth standard: Nurses must be recognized and must recognize others for the value each brings to the work of the organization (Barden,

2005). Recognition was important to 75% of the nurses in the healthy work environment study. A formalized process for recognition is essential for it to be effective. The CNS must be knowledgeable about recognition programs nationally (as with professional organizations), regionally (as with local chapters or statewide awards), or within the organization. The CNS must lead the recognition initiative to ensure that excellence in clinical practice, communication, patient–family relationships, and other key performance measures are recognized.

The final standard is authentic leadership: Nurse leaders must fully embrace the imperative of a healthy work environment, authentically live it, and engage others in the achievements (Barden, 2005). Authentic leaders are supported by their organization in developing skills and competency in skilled communication, true collaboration, effective decision making, meaningful recognition, and authentic leadership. Establishing and sustaining a practice environment that is supported by the concepts in the healthy work environment standards contributes to a hospital culture rich in safety, which contributes to an environment of patient safety.

Safety and Quality Organizations

The complexity of regulatory agencies and recommending organizations within health care is extraordinary. The CNS is frequently held accountable for compliance with multitudes of guidelines, competencies, rules, and regulations. In developing clinical programs for improvement, which may be in response to a regulatory requirement, the CNS must partner with the bedside nurse to collaborate with numerous disciplines to establish compliance strategies for each regulation or guideline.

Joint Commission accreditation is a nationwide seal of approval indicating that organizations meet high performance standards. The Joint Commission and Joint Commission International were designated in 1995 as the World Health Organization (WHO) Collaborating Centre for Patient Safety Solutions (WHO Collaborating Centre for Patient Safety Solutions, 2008).

There are numerous regulatory and recommending agencies that address healthcare safety and quality; many of their recommendations overlap and are quite similar given their shared evidence base. Key organizations include, but are not limited to, the Center for Medicare and Medicaid (CMS), Institute for Healthcare Improvement (IHI), AHRQ, National Patient Safety Goals (NPSG), Joint Commission, and National Quality Foundation (NQF).

Tools of the Trade

The World Wide Web has dramatically influenced patient care delivery. The role of the CNS in patient safety is inextricably linked to the use of electronically available tools in the form of assessment tools, guidelines, and other references, many of which can be downloaded without charge. Professional organizations, not-for-profit (NFP) recommending organizations, governmental agencies, regulatory bodies, and evidence-based practice Web sites offer many useful resources (refer to Tables 9-4 through 9-8).

Table 9-4 EXAMPLES OF WEB SITES WITH PATIENT SAFETY INFORMATION (PSI): PROFESSIONAL ORGANIZATIONS

Web Site	Contents	CNS Benefits
http://www.aacn.org/WD/HWE/Docs/HWEStandards.pdf *American Association of Critical Care Nurses (AACN)* Accessed: December 9, 2008	Healthy work environment standards: Six key factors in creating and sustaining a healthy work environment (HWE). Available to download the full document or the executive summary. Practice Alerts: Eleven succinct, dynamic evidence–based guidelines designed to close the research–practice gap and facilitate standardized practice.	Provides evidence-based guidelines that support the six key factors in creating a HWE. The CNS can operationalize these guidelines to meet the needs of the practice environment.
http://www.ons.org/publications/positions/patientsafety.shtml *Oncology Nursing Society (ONS)* Accessed: December 9, 2008	Position statement on patient safety	Oncology nurses can use this statement to formulate their own position statement on patient safety.
http://www.aorn.org/aboutaorn/whoweare/patientsafetyfirst *Association of periOperative Registered Nurses (AORN)* Accessed: December 9, 2008	Identifying, collecting, and developing clinical and educational resources to improve patient safety in the surgical setting. In addition: • General resources—links to numerous patient safety sites • AORN resources and journal article references	Resources on this site apply to perioperative, postoperative and procedural staff. These resources can be used to develop education programs, orientation programs, and patient safety programs.

(continues)

Table 9-4   (continued)

Web Site	Contents	CNS Benefits
	• List of patient safety journals and newsletters • Patient safety books and media • Joint Commission patient safety practices online • Journal scan • Position statement on patient safety • Nurse consultation opportunities • Correct sites surgery toolkit • National Time-Out Day	
http://www.anesthesiapatientsafety.com *American Association of Nurse Anesthetists (AANA)* Accessed: December 9, 2008	Site is designed to promote safe anesthesia patient care by educating the public. Contains need-to-know information for anesthesia patients: • "Patient Candor Essential for Safe Anesthesia Care", the full story discusses the importance of full disclosure to the anesthesia provider. • "New Anesthesia Standards for Office Surgeries", reflects the AANA new strict standards for office surgeries. • "Conscious Sedation", discusses which types of surgery and procedures can be done with conscious sedation.	This site contains extensive resources for patient education, which could be incorporated into a pre-op education program.

Table 9-4 (continued)

Web Site	Contents	CNS Benefits
http://www.aspan.org *American Society of Perianesthesia Nurses (ASPAN)* Accessed: July 23, 2006	Link to "Anesthesia and Your Child," provides a story and a coloring book for children who are about to have anesthesia to allay fears. Site contains resources for both the nurse and the patient/family. <ul><li>Link to ask a clinical practice question and numerous organizational committees, such as education and evidence-based practice</li><li>Nursing Core Curriculum for Perianesthesia Nurses</li><li>For patients, an extensive section on what to expect from the pre-admission interview through discharge</li></ul>	The pre-admission interview can begin the process of medication reconciliation, to comply with the Joint Commission National Patient Safety Goal on medication reconciliation.
http://www.aone.org/aone/pdf/Role%20of%20the%20Nurse%20Executive%20in%20Patient%20Safety%20Toolkit_July2007.pdf *American Association of Nurse Executives (AONE)* Accessed: December 9, 2008	The Role of the Nurse Executive in Patient Safety: 1. Lead cultural change 2. Provide shared leadership 3. Build external partnerships 4. Develop leadership competencies	The CNS can partner with the nurse executive to lead cultural change across disciplines, as well as develop and drive patient safety initiatives across the organization.

Table 9-5   EXAMPLES OF WEB SITES WITH PSI: NOT-FOR-PROFIT "RECOMMENDING" ORGANIZATIONS

Web Site	Contents	CNS Benefits
https://www.ecri.org/Pages/default.aspx *ECRI Institute* Accessed: December 9, 2008	Designated by AHRQ/World Health Organization as an evidence-based practice center. Administers: National Quality Measures Clearing House; National Guidelines Clearinghouse Complete list of technology assessments and evidence-based reports A "consumer reports" for medical devices MDSR—medical device incident and hazard information Publishes *Health Devices* journal	The CNS plays a key role in product selection. The technology assessment on the ECRI Web site can assist in assessing the safety of a technology, as well as offering a nonbiased comparison of different products that provide the same technology. The CNS can also seek out guidelines for a broad range of clinical issues.
http://www.ismp.org *Institute for Safe Medication Practices (ISMP)* Accessed: December 9, 2008	Extensive resources for staff and patients: • Education: newsletters, educational programs, self-assessments, patient safety video • Medication safety tools and resources: high-alert medication list, confused drug list, error-prone abbreviation list, do-not-crush list • "Pathways for Medication Safety", an extensive program for medication safety that can be downloaded for free • USP–ISMP Medication Error reporting system	Many tools will assist with compliance with Joint Commission NPSG to: • Improve the safety of using medications • Accurately and completely reconcile medications across the continuum of care "Pathways for Medication Safety" will guide the CNS in creating a

Table 9-5 (continued)

Web Site	Contents	CNS Benefits
	• Links to numerous patient safety sites • *Assess–ERR Medication System Worksheet* to facilitate medication use system evaluations (Figure 9-2)	medication safety program as a collaborative with pharmacy. Monthly newsletter contains information to improve medication administration process.
http://www.npsf.org *National Patient Safety Foundation (NPSF)* Accessed: December 9, 2008	National Patient Safety Foundation: • Create a core body of knowledge • Develop a culture receptive to safety • Raise public awareness • Foster communications Sponsors educational programs, patient safety fellowships; educational videos, newsletters Resources are available for patients, families, and caregivers	"When things go wrong…" is a document from the Harvard Hospitals to teach physicians and nurses what to do if something goes wrong. The CNS can use this in collaborative forums for physicians and nurses to discuss plans on how to respond when an adverse event occurs.

Table 9-6   EXAMPLES OF WEB SITES WITH PSI: GOVERNMENT AGENCIES

Web Site	Contents	CNS Benefits
http://www.ahrq.gov/clinic/ptsafety/pdf/ptsafety.pdf *Agency for Healthcare Research and Quality (AHRQ)* Accessed: December 9, 2008	"Making Healthcare Safer: Critical analysis of Patient Safety Practices (2001)." The aim of this extensive document was to collect and review existing evidence on practices relevant to improving patient safety. Eleven practices were identified and rated most highly in terms of strength of evidence.	These eleven practices can be integrated into a unit-based patient safety program.
http://www.ahrq.gov/qual/patientsafetyculture/hospsurvindex.htm *Agency for Healthcare Research and Quality (AHRQ)* Accessed: May 6, 2009	Hospital Survey on Patient Safety Culture (2004): how to administer the survey, how to analyze and interpret the results	The CNS can use this tool to begin an environmental assessment of the patient safety culture of the practice area.
http://www.psnet.ahrq.gov *AHRQ Patient Safety Network* Accessed: December 9, 2008	This resource is available as an e-mail from the AHRQ, which provides a continuously updated, annotated, and carefully selected collection of patient safety news, literature, tools, and resources. Also contains the "patient safety classics," including the most influential, frequently cited articles, books, and resources in patient safety.	Since this is automatically sent from the AHRQ, it keeps the CNS abreast of all the key recent patient safety literature.

Table 9-6 (continued)

Web Site	Contents	CNS Benefits
http://www.ahrq.gov/qual/errorsix.htm *Agency for Healthcare Research and Quality (AHRQ)* Accessed: December 9, 2008	Medical errors and patient safety: • Online journals • 41 patient safety documents for staff and patients • Patient Safety Task Force information • The Federal Quality Interagency Coordination QuIC Task Force: ensures that all federal agencies that purchase, provide, study, or regulate healthcare services are working in a coordinated way toward the common goal of improving the quality of care • Conferences and workshops	Teamwork is an essential component in patient safety. This site contains a link to: AHRQ's Medical Teamwork and Patient Safety: Competencies on knowledge, skill, and attitudes. The CNS can use those competencies to structure a team approach to a number of clinical initiatives; the development of a rapid response team is a good example. In addition to access to the online journals, the information contained in the patient safety documents is extensive.
http://www.ahrq.gov/about/nursing *Agency for Healthcare Research and Quality (AHRQ)* Accessed: December 9, 2008	Nursing activities associated with the AHRQ: • Nursing research • Research funding • Tools and resources; for example, palliative wound care at the end of life • List of 16 links for nursing resources • Keeping patients safe: Transforming the work environment for nurses	In assessing a clinical issue, this site provides links to the AHRQ Evidence-Based Practice Center, National Quality Measures Clearinghouse, and others. The CNS can utilize all these links to begin establishing a foundation of evidence for any clinical issue.

(continues)

Table 9-6 (continued)		
Web Site	**Contents**	**CNS Benefits**
http://www.webmm.ahrq.gov *AHRQ M&M: Morbidity and Mortality Rounds on the Web* Accessed: December 9, 2008	Case studies are presented from several disciplines, with reviews by content experts in that discipline	Case examples may be used to reinforce the importance of the NPGS. Recent select cases illustrate mistaken identity and a case of transition failure.
http://www.patientsafety.gov *National Center for Patient Safety* Accessed: December 9, 2008	Extensive Web site, sponsored by the Veteran's Administration, designed for patients and staff: • Culture change • Patient safety for patients • Alerts and advisory example: paper on anticoagulation vulnerability • FMEA (failure mode and effects analysis)/RCA (root cause analysis) process: Extensive discussion on FMEA as it relates to health care • Publications include "Topics in Patient Safety" • Patient safety resources, including information on the Patient Safety Reporting System (PSRS) and human factors resources • Toolkits on falls, hand hygiene, and ensuring correct patient surgery	This Web site contains volumes of useful information the CNS may use to address the patient safety culture within the practice environment: • PSAT • Use of the RCA process to evaluate factors involved in an error • Hand hygiene program • Falls prevention program • Patient safety workshop curriculum

Table 9-6 (continued)

Web Site	Contents	CNS Benefits
	• Patient Safety Assessment Tool (PSAT) that examines six elements of patient safety: management and leadership, patient safety management program, Joint Commission compliance, procurement and equipment management, recalls and VA alerts/advisories, patient safety policies, tools, and aids	
http://www.fda.gov *Food and Drug Administration (FDA)* Accessed: December 9, 2008	Product recalls Product safety News for health educators and students Online databases: Maude, MDR (medical device reporting), Medwatch	The CNS plays a key role in product selection and evaluation of new products. When the CNS has been asked to run a trial of a particular piece of technology or equipment, the FDA database can provide information on whether that particular technology/brand has been reported to the FDA as having been dysfunctional or caused injury to a patient or staff member.
http://www.va.gov/ncps/safetytopics.html *National Center for Patient Safety (NCPS)* Accessed: December 9, 2008	Hazard summaries: e.g., anticoagulation vulnerability Guidelines for completing a healthcare failure modes and effect analysis Guidelines for ensuring correct surgery	In leading an initiative on hand hygiene, this Web site has a PowerPoint presentation, posters, other media materials, and numerous

(continues)

Table 9-6 (continued)

Web Site	Contents	CNS Benefits
	Falls tool kit An extensive hand hygiene program Patient Safety Assessment Tool	tools for the CNS to use in this initiative, from calculating the amount of waterless soap to the time it takes to clean hands with the waterless soap.
http://www.guidelines.gov *AHRQ and American Medical Association* Accessed: December 9, 2008	AHRQ and American Medical Association national guidelines clearing house	CNSs challenged with a new patient population should start by going to the evidence to see what has already been published. Guidelines on this site are evidence based.

Table 9-7   EXAMPLES OF WEB SITES WITH PSI: REGULATORY AGENCIES

Web Site	Contents	CNS Benefits
http://www.ccforpatientsafety.org *WHO Collaborating Centre for Patient Safety Solutions* Accessed: December 9, 2008	Patient Safety Practices Resources, patient safety tools, cases studies • Tools/resources including a link to approximately 40 patient safety Web sites • Awards • Case studies • Patient safety good practices • Articles/newsletter Facilitates finding patient safety goals and practices by using drop-down menus • Causes of adverse events/types of events • U.S. national patient safety goals/international patient safety goals Patient safety link, newsletter Links to patient safety practices, products and services, and resources. Archives available online Official newsletter: *Collaboration* (quarterly; electronic)	The CNS observes that the culture of safety is not ingrained in the practice area. There is a sample outline for a patient safety program. In investigating a sentinel event via the root cause analysis mechanism, this site walks the CNS through the causes of adverse events and types of adverse events that might be uncovered. Solution sets for look-alike, sound-alike medication names, patient identification, communication during hand-offs, and performance of correct procedure at correct body site.

Table 9-8 EXAMPLES OF WEB SITES FOR EVIDENCE-BASED PRACTICE

Web Site	Contents	CNS Benefits
http://www.ohsu.edu/epc *Oregon Evidenced-Based Practice Center* Accessed: December 9, 2008	OHSU is an evidenced-based practice center that conducts systematic review of healthcare topics for federal and state agencies and private foundations. These reviews report the evidence from clinical research studies and the quality of that evidence for use by policy makers in decisions on guidelines	The CNS is the leader in the introduction of the concepts of evidenced-based practice. Either of these Web sites provides guidance on "where to start" in introducing evidence-based practice at the bedside.
http://www.joannabriggs.edu.au/about/home.php *Joanna Briggs Institute* Accessed: December 9, 2008	International Research and Development Unit, which provides a collaborative approach to the evaluation of evidence derived from a diverse range of sources, including experience, expertise, and all forms of rigorous research	

Educating New and Experienced Nurses: Electronic Resources for the CNS

Patient safety as a discipline is a relatively new phenomenon. Many nurses, as well as other healthcare providers, did not explore the science of safety and error reduction or the relationship of culture to patient safety during formal nursing education experiences. Nurses may be inclined to consider patient safety as closely aligned with the traditional five rights of medication administration. These five "rights" include right patient, right drug, right dose, right route, and right time. Many nurses will recall learning these rights by rote as students, and new orientees were often drilled about these rules during clinical experiences involving medication or treatment deliveries. Nurses may continue to view these five rights as the gold standard of error prevention; however, these five rights are best viewed as the desired outcomes of safe medication practices (Federico, 2007). They do not offer strategies for nurses interested in achieving these goals other than a rather bewildering perception that error is the result of individual performance and good nurses do not make mistakes (Federico, 2007). Given that nurses do not come to work intending to commit errors, opportunities for error and accident reduction must be more broadly based than relying on drilled processes.

CNSs interested in using creative, evidence-based resources for educating new-to-practice nurses as well as more experienced staff without much formal exposure to health safety and quality topics will appreciate the opportunities available through Quality and Safety Education for Nurses (2007), a comprehensive resource funded by the Robert Wood Johnson Foundation (see Exemplar 9-2).

Exemplar 9-2

Promoting Safety by Influencing New-to-Practice Nurses

Geralyn Altmiller, EdD, MSN, APRN

Quality improvement and patient safety initiatives are much broader and more evidence-based than suggested by simplistic and systematized rules historically emphasized in basic nursing education. Recognizing the need for change, the Robert Wood Johnson Foundation spawned a national movement to change the way that nurses are prepared for patient care delivery by funding the Quality and Safety in Nursing Education (QSEN) grant through the University of North Carolina, Chapel Hill (2005). The grant provided 15 pilot schools across the nation with the opportunity to integrate practices for quality improvement and patient safety standards into their nursing curricula. As this national movement to improve preparation in prelicensure education of all nurses grows, recently graduated nurses are entering the workforce with varying degrees of competency in addressing patient safety concerns.

The CNS has a particularly important role in bridging the gap between prelicensure nursing education and the first work position of new-to-practice nurses. Providing resources and opportunities that connect practitioners to nationally accepted standards and by supporting and developing safety initiatives, CNSs model the transformation of nursing practice into a higher quality, safer endeavor.

The Institute for Healthcare Improvement (IHI) Web site (n.d.) contains a wealth of resources to assist the CNS as she or he supports those new to the profession of nursing. One such resource is Transforming Care at the Bedside (TCAB) (IHI, 2003), an initiative developed to connect nursing education to the vision of improving bedside care for the patient. Using the easily downloadable TCAB storyboard (IHI, 2008b), the CNS can connect the newly graduated nurse to the new skill sets being implemented across the nation to provide patient-centered care. The storyboard promotes personal accountability and situational awareness as tools to avoid codes, reduce readmission rates, prevent falls, and improve patient satisfaction.

At the same Web site, CNSs may access the 5 Million Lives Campaign (IHI, 2008a). This initiative works toward preventing 5 million incidents of medical harm by asking healthcare institutions to adhere to 12 safety-focused interventions. By clicking the Materials tab, the CNS has access to free slide presentations that demonstrate strategies for implementing the 12 interventions, along with blueprints for educational presentations to staff, updates on the latest prevention interventions, and related articles.

An important role of the CNS is to introduce the new language of safety and quality care improvement to the new-to-practice nurse or to the uninitiated seasoned professional. Value-added nursing care, which is the care that directly contributes to an improved outcome for the patient (such as rounding on the unit), or *workarounds*, the term that identifies routes to circumvent the established work system (obtaining meds from another patient's drawer rather than the pharmacy), may be terms more commonly used in the work environment but missing from some aspects of nursing education at present, thereby creating a communication barrier for the new graduate RN. To bridge that gap, the Agency for Healthcare Research and Quality (AHRQ) provides a Glossary (n.d.) of current terms as a resource on its Web site.

Many times new-to-practice nurses are uncomfortable communicating with other members of the healthcare team, particularly when they believe a patient concern is not being attended to. Improving communication skills can be facilitated by the CNS using helpful tools available through the AHRQ such as *TeamSTEPPS* (AHRQ, 2005). The *TeamSTEPPS* site contains free slide show downloads for presentations as well as short vignettes in high-resolution video that are designed to familiarize healthcare workers with current trends in communication techniques and risk-reduction practices. On the Web site, there are many examples of safe communication practices that can be used to increase the attention of other healthcare team members such as CUS (I'm Concerned, Uncomfortable, Safety) or DESC (Describe the situation, Express feelings about the situation, Suggest other alternative actions, Consequences of current actions are stated).

The Joint Commission is an organization that is frequently discussed in healthcare settings but many new-to-practice nurses do not have a clear understanding of what the Joint Commission does or how it functions within the healthcare setting. It is a national organization that accredits healthcare facilities. In doing so, hospitals are graded based on their ability to demonstrate that they follow the standards set by the Joint Commission to maintain a highly reliable practice setting. Not only does this accreditation assure the public that the hospital is meeting standards, but it provides a measure that insurance companies use to determine their willingness to refer members to that facility. The CNS promotes compliance of the standards when she or he helps staff members understand the value of accreditation and the pivotal role of nurses in the process.

Familiarizing new-to-practice nurses with the Joint Commission Web site (n.d.) promotes a sense of personal accountability for system improvement to ensure patient safety. The Patient Safety tab provides concrete information regarding the current National Patient Safety Goals, abbreviations that are not acceptable due to high error potential, and extensive materials that can be used to demonstrate and promote patient safety practices. The Sentinel Event tab provides a root cause analysis framework that presents a step-by-step walk through the process. Using this resource, the CNS demonstrates to the new graduate that there are usually multiple factors that contribute to error. The root cause analysis specifically identifies those factors and frequently reveals that error is attributed to systems failure. The CNS empowers the new-to-practice nurse when that individual recognizes that reporting an adverse event can lead to quality improvement because only then can the root cause be identified and the system or process be corrected to reduce risk.

In addition, the Joint Commission Sentinel Event tab highlights current alerts. Most notable is the alert that workplace intimidation and aggression is a threat to patient safety. The Joint Commission has mandated that all healthcare systems address hostile work environment behavior by January 2009 as a risk-reduction strategy. Many times, new-to-practice nurses are the most vulnerable to intimidation by peers in the workplace as they have known knowledge deficits. Intimidation interferes with their acquisition of knowledge and skill development. Cognitive rehearsal of shielding responses (Griffin, 2004) has been an effective strategy that the CNS can teach new-to-practice nurses. It enables them to recognize that the intimidating behavior is a result of stress and frustration and not a personal affront, thereby allowing the new graduate to respond in an intellectual manner rather than respond emotionally.

The unfolding case study is a learning strategy that has been promoted by QSEN (2007) to increase critical thinking in undergraduate nursing education. This approach can be used by the CNS to promote critical thinking in new-to-practice nurses by stimulating real-world decision making. The CNS can access descriptions of actual workplace adverse events on the AHRQ's Patient Safety Network (n.d.) by clicking the Patient Safety Primers tab. Based on these descriptions, the CNS can develop unfolding case scenarios that cultivate critical thinking and decision-making skills. The CNS can utilize the unfolding case study method as a strategy to inform new-to-practice nurses of the available resources at the institution that should be utilized to achieve a positive outcome for patients in similar situations.

Lastly, the CNS functions as a bridge between research and practice. Many new-to-practice nurses have a familiarity with evidence-based practice but are not sure how it is implemented in the clinical setting. The Cochrane Collaboration (n.d.) is an international database that the CNS can access to retrieve the latest information regarding appropriate interventions. AHRQ's National Guideline Clearinghouse (2008) provides recommendations and rating schemes of the strength of evidence for specific diseases and health problems. The CNS can promote the use of these sites with new-to-practice nurses as a means to determine the appropriate care required for their patients.

There are many resources available to the CNS working with new-to-practice nurses that will support a smooth transition from the prelicensure educational setting to the work environment. The CNS needs to recognize the significant role he or she plays in the transformation that occurs when a nurse enters the workforce and is confronted with the challenges to provide high-quality, safe patient care in a rapid-paced, constantly evolving profession. A toolkit of resources (see Table 9-9) is an invaluable asset.

Table 9-9   TOOLKIT OF INTERNET RESOURCES FOR THE CNS WORKING WITH NEW-TO-PRACTICE NURSES

Resource	Web Site Address
AHRQ: Glossary	http://www.webmm.ahrq.gov/glossary.aspx
AHRQ: National Guideline Clearinghouse	http://www.guideline.gov/compare/synthesis.aspx
AHRQ: Patient Safety Network	http://psnet.ahrq.gov
AHRQ: TeamSTEPPS	http://dodpatientsafety.usuhs.mil/index.php?name=News&file=article&sid=31
The Cochrane Collaboration	http://www.cochrane.org
IHI: Transforming Care at the Bedside	http://www.ihi.org/IHI/Programs/StrategicInitiatives/TransformingCareAtTheBedside.htm
IHI: Transforming Care at the Bedside Storyboard	http://www.ihi.org/NR/rdonlyres/F81270CD-B8BC-47D5-B2A6-BDA550096AA9/4252/TCABStoryboardFall2006FINAL.pdf
IHI: 5 Million Lives Campaign	http://www.ihi.org/IHI/Programs/Campaign
QSEN Teaching Strategies	http://qsen.org/teachingstrategies/search_strategies#results
The Joint Commission	http://www.jointcommission.org

Case Study: Development and Implementation of a Rapid Response Team

The majority of hospitalized patients experience antecedent physiologic abnormalities prior to cardiopulmonary arrests. When these abnormalities occur outside an intensive care unit, they are often unrecognized or are not responded to in a timely, appropriate manner by the hospital care team. This may be partially due to a reduced awareness of the importance of these physiologic abnormalities in the spectrum of disease or perhaps due to competing clinical responsibilities on the part of the physician or nurse practitioner. This scenario becomes increasingly complex in academic medical centers, as the most junior-level physicians typically perform the triage, clinical management, and communication around these critical events.

A rapid response team (or medical emergency team) is a team of critical care clinicians who can respond to the bedside of a deteriorating patient before a catastrophic event (e.g., cardiac or respiratory arrest) occurs. The goal of the team is to reduce the number of cardiac arrests and unanticipated intubations outside the ICU through clinical staff members' heightened awareness to signs of physiologic deterioration and through the development of a mobile team that can provide immediate critical care to the bedside.

The IHI *Save 100,000 Lives* campaign had designated the development of a rapid response team as one of the six interventions to decrease unanticipated mortality. The subsequent *5 Million Lives* campaign, launched in December 2006, continues to advocate for rapid response teams and the other five original interventions while also adding new interventions selected to reduce harm (IHI, 2008a). IHI provides many useful, effective, and cost-efficient resources for CNSs interested in beginning programs designed to improve healthcare safety. It is an "absolute must" Web site that should be easily accessible to CNSs and professional staff.

Kleinpell and Gawlinski (2005) have developed a nine-step process to guide the CNS in planning and implementing an outcomes-driven initiative. Table 9-10 describes an example of a process to establish a rapid response team, one of the recommendations of the IHI *Save 100,000 Lives* campaign and continued with the *5 Million Lives* campaign. The model can be used to develop other safety-related interventions, such as programs to decrease central line infections and ventilator-associated pneumonia (IHI, 2008b).

Skill breadth, competence, and familiarity with multiple roles uniquely positions the CNS to play a pivotal role in patient safety. The CNS is able to integrate knowledge of patient safety with evidence-based practice to improve outcomes (Phillips, 2005). The role of the CNS in patient safety will continue to expand exponentially; thus, the introduction of the CNS into the world of patient safety is just the beginning of a successful journey toward creating a culture of safety, integrated with evidenced-based practice to produce the highest quality of care possible.

Table 9-10 DEVELOPING A RAPID RESPONSE TEAM

Steps in the Process	Interventions
Find/Identify outcome variables that the CNS can impact. CNS Skills/Roles: Collaborator, clinical leader, research (Hamric, 1989)	1. Decrease codes/airway emergencies outside the ICU. 2. Decrease unplanned transfers to the ICU. 3. Improve nurse/caregiver satisfaction by providing a support system for the staff to call when their patient is in distress.
Organize a team: Who are the key stakeholders? CNS Skills: Change agent, collaborator, role model (Hamric, 1989)	1. Engage senior leadership: physicians, nursing, administration. 2. Other stakeholders: nursing, house staff and training directors, respiratory therapy, pharmacy.
Clarify current knowledge of the practice issue to be resolved. CNS Skills/Roles: Research, collaborator, patient advocate, change agent (Hamric, 1989)	1. Preparation phase includes accurate collection of baseline levels of serious adverse events and cardiac arrests. 2. What percent of codes or airway emergencies occur outside the ICU? 3. What percent of codes or airway emergencies are accompanied by clinical antecedents? 4. Were the clinical antecedents recognized? 5. What is the understanding of the staff of early detection of physiologic deterioration? 6. What communication strategies are utilized to accurately and concisely get the message across? 7. SBAR (situation, background, assessment, recommendation).

Table 9-10 (continued)

Steps in the Process	Interventions
Understand sources of variation. CNS Skills/Roles: Research, consultant, educator, patient advocate (Hamric, 1989)	1. When clinical deterioration is recognized, how is that clinical presentation responded to by the nurse? House staff? 2. What barriers prevent the bedside practitioner from calling for help (calling the attending physician) when his or her gut instinct suggests it is the right thing to do?
Select practices and strategies for improvement. CNS Skills/Roles: Clinical leader, educator, change agent (Hamric, 1989)	1. Establish a trigger tool to provide the staff with a concrete reference for when to call the team. Include at least one caveat that relates to that "gut feeling." 2. Design the team based on currently available personnel. Team construction varies from hospital to hospital. Teams are as simple as the ICU charge nurse and respiratory therapist to as complex as an eight-member team led by an intensivist. 3. Develop protocols for practice if needed. 4. Define team role during activation. 5. Provide team leadership. 6. Assess, intervene, stabilize, arbitrate to appropriate level of care. 7. Communicate, communicate, communicate! 8. Establish a feedback mechanism for the response team to feedback information to the teams that made the calls.
Plan for implementation. CNS Skills/Roles: Clinical leader, role model, educator, consultant (Hamric, 1989)	1. Develop educational curriculum. 2. Bedside practitioners. 3. Responding team.

(continues)

Table 9-10   (continued)

Steps in the Process	Interventions
Plan for implementation. (continued)	4. Physicians, nurses, therapists, technicians, virtually anyone who comes in contact with the patient, page operators.
	5. Data management.
	6. Documentation while on the scene.
	7. Why team was called, who called, interventions, outcomes, communication with attending physician.
	8. Log and analyze calls and "missed opportunities."
	9. Public relations (need at least five venues to get the word out).
	10. Posters, flyers.
	11. Grand rounds for nursing, medicine, any department.
	12. Present at departmental meetings.
	13. Discuss at unit-based meetings.
	14. "Roadshow," or traveling inservice, bringing the information to the staff on the floors.
Do the interventions according to the plan. CNS Skills/Roles: Research, education, change agent, role model, expert practitioner (Hamric, 1989)	1. Operationalize team as planned.
	2. Phase I or pilot for a defined period of time.
	3. Analyze each call to identify areas of opportunity.
	4. Clinical review: Why were calls placed? What happened at the bedside?
	5. Operational review: Did everything go as planned? Did the team show up? Did the equipment work? Did you need something that you didn't have? Did you need someone who was not available?

Table 9-10 (continued)	
Steps in the Process	**Interventions**
Check/analyze/review data CNS Skills/Roles: Collaborator, researcher (Hamric, 1989)	1. Review data from each event for clinical and operational efficiencies. 2. Compare preintervention/postintervention data for changes in rates of codes outside the ICU, unanticipated transfers to the ICU, and unanticipated mortality.
Put improvement into effect, hold gains, and establish lessons learned. CNS Skills/Roles: Change agent, collaborator, clinical leader, role model, patient advocate (Hamric, 1989)	1. Evaluate process and make appropriate changes to trigger tool, documentation tool, team notification process, or team activities at the bedside. 2. Continue to review data to establish success of program. 3. Involve staff in satisfaction survey to ascertain the effect on nursing satisfaction.

Source: Kleinpell and Gawlinski, 2005; Phillips, 2005.

References

American Association of Critical-Care Nurses (AACN). (2002). *Scope of practice and standards of professional performance for the acute and critical care clinical nurse specialist.* Aliso Viejo, CA: Author.

American Association of Critical-Care Nurses (AACN). (2005). *AACN standards for establishing and sustaining healthy work environments. A journey to excellence.* Retrieved July 7, 2006, from http://www.aacn.org/aacn/pubpolcy.nsf/Files/HWEStandards/$file/HWEStandards.pdf

Agency for Health Research and Quality (AHRQ). (2001). Patient safety practices: Practices rated by strength of evidence. In *Making health care safer: A critical analysis of patient safety practices* (Evidence report/technology assessment Number 43, AHRQ Publication No. 01-E058). Retrieved July 23, 2006, from http://ahrq.gov/clinic/ptsafety/pdf/ptsafety.pdf

Agency for Health Research and Quality (AHRQ). (2003) Chapter 2: Efforts to reduce medical errors: AHRQ's response to senate committee on appropriations. In *Patient safety initiative: Building foundations reducing risk.* Retrieved July 23, 2006, from http://www.ahrq.gov/qual/pscongrpt/psini2.htm

Agency for Health Research and Quality (AHRQ). (2008a). Appendix B. *High reliability organization learning network operational advice from the Exempla Healthcare site visit.* Retrieved December 8, 2008, from http://www.ahrq.gov/qual/hroadvice/hroadviceapb.pdf

Agency for Health Research and Quality (AHRQ). (2008b). *Transforming hospitals into highly reliable organizations.* Retrieved December 8, 2008, from http://www.ahrq.gov/qual/hroadvice/hroadvice1.htm

Agency for Health Research and Quality (AHRQ). (2008c). *Patient safety culture surveys.* Retrieved December 8, 2008, from http://www.ahrq.gov/qual/hospculture

Aspden, P., Corrigan, J. M., Wolcott, J., & Erickson, S. M. (Eds.). (2004). *Committee on Data Standards for Patient Safety. Patient safety: Achieving a new standard for care.* Washington, DC: National Academies Press.

Barden, C. (Ed). (2005). *AACN standards for establishing and sustaining healthy work environments.* Retrieved July 23, 2006, from http://www.aacn.org/aacn/pubpolcy.nsf/Files/HWEStandards/$file/HWEStandards.pdf

Centers for Medicare and Medicaid Services (CMS) and Joint Commission. (2008). *Specifications Manual for National Hospital Inpatient Quality Measures Discharges 10-01-08 (4Q08) through 03-31-09 (1Q09).* Retrieved October 26, 2008, from http://www.jointcommission.org/NR/rdonlyres/304A9AA7-0C23-46F8-A94C-A14C25744690/0/NHQM_v25b_pdf_add76513.zip

Cook, A. F., Hoas, H., Guttmannova, K., & Joyner, J. C. (2004). An error by any other name. *American Journal of Nursing, 104,* 32–43.

De Rosier, J., & Stalhandske, E. (2006). *Veteran's Administration Center for Patient Safety: Veterans Health Administration: Root cause analysis (RCA).* Retrieved July 23, 2006, from http://www.va.gov/ncps/Cogaids/RCA/index.htm#

Duwe, B., Fuchs, B., & Hansen-Flashen, J. (2005). Failure mode and effects analysis application to critical care medicine. *Critical Care Medicine, 21*, 21–30.

Federico, F. (2007). *The five rights of medication administration. Topics. Medication systems. Improvement stories.* Retrieved November 3, 2008, from http://www.ihi.org/IHI/Topics/PatientSafety/MedicationSystems/ImprovementStories/FiveRightsofMedication Administration.htm

Friersen, M. A., Farquhar, M. B., & Hughes, R. G. (2006). *The nurse's role in promoting a culture of patient safety. Center for American Nurses.* Retrieved July 23, 2006, from http://www.ana.org/mods/mod780/role.pdf

Hamric, A. B. (1989). History and overview of the clinical nurse specialist. In A. B. Hamric & J. B. Spross (Eds.). *The clinical nurse specialist in theory and practice.* Philadelphia, PA: W. B. Saunders.

HealthGrades. (2006). *Third annual patient safety in America study.* Retrieved December 8, 2008, from http://www.healthgrades.com/media/dms/pdf/patientsafetyinamerican hospitalsstudy2006.pdf

Helmreich, R. (2005). *Culture of safety. Risk and quality management strategies: HRC supplement A.* Retrieved December 8, 2008, from http://www.ecri.org/Documents/Patient_Safety_Center/HRC_CultureofSafety.pdf

Institute for Healthcare Improvement (IHI). (2008a). *Protecting 5 million lives from harm PowerPoint.* Retrieved December 8, 2008, from http://www.ihi.org/NR/rdonlyres/7AE7044B-C006-4A5F-896E-

Institute for Healthcare Improvement (IHI). (2008b). *Protecting 5 million lives from harm.* Retrieved December 8, 2008, from http://www.ihi.org/IHI/Programs/Campaign/Campaign.htm?TabId=1

Institute for Safe Medication Practices. (2006). *Assess-ERR medication system worksheet.* December 8, 2008, from http://www.ismp.org/Tools/AssessERR.pdf

Joint Commission. (2006). *National patient safety goals, 2007.* Retrieved July 23, 2006, from http://jointcommission.org/Patientsafety/NationalPatientSafetyGoals/07_hap_cah_npsgs.htm

Kleinpell, R., & Gawlinski, A. (2005). Assessing outcomes in advanced practice nursing practice. *AACN Clinical Issues, 16*, 43–57.

Kohn, L., Corrigan, J., & Donaldson, M. (Eds.). (2000). *To err is human: Building a safer health system.* Washington, DC: National Academies Press.

Leapfrog Group. (2007). *Our mission: The Leapfrog Group mission statement.* Retrieved October 20, 2008, from http://www.leapfroggroup.org/about_us/our_mission

Leonard, M., Graham, S., & Bonacum, D. (2004). The human factor: The critical importance of effective teamwork and communication in providing safe care. *Quality and Safety in Healthcare, 13*(Suppl. 1), i85–i90.

National Association of Clinical Nurse Specialists (NACNS). (2004). *Statement on clinical nurse specialist practice and education* (2nd ed.). Harrisburg, PA: Author.

Oncology Nursing Society. (2003). *The role of the advanced practice nurse in oncology care.* Retrieved July 24, 2006, from http://www.ons.org/publications/positions/Advance Practice.shtml

Phillips, J. (2005). Neuroscience CC: The role of the APN in patient safety. *AACN Clinical Issues, 16*, 580–591.

Pronovost, P. J., Thompson, D. A., Holzmueller, C. G., Lubomski, L. H., & Morlock, L. L. (2005). Defining and measuring patient safety. *Critical Care Clinics, 21*, 1–19.

Quality and Safety Education for Nurses. (2007). Home page. Retrieved November 3, 2008, from http://www.qsen.org

Reason, J. (1990). *Human error.* New York: Cambridge University Press.

Sora, J., & Nieva, V. (2003). Safety culture assessment: A tool for improving patient safety in healthcare organizations. *Quality and Safety in Healthcare, 12*(Suppl. 2), ii17–ii23.

Tucker, A. L., & Edmondson, A. C. (2002). When problem solving prevents organizational learning. *Journal of Organizational Change Management, 15*, 122–138.

Volker, D. L., & Clark, A. P. (2004). Taking the high road: What should you do when an adverse event occurs, Part II. *Clinical Nurse Specialist, 18*, 180–182.

White, S. V. (2004). Patient safety issues. In J. Byers & S. White (Eds.), *Patient safety: Principles and practice.* New York: Springer.

Wolf, Z. (2007). Pursuing safe medication use and the promise of technology. *Medical-Surgical Nursing Journal, 16*, 92–100.

World Health Organization Collaborating Centre for Patient Safety Solutions. (2008). About us. Retrieved November 3, 2008, from http://www.ccforpatientsafety.org/31588

Zuzelo, P., Gettis, C., Hansell, A., & Thomas, L. (2008). Describing the influence of technologies on registered nurses' work. *Clinical Nurse Specialist, 22*(3), 132–240.

Exemplar 9-2 References

Agency for Healthcare Research and Quality (AHRQ). (2005). *TeamSTEPPS.* Retrieved July 9, 2008, from http://dodpatientsafety.usuhs.mil/index.php?name=News&file=article&sid=31

Agency for Healthcare Research and Quality (AHRQ). (2008). *National guideline clearinghouse.* Retrieved on July 30, 2008, from http://www.guideline.gov/compare/synthesis.aspx

Agency for Healthcare Research and Quality (AHRQ). (n.d.). *Patient safety network.* Retrieved July 30, 2008, from http://psnet.ahrq.gov

Agency for Healthcare Research and Quality (AHRQ). (n.d.) *Web M&M: Glossary.* Retrieved July 28, 2008, from http://www.webmm.ahrq.gov/glossary.aspx

Cochrane Collaboration. (n.d). *Homepage.* Retrieved July 30, 2008, from http://www.cochrane.org

Ebright, P. R. (2004). Understanding nurse work. *Clinical Nurse Specialist, 18*, 168–170.

Griffin, M. (2004). Teaching cognitive rehearsal as a shield for lateral violence: An intervention for newly licensed nurses. *Journal of Continuing Education in Nursing, 35*(6), 257–263.

Institute for Healthcare Improvement (IHI). (2003). *Transforming care at the bedside.* Retrieved July 8, 2008, from http://www.ihi.org/IHI/Programs/StrategicInitiatives/TransformingCareAtTheBedside.htm

Institute for Healthcare Improvement (IHI). (2006a). *5 Million Lives campaign.* Retrieved July 30, 2008, from http://www.ihi.org/IHI/Programs/Campaign

Institute for Healthcare Improvement (IHI). (2006b). *Transforming care at the bedside storyboard.* Retrieved July 8, 2008, from http://www.ihi.org/NR/rdonlyres/F81270CD-B8BC-47D5-B2A6-BDA550096AA9/4252/TCABStoryboardFall2006FINAL.pdf

Institute for Healthcare Improvement. (n.d.). *Homepage.* Retrieved July 30, 2008, from http://www.ihi.org/ihi

Joint Commission. (n.d.) *Homepage.* Retrieved July 30, 2008, from http://www.jointcommission.org

Quality and Safety in Nursing Education (QSEN). (2005). *Overview.* Retrieved July 8, 2008, from http://qsen.org/about/overview

Quality and Safety in Nursing Education (QSEN). (2007). *Search teaching strategies.* Retrieved July 30, 2008, from http://qsen.org/teachingstrategies/search_strategies#results

The Basics of Nursing Business

Patti Rager Zuzelo, EdD, MSN, RN, ACNS-BC

Mary Beth Kingston, MSN, RN, NEA-BC

Nursing administration is a specialty that requires the juxtaposition of business savvy and regulatory expertise with an understanding of clinical practice demands. CNSs have a systems perspective and an understanding of modes of influence that make them valuable to nurse managers and nurse executives. In fact, many CNSs consider administrative job opportunities at some point in their professional careers. It is not uncommon to find nurse executives educationally prepared as CNSs but practicing as administrators.

Arguably, nurse executives require formal expertise in business and nursing administration; however, the many opportunities available to nurses combined with the shortage of nurses prepared at the graduate level in nursing administration promote the wide range of academic and clinical backgrounds found in the ranks of nurse administrators. Perhaps this diversity is a strength and no different than the diversity found in the physician–executive group.

CNS practice requires a basic grasp of healthcare business principles and a clear understanding of the healthcare system. This knowledge is required for rational, effective practice in multidisciplinary settings with outcomes emphases and tight fiscal constraints. Basic familiarity with health care and nursing "business" is critical for CNSs who are expected to develop new programs and improve clinical processes. Basic business acumen is also useful for the CNS who envisions future employment in nursing administration.

The Context of CNS Practice: An Overview of the U.S. Healthcare System

A variety of well-written resources are available on this subject. Shi and Singh (2005) provide an overview of the U.S. healthcare system that is concise and essential. CNSs are advised to understand different types of managed care organizations (MCOs), including health maintenance organizations (HMOs), preferred provider organizations (PPOs), and exclusive provider organizations (EPO). It is also helpful to appreciate the characteristics of point-of-service plans that allow for more patient choice than HMOs but at greater cost to enrollees.

MCOs are part of a larger group referred to as third-party payors because they are connected to two other key parties of interest in health care, the patient and the provider (Shi & Singh, 2005). Other members of the third-party payor group include insurance companies, Blue Cross/Blue Shield, Medicare, and Medicaid. Each third-party payor pays differently, depending on its reimbursement method and contractual arrangement.

Fee-for-service is a rare arrangement when compared to other forms of reimbursement. Providers determine charges, bills are generated, and insurers pay. The higher the charges, the greater the net revenue. Diagnosis-related groups (DRGs) were an early strategy for curtailing the spiraling costs associated with fee-for-service arrangements.

Third-Party Payors

The "payor mix" of an institution is a critically important variable in the assumptions underlying institutional budgets. CNSs need to have a general sense of the payor mix of their practice and of the employing institution, network, or practice as this mix directly influences the amount and variability of revenue streams available for all types of services, including educational programs, equipment, and the affordability of staffing mix and nurse-to-patient ratios.

Managed Care Organizations

HMOs are the earliest forms of MCOs and continue as a popular arrangement. The goal of HMOs is to reduce costs while providing quality care. Care is coordinated through the primary care provider, who serves as a "gatekeeper" to services and safeguards against unnecessary tests or treatments. HMOs offer services to maintain or improve health status, recognizing that it is more cost effective to avoid illness than to treat illness. Preventive services such as smoking cessation, weight management, physical fitness, and routine wellness visits are examples of services designed to reduce the risk of disease and to intervene early when illness occurs.

HMOs usually pay providers a fee per person on a contracted basis. This fee is referred to as "capitation." Enrollees are restricted to service providers, including hospitals, physicians, laboratories, and other diagnostic service facilities within the network. There are a variety of HMO models with differing physician arrangements; for example, staff models with HMO-salaried providers, group models with contracted physicians within a group practice rather than employed physicians, network models with a variety of contracted medical groups, and the independent practice association (IPA) model, in which the IPA shares risk and assumes responsibility for utilization and quality management (Shi & Singh, 2005).

PPOs offer enrollees more choices and increased control over their utilization of specialists. Enrollees can opt for out-of-network service providers, albeit at a higher cost, through preestablished copayments (Shi & Singh, 2005). PPOs are more expensive on average than HMOs (American Association of Preferred Provider Organization, 2004) and do not use capitation arrangements. They typically work on a contractual arrangement with providers in a modified fee-for-service approach. PPOs are the most common form of health coverage having 60% of insured employees as members, whereas HMOs have approximately 20% of covered workers, despite the lower costs of HMO programs (Kaiser Family Foundation, 2006).

EPOs are similar to PPOs, but enrollees cannot receive reimbursed care from a provider outside of network (Bureau of Labor Statistics [BLS], 2002). This arrangement prioritizes cost savings. Providers serve as gatekeepers, similar to the HMO arrangement.

Private Health Insurance

Blue Cross/Blue Shield plans are nonprofit and cover hospital and physician services. In addition to Blue Cross and Blue Shield, other private health insurance plans may be purchased privately as an individual or family member or purchased as an employee participating in an employer-provided plan. Private health insurance plans are offered in a variety of forms, including MCOs, indemnity, or fee-for-service.

Public Health Insurance

The Centers for Medicare and Medicaid Services (CMS) are responsible for Medicare and Medicaid programs. CMS is organized within the Department of Health and Human Services (DHHS) and has a strategic plan that includes objectives related to regulatory, budgetary, and quality responsibilities for a variety of stakeholders (CMS, n.d.) (Table 10-1). CNSs need to have a basic understanding of CMS and its programs, given that many hospitals and healthcare practices are significantly influenced by regulations and reimbursements controlled by CMS.

Title 18 of the Social Security amendment of 1965 provided for Part A and Part B of Medicare, whereas Title 19 established the Medicaid program. Medicare provides publicly financed health insurance to elders, regardless of income. Some disabled people and individuals with end-stage kidney disease are also covered (Shi & Singh, 2005). Prescription benefits have been added via Part D benefits, and most people pay a monthly premium for this coverage (CMS, 2005). Medicaid covers eligible poor. Both programs are financed by the government, but healthcare services are provided by private healthcare entities.

Medicare Parts A and B cover different types of benefits. In general, Part A covers hospitalization and short-term nursing home stays following hospitalization. Part B covers physicians' bills and other outpatient services. Elders pay part of the premium expense of Part B, whereas Social Security taxes pay for Part A.

Federal expenditures have dramatically increased since the inception of these programs. The United States spent $1.9 trillion on health care in 2004, an average of $6280 per person. The health spending share of gross domestic product in 2004 was

Table 10-1   CMS MISSION, VISION, AND KEY OBJECTIVES

Mission: To ensure effective, up-to-date healthcare coverage and to promote quality care for beneficiaries.
Vision: To achieve a transformed and modernized healthcare system.
CMS will accomplish our mission by continuing to transform and modernize America's healthcare system.
Strategic Action Plan Objectives:
  • Skilled, committed, and highly motivated workforce
  • Accurate and predictable payments
  • High-value health care
  • Confident, informed consumers
  • Collaborative partnerships

Source: Centers for Medicare and Medicaid Services, n.d.

16% (CMS, 2006) and increased to 16.3% in 2007 (CMS, 2008). Growth in healthcare spending is predicted to annually increase by 6.7% during the period of 2007–2017 (CMS, 2008). As healthcare costs climb, federal, state, and local governments exert more stringent controls over reimbursements. Simultaneously, healthcare consumers and practitioners demand increasingly sophisticated and expensive technologies and services.

The struggle between cost and reimbursement has significant influence on the "bottom line" of healthcare organizations. Understanding this struggle is important for well-informed CNS practice. There is concern that CNSs may have inaccurate or inadequate understanding of CMS programs (Zuzelo et al., 2004) and that this knowledge deficit may disadvantage the public by artificially limiting the accessibility of CNSs to healthcare service recipients.

CNSs need to appreciate the context in which healthcare services are provided in the United States. A basic familiarity with various insurance models, differences between Medicare and Medicaid programs, and the effect of payor mix on healthcare organizations' budgets will assist the CNS in understanding the challenges confronting healthcare organizations and society.

Although CNSs are not ordinarily involved in budget and business processes at organizational or network levels, they are occasionally involved in these activities at the unit or department level or by service line. CNSs participate in capital budget development through product evaluations and recommendations. Nurses often ask CNSs to explain budget processes, and it is not uncommon for program administrators to solicit CNS input regarding basic operating and capital budget needs. This chapter explains key concepts of nursing budgets and, related to capital budgets, provides strategies and tools for product evaluation.

The Budget Process

Mary Beth Kingston, MSN, RN, NEA-BC

The degree of the CNS's involvement in the budget process varies depending on the organization. CNS exclusion from the process can represent a missed opportunity for nursing administration. The experience and expertise, as well as the clinical focus of the CNS, has the potential to add value to many facets of the budget process, including resource planning for new clinical programs, identification of quality-of-care issues, and comparison of equipment and clinical supply items. For the CNS to have a positive impact, knowledge of the general process and principles of the nursing budget is essential.

The budget is an annual process of identifying anticipated revenues and expenditures for an organization. It provides a framework to allocate resources that support ongoing operations and programs. Additionally, the budget serves as a monitoring and evaluation tool throughout the fiscal year (Table 10-2). The fiscal year (FY) is defined by each organization. The FY can correlate with the calendar year (January through December), but more often follows a July through June or October through September time frame.

Budgeting has often been described as an organization's best guess regarding future performance and expenses. However, the budget is based on a careful review of factors that might influence revenue and expenditures. The organization's strategic plan provides the framework for beginning the review process. The external environment, prior year performance, new programs, additional physician practices, and marketing initiatives are carefully reviewed. Additional sources of information include projected salary and price increases and regulatory changes.

The organization may start the budgeting process in a number of ways. In zero-based budgeting (ZBB), each budget request is justified every cycle regardless of prior history. Use of ZBB requires that managers justify why they should spend the organization's resources in the manner proposed. Each planned activity or project must include an analysis of cost, benefit, alternatives, and measures of performance. One major drawback to ZBB is the amount of time required to review and justify, at times, routine operational costs in great detail on an annual basis.

Table 10-2 FUNCTIONS OF A BUDGET

Budget Functions

1. Identify anticipated revenues.
2. Identify planned expenditures.
3. Provide a framework for resource allocations.
4. Monitor spending.
5. Evaluate accuracy of allocation decisions.
6. Evaluate fiscal responsibility.

Historical, or baseline, budgeting begins with the organization's historical data and builds on the readily available past performance of its operations. Historical budgeting works well in organizations with predictable operations. This method of budgeting saves time and is less likely to result in an omission of a key event, trend, or expense. Alternatively, it may also result in inclusion of items that no longer have relevance. In practice, many healthcare organizations use a combination of methods, relying on historical or baseline data combined with assessment of trends. A ZBB approach is frequently used when proposing new programs and initiatives (Table 10-3).

Types of Budgets

There are several types of budgets: operating budgets, revenue budgets, expense budgets, and capital budgets.

Operating Budget

The operating budget is the financial plan for the organization's day-to-day activities. It details the immediate goals for revenues, volumes, and expenses. The operating budget is extremely detailed and is used for monitoring throughout the year. The revenue and expense budgets make up the operating budget.

Revenue Budget

The revenue budget is the projected income for the fiscal year. The primary source of revenue in a healthcare organization is the delivery of healthcare services. Volume projections in each department drive the revenue budget. The definition of volume or

Table 10-3	BUDGET APPROACHES: ZERO-BASED BUDGET VERSUS HISTORICAL BUDGET		
Budget Type	**Description**	**Advantages**	**Disadvantages**
Zero-based budget	Start at zero. Justify each expense and revenue source.	1. Tight control over resources 2. Dollars allocated based on need rather than history	1. Time-consuming 2. Justifying routine, required expenses
Historical budget	Begin with previous budget. Build on past performances.	1. Works well in predictable situations 2. Saves time 3. Less likely to omit key events or trends	1. May budget for irrelevant items 2. May not scrutinize expenses as thoroughly

"units of service" varies with the specific patient care area, but includes visits in the emergency department, patient days in the inpatient areas, procedures in the surgical suite, and numbers of tests in the laboratory.

Volume is a major factor in calculating anticipated revenue, but there are other primary considerations. Federal and state reimbursement changes and contractual relationships with payors have a significant effect on revenue projection. Assumptions are also made regarding the acuity level of patients, specifically the case mix index (CMI) that affects Medicare reimbursement. The CMI is a marker of the severity of a patient's illness and is tracked by Medicare.

In the inpatient areas, the length of stay (LOS) and number of patient days affects revenue projections from admissions. LOS varies by specialty area and is influenced by historical data and the organization's ability to move patients to the appropriate level of care at the right time. LOS is typically longer on an inpatient behavioral health or rehabilitation unit as compared to a general surgical patient care area. If an organization has the ability to move patients from an acute care area to a skilled or long-term nursing facility, then the LOS may be reduced.

The number of patient days is another key revenue budget metric. The number of budgeted admissions multiplied by the LOS results in total number of patient days (Figure 10-1). The number of patient days has a direct effect on patient revenue, as well as expense. Many payors reimburse based on a case rate or diagnosis. In this instance, a prolonged LOS results in additional expense without corresponding revenue. If a payor pays a per diem rate, then an increased LOS might enhance revenue. Patient days are also an important metric in determining the nursing expense budget.

Expense Budget

The expense budget includes salaries, supplies, fees, purchased services, repairs, maintenance, consulting, education, insurance, depreciation, and many miscellaneous items. Healthcare expenses, particularly in nursing, are largely made up of salary expenses.

Salary Expenses

Salary expense can be divided into productive and nonproductive time. Productive time is time actually worked, and nonproductive time includes sick, holiday, vacation, orientation, and education hours. Productive hours include direct time or time spent in caregiving activities. Indirect hours include unit secretarial, nurse manager, and educator time.

Direct caregiver hours are usually classified as variable. These hours adjust to the patient care volume. Areas with minimum staffing requirements and those that have

---

Admissions × Length of Stay = Patient Days

20,000 annual admissions × 6.0 days LOS = 120,000 patient days

Figure 10-1 Number of patient days with example.

difficult-to-predict daily volume, for example, EDs or labor and delivery services, cannot routinely flex their direct care staff. Fixed hours are those required to run the unit regardless of fluctuating volume and census and include positions such as the unit secretary, housekeeper, and nurse manager.

Nonsalary Expenses

Supplies are second in importance to salary in the healthcare organization's budget. Supply expenses can also be categorized as fixed versus variable. Patient care supplies and forms usually fluctuate or vary with patient days. Expenses that are fixed include phone services and electricity. Many organizations have joined group purchasing programs to take advantage of reduced supply prices when purchased in quantity. Supply costs can often be a large component of the budget, particularly in surgical areas.

The Bottom Line

The bottom line or net income from operations is commonly measured as net patient revenues minus the total operating expenses (Figure 10-2). The organization's operating margin is the percentage of profit realized from the operations of its day-to-day business. Profit can be defined simply as the difference between net expenses and net revenue.

Capital Budget

The capital budget is developed separately from the operational budget and pertains to the organization's plan for investments in building or plant and major equipment. The capital budget is driven by the organization's strategic plan and is composed of two components: equipment purchases, building plans, and plant maintenance that occur within the annual budget cycle, and those that exceed 1 year in length. Typically a defined dollar amount determines whether an item is defined as capital. The amount varies, but is usually $500 or greater.

The annual capital budget begins with identification of equipment needs or building/renovation projects for the upcoming year. Patient care equipment needs may be unit based, program specific, or they may cut across clinical specialty lines. The initial list in nursing is often generated at the department level and should be developed by the nurse manager or director with significant input from the CNS, as well as the nursing staff. Examples of capital items are critical care monitoring equipment, dialysis machines, scales, hospital beds, and mattresses. Identification and communication of need are crucial steps, and the CNS can play a major role in this area. Identifying and evaluating products as part of the capital budget process are important CNS responsibilities, depending on the type of CNS practice.

Communication with other departments is particularly important when developing the capital budget. Determining which department is responsible for capital pur-

---

Net patient revenues − Total operating expenses = Bottom line

Figure 10-2 The bottom line.

chases may be confusing. For example, stretchers are purchased by the transport service for general use, yet the emergency department, operating room, and radiology purchase stretchers for their specific areas.

Many capital requests from other departments affect nursing practice and patient care, particularly related to renovating existing patient care areas. Capital requests may require renovation, and this need must be noted early and identified as an associated cost (Figure 10-3). For example, if monitoring equipment is purchased and the current electrical outlets are inadequate or in difficult-to-reach locations, renovation needs must be taken into account and communicated to the facilities and maintenance director (Figure 10-4).

Once items for a specific area are identified, the manager generally identifies the following information:

- Describes the item or equipment
- Identifies the number of items needed and whether this is a replacement or addition
- Lists the date or quarter of the fiscal year the purchase will take place
- Prioritizes each item

The manager typically works with the purchasing department to provide supporting documentation. The CNS often plays a role in comparing different vendors' products and networking with others to learn about new technology and efficacy.

Building the Nursing Budget

Nursing expenses are primarily based in the salary or personnel budget. The foundation of the salary budget is the full-time equivalent or FTE (Figure 10-5). It is important to note that the FTE is not a person, merely a time equivalent. Nursing job requirements for being considered a full-time employee vary widely, particularly with 12-hour shifts and increasing flexibility in scheduling. A nurse who works three 12-hour shifts per week is considered full time in many organizations, but the budget will reflect the position as a .9 FTE (Figure 10-6).

The number of FTEs required to provide care is determined in a number of ways. Nursing units begin with a standard and then match the standard to the projected volume. Inpatient units often utilize nursing hours per patient day (NHPPD) as the standard or metric; the number of hours of care divided by the number of patient days (Table 10-4). The required nursing hours are based on a variety of factors, including the type of unit, acuity of the patient population, and patient outcomes.

In specialty areas that do not utilize NHPPD, other standards are utilized. In the emergency department, nursing hours per patient visit is the metric. In the operating room, the number of staff required is case dependent, but also determined by a standard FTE per room.

Establishing the number of direct-care FTEs is not the final step in building a nursing budget. Not all of an FTE's 2080 hours per year are productive or worked hours. Replacement time must be built in to provide coverage for nursing staff during

CAPITAL EQUIPMENT REQUEST
CAPITAL JUSTIFICATION WORKSHEET

( ) MEDICAL   ( ) ADMINISTRATIVE   ( ) COMPUTER   ( ) RENOVATION*

ITEM DESCRIPTION/USAGE

CHECK OR ANSWER ALL THAT APPLY

PRIORITY RATING	REASON FOR REQUEST	ESTIMATED COST
( ) URGENT & NECESSARY (less than 6 months) ( ) NECESSARY (6 months to 1 year) ( ) ECONOMICALLY DESIRABLE ( ) OTHER - EXPLAIN	( ) NEW SERVICE ( ) REPLACEMENT ( ) IMPROVED SERVICE ( ) CODE/REGULATION REG. ( ) EXPENSE SAVINGS ( ) INCREASED VOLUM/PROD. ( ) RENOVATION ( ) OTHER	$_____ PURCHASE PRICE $_____ INSTALLATION* $_____ SHIPPING $_____ RENOVATION* $_____ TRIAL RUN $_____ TRAINING $_____ OTHER $_____ (LESS TRADE IN)

REPLACEMENT/DISPOSITION	REASON FOR REQUEST	
( ) RETAINED - AGE _____ ( ) DISPOSAL - AGE _____ ( ) OTHER - EXPLAIN _____	#OF TEST #OF PATIENTS #OF FTE'S	$_____ NET COST WARRANTY PERIOD EQUIPMENT ONLY

ESTIMATED INCREMENTAL REVENUES, EXPENSES & COST SAVINGS

ADDITIONAL OPERATING EXPENSES   ADDITIONAL REVENUES & EXPENSE SAVINGS

Item	Fiscal YR 2003	Annual	Item (LIST)	Fiscal YR 2004	Annual
Salaries					
Benefits 20%					
Supplies					
Insurance					
Service Contr.					
Other					
TOTAL			**SAVINGS**		

REMARKS

REVIEWED WITH VP INFORMATION SYSTEM?   ( ) YES   ( ) NO
REVIEWED BY: (Signature VP Information Systems)

REVIEWED WITH FACILITIES MANAGEMENT (INSTALLATION, UTILITIES, RENOVATION/ALTERATION)? FORM A-40 ATTACHED. ( ) YES ( ) NO

PLEASE ATTACH BUSINESS PLAN WHERE APPROPRIATE: EXAMPLE: NEW/IMPROVED SERVICE, INCREASED
REVENUE OR REVENUE JUSTIFIED ETC.   BUSINESS PLAN ATTACHED? ( ) YES ( ) NO

SUBMITTED BY: DEPT. NAME _____   DEPARTMENT HEAD SIGNATURE _____

                     DEPT. # _____

Campus Location

REVIEWED BY: VICE PRESIDENT _____   DATE: _____

PREVIEWED BY: range# _____
(office use only)   ADMINISTRATOR _____   Ranking _____

March 24, 2006   **PLEASE ATTACH DOCUMENTATION FOR EACH REQUEST TO THIS FORM!**

Figure 10-3 Capital budget request form.

Source: © 2006. Albert Einstein Healthcare Network. Reprinted with permission.

Albert Einstein Healthcare Network
Capital Request Form

SPACE, BUILDING & RENOVATION REQUEST

Capital Project # _____

To be completed by Department Head

DEPT. # _____	PROJECT DATE REQUESTED _____
DEPARTMENT NAME _____	PHONE# _____
Campus Location	Building Floor

1. Request for:

_____	Renovation of Area	_____	Relocation of Dept/ Equipment	_____ Additional Space*
_____	Reconfiguration of Area	_____	Installation of New Equipment	_____ Other

2. Description of Work: _____

_____

_____

_____

3. Justification for Work. _____

_____

_____

Signature of Department Head: _____ Date _____

Signature of Vice President: _____ Date _____

To be completed by Director Facilities Management

4. Cost Estimate Breakdown   Projected Length of Project _____

A. Project can be accomplished:

_____ With in-house labor and materials.
_____ Through outside contracting.
_____ Through a combination of in-house effort and contracting.
_____ DOH Approval/Notification required

B. Costs

Material Costs:	$ _____
Contractor Costs:	$ _____
In-House Labor Costs	$ _____
I. S. Costs (cabling/terminations)	$ _____
Other Costs	$ _____
Total Project Estimate	$ _____

Comments: _____

_____

_____

Signature of Vice President Facilities: _____ Date _____

Administrative Use Only

Ranking: _____ Approved _____ Denied _____ Deferred _____

Administrator Signature: _____ Date _____

PLEASE ATTACH DOCUMENTATION FOR EACH REQUEST TO THIS FORM!

March 24 2006

Figure 10-4 Space renovation form.

Source: © 2006. Albert Einstein Healthcare Network. Reprinted with permission.

> **40 hours per week × 52 weeks/year = 2080 hours 1 FTE**

Figure 10-5 Full-time equivalent (FTE) calculation.

> **36 hours per week × 52 weeks/year = 1872 hours**
> **1872 HOURS/2080 HOURS = .9 FTE**

Figure 10-6 Three 12-hour shifts per week employee.

Table 10-4	SAMPLE CALCULATION OF REQUIRED FTES BASED ON A STANDARD NHPPD
	Projected patient days = 7,300 patient days (equates to an Average Daily Census (ADC) of 20 patients.
	7300 patient days divided 365 days/year = 20 patients/day)
	NHPPD standard = 7.0
	(*Patient days × NHPPD standard = Total number of direct-care hours required*)
	7300 patient days × **7.0** NHPPD = 51,100 direct-care hours
	51,100 direct-care hours /2080 (1 FTE) = 24.56 required FTEs

vacation and sick, holiday, education, and orientation time. The replacement factor is based on the average benefit time, and this varies from organization to organization.

How Is Benefit Time Determined?

Benefit time is calculated by subtracting the number of benefit hours from the total FTE time (Table 10-5). In practice, there is individual variability with factors such as seniority playing a role in the amount of vacation time. Most organizations use an average to calculate time. It is important to recognize that on units with high percentages of senior staff, organizational averages may not be the best barometer for calculating benefit time.

Staffing Patterns and Ratios

A nursing budget can also be built by starting with a staffing pattern. Staffing patterns relate to NHPPD, but the budgeting process starts a bit differently depending on the metric. Recently, nurse–patient ratios have been a topic of debate and discussion. For example, California has a legislated 1:5 nurse (RN)–patient ratio on medical–surgical units, and the number of FTEs is based on this metric (Table 10-6). When using a staffing pattern to build the budget, LPN and assistive staff would be added to the matrix.

Table 10-5	BENEFIT TIME CALCULATIONS

Benefit Time

Vacation time = 4 weeks vacation annually or 160 hours

Sick time = average 6 days annually or 48 hours

Holiday time = 6 days annually or 48 hours

Personal days = 3 days annually or 24 hours

Educational time = 4 days annually or 32 hours

TOTAL = 312 hours

2080 hours (1 FTE) − 312 hours of benefit time = **1768 hours actually worked**

In this scenario, 312 hours, or 15% of total hours, will need to be replaced per FTE.

FTEs × 15% = total number of direct-care FTEs required

Again, indirect salaries need to be added, including medical clerks, nurse manager, clinical nurse specialist, and any other support staff that are in the nursing budget. A replacement factor must be built in for the medical clerks, but is not included for the nurse manager or clinical nurse specialist.

Once FTEs are determined, the type of hours or who will be filling the FTEs is a key decision. The following areas must be considered:

- Skill mix (percentage may already be determined by standard or history)
- Special programs, such as weekend rates/shift differentials
- Use of supplemental staff

Skill Mix

Skill mix refers to the proportion of licensed to nonlicensed caregivers in a patient care delivery model. Some organizations use an RN/LPN to nursing assistant/technician

Table 10-6	USING STAFFING RATIOS TO BUDGET FTES

Assumptions

Unit census = 20 patients

Nurse-to-patient ratio = 1:5

Number of required staff = 4

Three 8-hour shifts = 12 staff

Replacement factor 15% (see Table 10.5) = 12 staff × .15 replacement factor = 1.8 FTE

Total number of required staff:

12 FTEs + 1.8 FTEs = 13.8 FTEs

ratio and others use an RN to LPN/nursing assistant technician ratio. Ideally, the skill mix should be determined by carefully examining the patient population being served and identifying skills and tasks required to provide care. In practice, many factors affect skill-mix determinations.

Available RN supply affects skill mix. During times of RN shortage, skill-mix percentages often decrease due to inability to fill positions. Skill mix can also affect cost. Higher skill mix equals higher salary dollars. When developing the budget, the manager most often follows the historical trend for skill mix, unless a justification for change is submitted. The CNS can assist in identifying whether a change in skill mix is required based on the assessed needs of the patient population being served.

Typically, the historical pattern for skill mix varies based on the patient population and level of care. Critical care units tend to have a very high RN mix, and long-term care facilities have a lower RN mix. Nursing research has begun to focus on the impact of skill mix on patient outcomes.

Cho, Ketefian, Barkauskas, and Smith (2003) found that a 10% increase in RN proportion was associated with a 9.5% decrease in the incidence of pneumonia. Sovie (2001) noted that during hospital restructuring efforts, RNs were fewer in number, with an increase in unlicensed assistive personnel. The increased RN hours worked per patient/day was associated with lower fall rates and higher patient satisfaction levels with pain management. However, findings did not generate specific staffing recommendations. The CNS working with the manager can track outcome data on individual units and identify correlations with staffing to determine whether changes are required.

Incentives/Differentials

Organizations differ on how specific program incentives and differentials are captured. If shift differential or weekend program salary rates are not incorporated into the budget, then the unit will be over budget during the year, even though the hours of care remain constant.

The manager is responsible to identify the percentage of staff working hours requiring pay above the base salary rate. During times of nursing shortages, incentive programs such as sign-on bonuses, additional differentials for night shift, and retention bonuses proliferate. Targeted incentives can be beneficial during unanticipated volume increases or nursing shortages, but can be difficult to administer and maintain.

Sign-on bonuses for new hires often create resentment among long-term staff. "Sunsetting" or ending very rich programs can feel like a pay reduction or "takeaway" to staff. The CNS is instrumental in identifying workplace issues that promote retention and a satisfying work environment. Carefully reviewing past history and judicious use of supplemental staff are strategies that can reduce the need for incentives. If programs are in place or anticipated during the year, they must be included during the budgeting process.

Supplemental Staff

Workload increases, staff vacancies due to resignations or leaves of absence, or increases in required staff numbers related to new programs lead to supplemental staffing strategies. Supplemental staff can include internal nursing pools, temporary staff provided by an external agency, increased hours for part-time staff, and overtime. With the exception of part-time staff increasing hours to full-time status, these options increase salary costs due to the higher associated hourly rate.

Supplemental staff salaries are frequently the cause of a major variance in the nursing budget. It is crucial that the manager realistically project supplemental staff needs and closely monitor these costs. Obviously, filling vacant positions reduces the need for supplemental staffing.

Using per diem pool staff has become a major strategy for many organizations. Per diem staff usually have a minimum requirement of hours, no or reduced benefits, and a significantly higher hourly rate. In units with high vacancy rates, an interesting shift may occur. Nurses who have benefits through their spouses or do not need benefits coverage shift from full-time positions to per diem. They receive a higher hourly rate, often work up to full time, and have a reduced holiday and weekend commitment. In this case, the manager depends on the per diem staff for regular hours and does not have the flexibility of the per diem pool to cover high-volume needs or replacement for leaves and sick calls.

With a fairly consistent average daily census, a wise strategy is to hire full- and part-time staff into budgeted positions utilizing per diem staff for flexibility. An exception is in units with a widely fluctuating census, such as in neonatal intensive care units. In this type of unit, allotting a percentage of FTEs to per diem or pool staff is an important strategy for efficient resource management. When the census increases, per diem staff can increase their hours. If a decrease in census is sudden and prolonged, the number of full-time staff required to use nonproductive time may be minimized.

Additional sources of premium pay are overtime and temporary staffing. Overtime can be incidental, short times to complete work, or additional shifts. A number of organizations do not budget overtime, but inevitably a late sick call will result in the request for a staff member to stay, even if it is for a short time. Historical data is important in budgeting overtime; however, scheduling practices can often play a role. Prescheduling overtime or schedules that consistently create an overtime situation, such as scheduling staff for four 12-hour shifts within a week, are often reasons for an overage or increase in overtime pay.

Temporary or agency help also provides a degree of flexibility, particularly during times of sustained volume. For example, if an organization has historical data that identifies an increase in the average daily census of 20 patients during the month of January, utilizing temporary staff might be a viable strategy.

Temporary supplemental staffing agencies can provide local individuals on a day-to-day basis, provide a "block" agreement for a longer time frame, or provide a consistent individual for a specific time period. Again, the hourly rate is significantly higher than the average staff nurse salary and can have a negative impact on the bottom line.

The Demand for Close Observation

Many organizations wrestle with the need for close observation, also known as one-to-one or *sitter* care. The CNS can play a major role in establishing sitter criteria and working with staff to identify appropriateness of one-to-one observation. Clearly, this type of monitoring is required for suicidal patients and in specific clinical situations. Sitters are frequently utilized to prevent falls, inadvertent tube removals, elopement, and wandering. Additionally, with the focus on restraint-free environments, the use of sitters has increased. It is important to review past history and assess the needs of the patient population during the budget process. Working with physicians and other members of the healthcare team to identify appropriate alternatives to one-to-one care is a key strategy.

Justification Considerations for Nursing Staffing

It is important to note that although NHPPD and staffing patterns can be used to build the nursing budget, these figures are calculated averages. Staffing in patient care areas on a daily basis must take into account the population of patients and the roles and responsibilities of the care providers.

In *Principles for Nurse Staffing* (American Nurses Association, 1999), four critical factors are identified in determining nurse staffing:

- Number of patients
- Level of intensity
- Environment, including availability of technology
- Level of participation and experience of those providing care

Often the NHPPD is budgeted based on the prior year, and nursing leadership needs to make the case for an adjustment or increase. In recent years, there has been a concerted effort to benchmark nursing staffing data. Participation in national benchmarking initiatives, such as the National Database of Nursing Quality Indicators (NDNQI), has been increasing.

The NDNQI compares an organization's actual nursing care hours by specialty to the median of other participating hospitals on a quarterly basis. Nursing hours as reported by the NDNQI are the direct-care provider hours and do not include indirect time. Nurse-sensitive quality indicators, such as the development of nosocomial pressure ulcers and fall rates, are also benchmarked in the NDNQI database. Comparison of data, including patient care outcomes and nurse-sensitive quality data, can provide a powerful tool when preparing budget justification for changes in nursing hours of care.

A number of investigators have studied the relationship between nurse staffing and patient outcomes. Aiken, Clarke, Sloane, Sochalski, and Silber (2002) noted that in hospitals with high patient-to-nurse ratios, surgical patients experience higher risk-adjusted 30-day mortality and failure-to-rescue rates than hospitals with lower ratios. Cho et al. (2003) found that an increase of 1 hour worked by RNs per patient day was associated with an 8.9% decrease in the incidence of pneumonia. The body of nursing research examining nurse staffing and outcomes is building, and the CNS can play a role in continuing to examine this relationship.

Variance Reporting

Budget monitoring during the year usually occurs on a monthly basis. Actual revenue and expense reports are compared to the budget figures. Identifying a variance is the first step, but analysis is essential to make needed adjustments. Factors that contribute to a positive or negative variance are many and cannot always be controlled. A report describing the reason for a discrepancy is consistently required for a variance of 5% or more.

FTEs, actual dollars spent, and revenues vary with patient volume, but NHPPD and other standards remain constant. Supplemental staffing costing premium pay is a common area of negative variance in nursing. A unit could be well within the budgeted NHPPD or other standard, but have a negative dollar variance due to higher hourly rates.

Another metric that is used is the nursing costs per patient day. Cost per patient day encompasses the total salary and supply costs for a specific unit and divides it by the number of patient days. The higher salaries of supplemental staff or unusual supply usage are reflected in the total cost. A unit or department may end the month or even the year within budget, but not have flexed appropriately to the units of services. It is also possible in a variable budget context to be over budget and justify this variance as due to volume increases. Cost per patient day is an important metric that often demonstrates failure or success in adjusting staff and associated expenses to volume fluctuations.

Additional reasons for negative volume variances (over the budget) include unusually high sick calls, use of nonproductive time for vacation, unanticipated leaves of absence, high patient acuity, and supply costs for specific patient populations; for example, gowns and gloves. Righting course may be necessary, but not at the expense of providing the agreed-upon standard (NHPPD, hours per visit) of care.

Although CNSs are not the architects of the hospital or nursing budgets, their clinical experience and expertise has the potential to inform many budget projections and decisions. CNSs are particularly needed as contributors to the capital budget process. CNSs participate in product and equipment identification and evaluation. They influence the quality of the care environment and efficiency of the work environment by assisting in the provision of cost-effective, quality devices and products that improve nursing care processes and positively affect outcomes.

Preparing for the Capital Budget: Product Evaluation

Patti Rager Zuzelo, EdD, MSN, RN, ACNS-BC

CNSs are often involved in evaluating and selecting products and medical devices that are used in a variety of clinical settings. There is little in the literature to guide CNSs through this decision-making process. A review of published nursing literature reveals that perioperative nurses recognize that nursing input is crucial to good product and device decisions, particularly because nurses are the highest-volume end users of hospital products (Carroll, 1992).

There are more products than ever from which to choose. In 1992, Berkowitz, Diamond, and Montagnolo observed that in the early 1980s, there were more than 6000 distinct types of medical devices and an estimated 750,000 brands, models, and sizes produced by approximately 12,000 manufacturers worldwide. The number and varieties can only have increased over the past 25 years.

Selecting the right product and most appropriate technology requires much effort. Fiscal resources are limited, so product and device decisions have to be good. Most hospitals' capital equipment budgets are smaller than the amount of total requests, so competition for dollars is fierce between equally worthy projects. The goals of product evaluation include selecting products and devices that (1) meet specific performance criteria, (2) are safe for both patients and staff, (3) encourage positive patient outcomes, and (4) are cost-effective for all stakeholders (Halvorson & Chinnes, 2007).

Trade shows and conferences are good venues for exploring new products. The American Association of Critical-Care Nurses (AACN) and Association of peri-Operative Registered Nurses (AORN) have two of the largest exhibition halls for nursing conferences (Carroll, 1992). Most clinically focused national conferences have vendors available to share product updates and demonstrate new technologies. CNSs should make certain to visit vendors and keep current with new product opportunities. Although some products and devices may initially appear cost prohibitive, careful analysis may reveal that new equipment could reduce expenditures related to high-ticket patient care concerns such as length of stay, complications, nurse injuries, and patient safety enhancements.

Malloch (2000) suggested that CNSs making purchasing decisions need three new competencies specific to product evaluation: end-user accountability, evidence-based product selection, and nursing commercial competence. End-user accountability relates to achieving specific results. Evidence-based product selection means that CNSs need to collect important end-user clinical information from the staff who preview the product or equipment. Nursing commercial competence is balancing clinical intent with economic impact. Malloch emphasized that CNSs need to consider the real value of different choices by analyzing alternatives and their consequences. Environmental impacts associated with products and devices are also worthy of consideration. Disposability and whether an item can be recycled should be taken into account.

CNSs and staff may be inclined to think of price as the most important purchase consideration. Certainly, given constrained resources, product and device costs are important considerations. Contino (2001) identified that there are two ways to consider costs when purchasing equipment. These include the payback period, defined as the number of years required to recover the original investment, or the internal rate of return, calculated to determine whether the generated revenue will cover the purchase cost. CNSs should understand that there are other components affecting supply costs besides price. These factors include needed technological changes, theft, and meeting the recommendations of regulatory agencies (Lyons, 1992).

AORN has established guidelines for evaluating and selecting products and medical devices used in perioperative settings (AORN, 1998). These guidelines call for products to meet safe, identified needs and promote quality patient care. CNSs should consider developing similar guidelines for other practice areas as a reasonable way to ensure consistency and quality in decision making.

Opportunities for Staff Engagement in Product Decisions

CNSs should consider including staff in product selection and evaluation processes. Evaluation projects offer staff opportunities to learn the research process by devising small-scale studies that are practical and interesting. Pelter and Stephens (2008) designed an experimental study to compare first-attempt success rates, patient comfort, and insertion time between urinary catheterizations using a new device designed to facilitate urethral catheterization versus catheterization procedures without the new device. Consenting patients were randomly assigned to one of the groups. The nurses conducting the urethral catheterization procedure also received informed consent. Two-tailed student t-tests and Chi-square tests were used for statistical analysis. A small sample size limited the generalizability of the results; however, study findings did suggest that while the device had little influence on the dependent variables, findings indicated that nurses are challenged by urethral catheterization and some find that this is a difficult procedure to master.

This study (Pelter & Stephens, 2008) provides a simple but elegant example of an opportunity to engage staff in research while evaluating devices in the clinical setting. The basic setup of this particular project may be applied to a variety of product evaluation opportunities. For example, nurses could brainstorm outcomes or dependent variables of interest related to hygiene products, dressings, airway-securing devices, or any number of other devices, products, or systems and then use basic experimental or quasi-experimental designs to answer relevant questions. Research questions may relate to comparing different products as part of the purchase decision, determining whether a product is successfully addressing a particular clinical concern, or looking at already established products to ascertain whether implementation processes require improvement.

Theft Concerns

Lyons (1992) noted that theft affects annual nonsalary inflation by as much as $1000 to $2000 per occupied bed. Stolen items may include linens, equipment, instruments, stationery, printer cartridges, toiletries, and medications. Services may also be stolen, including laboratory tests or radiology procedures. Lyons noted that employees may steal these services for themselves or others.

It may be wise for CNSs to consider the possibility of item attractiveness and thievery when considering products and devices. Some equipment requires chargeable housing that is not easily stolen. Other devices are simply not appealing to would-be thieves due to their limited practicality outside the healthcare setting. If a new product or device has a high theft appeal, CNSs may need to consider the additional expenses associated with storing the equipment or product and tracking its use.

Safety Concerns

CNSs should consider searching for reports of adverse events (AE) involving medical devices as a step in product evaluation. The Food and Drug Administration (FDA) maintains a publicly available medical device reporting Manufacturer and User Facility Device Experience (MAUDE) database (Hankin, Schein, Clark, & Panchal, 2007). MAUDE data consists of voluntary reports submitted since 1993 and also includes user facility reports beginning in 1991, distributor reports since 1993, and manufacturer reports since 1996 (Center for Devices and Radiological Health [CDRH], 2008a).

The online database provides access to information on medical devices that may have malfunctioned or caused serious injury or death. The CDRH advises that MAUDE is not intended for AE rate comparisons or to evaluate AEs between devices (CDRH, 2008a). The Medical Device Reporting (MDR) database is also made available to the public by the CDRH. The MDR database contains information from the earlier CDRH database, the device experience network (DEN). There are over 600,000 reports catalogued up to June 1993 in the MDR with subsequent recording in MAUDE (CDRH, 2008b).

CNSs may not be aware of the richness of data made available through CDRH. A quick scan of its home page reveals information on breast implants, contact lenses, personal protective equipment, point-of-care blood glucose meters, and many other categories and types of devices (CDRH, 2008c). The available information has tremendous implications for CNS practice across all types of clinical settings and regardless of specialty or population.

Hankin et al. (2007) used MAUDE to explore the AEs involving intravenous (IV) patient-controlled analgesia (PCA). Data file extrapolation revealed 2009 individual IV PCA-related MAUDE medical device events reported from January 1, 2002, through December 31, 2003. These events included manufacturer-confirmed device malfunctions. CNSs should consider the implications of this data on practice and policies and include such information during device in-servicing and education programs.

The What-If and More-Is-Better Syndromes of Materials Management

It is important to remember that there is usually more than one way to perform a procedure or more than one product to accomplish a job (Lyons, 1992). The best product, defined in any number of ways, is not always needed. An average product may work just as well and suit the needs of the organization quite satisfactorily. The problem is that CNSs may equate average with cheap. Lyons (1992) directs material managers to assist CNSs in understanding that quality can be defined as meeting the requirement or the need. Average products may be the better choice.

Lyons (1992) emphasized that need must be separated from want. The "what-if" syndrome tends to encourage practitioners to think of every possible scenario, no matter how unlikely, and then to look for equipment or products that can address these unlikely situations (Exemplar 10-1). This type of thinking drives up projected costs that may lead to rejection of the proposed capital budget expenditure.

Exemplar 10-1

The "What-If" Syndrome of Materials Management

Several medical intensive care unit (MICU) nurses attended a regional critical care conference. During the conference's trade show, the nurses came across a new automatic blood pressure cuff system. This system was very appealing for a number of reasons, but in particular, it had a safety feature for cuff size and placement that the nurses believed would help to ensure the accuracy of MICU vital signs assessment.

The conference attendees brought information back to their colleagues. The nurses were enthusiastic about the product, as there had been recent problems with assessment inaccuracies related to incorrect cuff fit and placement that had compromised patient assessment data and affected care. The nurses evaluated the project per the recommended checkpoints and concluded that the equipment should be submitted for review during the capital budget request period. As the nurses developed their proposal, they discussed the number of automatic cuffs that would be required on the unit. Some nurses believed that each room required this new system. Others were concerned that "extras" were required because equipment "always walks." Each estimated figure cost more due to the increasing numbers of requested cuffs. The CNS was consulted for assistance with the capital budget request.

The CNS began the consultation process by reviewing the nurses' rationale for requesting this particular blood pressure monitoring system. Other brands of automatic cuffs were available and were considerably less expensive. The CNS asked the staff to identify the "typical" types of patients who required such sophisticated technology. The CNS encouraged the staff to think in terms of "must have" rather than "nice to have." The nurses believed that patients with small upper arm circumferences and patients with above-average arm circumferences required these cuffs, in other words, patients who were outliers specific to arm circumference size. The CNS worked with the staff to isolate the approximate number of MICU patients who met these criteria on an average shift. The nurses agreed that approximately two patients per shift were difficult to fit with the standard automatic blood pressure system, leading to accuracy concerns. After further guided discussion, the staff identified a simple strategy for confining the equipment on the unit to prevent loss. The nurses also developed guidelines for staff to consider when deciding whether to use manual, standard automatic, or specialized automatic blood pressure cuffs.

The staff group decided to requisition the budget for two of the new, specialized automatic blood pressure cuffs. They realized that their opportunity for expenditure approval was better with a tight proposal that clearly avoided the "more-is-better" syndrome. Although there was no guarantee that the equipment request would be approved, the nurses felt confident that if the request was denied, it would be denied due to funding limitations or competing priorities rather than due to an unrealistic needs assessment.

The more-is-better syndrome encourages the belief that if one is good, two must be better (Lyons, 1992). CNSs must assist staff in identifying exactly what is needed in terms of the number of products or the frequency of equipment use. Determining an accurate measure of "need" is important for calculating direct and indirect costs. Need does not have to pertain to number of units. It may also apply to the features of technological products (Exemplar 10-2).

Exemplar 10-2

The "More-Is-Better" Syndrome of Materials Management

The surgical trauma unit nurses and physicians were interested in replacing the unit's cardiac monitors. The biomedical engineering department agreed that it was time to replace the aging system. The staff contacted several reputable vendors and began to explore monitor options.

As the group was introduced to increasingly sophisticated equipment options, the nurses and physicians began to acquire the "more-is-better" syndrome. They were surprised and impressed with the various technological advances and were amenable to the sales representatives' premise that their patients deserved the best. The monitors were capable of powerful analyses, and the data collection and alarming options were impressive. After a few months of investigation, the group began to think about fiscal and clinical practice realities and asked a critical care CNS to offer an unbiased opinion.

The CNS preliminarily collected historical data from the staff and physicians to explore the capabilities of the current monitoring system and to contrast these opportunities with the functions that were actually used on a regular basis. The multidisplinary group was surprised to learn that the old monitoring system was not used to peak efficiency. Certain capabilities, including ST segment monitoring and historical trending data, were rarely used for nursing assessment or medical management, despite the perceived importance of the functions. The CNS emphasized to the group that if monitoring capabilities were identified in policies and procedures as essential to quality of care and a required part of routine assessment, the nurses and physicians were potentially inviting risk or compromising care by failing to follow the established protocols that they had developed!

The CNS began the group process by meeting with the physicians and nurses to determine what monitoring functions were critical to patient care. The CNS emphasized that unless equipment features are consistently used, they may become more of a care liability than benefit. Staff was asked to prioritize equipment functions. Physicians were involved in discussions specific to detailing the information that they really would use for patient care management. Nurse educators were asked to review the equipment options from the perspective of teaching and learning.

The CNS compiled this information and developed a list of desired monitoring capabilities that could be reasonably taught and would be valued and consistently utilized by nursing and medical staff. This list was reviewed by the prospective users and was validated for accuracy. Vendors were asked to respond to this list. Equipment was selected based on the match between price and capabilities.

This experience revealed to practitioners that more is not always better. There is no value in paying for equipment capabilities that are not desirable or are underutilized. Liabilities may increase if monitoring capabilities are available but not used by staff in the intended way. Educational needs should be considered as well. If orientation and inservicing demands are too complex or rigorous, the likelihood of staff using the equipment correctly is reduced. The CNS cautioned the group that neither more nor less is better. Rather, it is wisest to get exactly what is needed at an affordable price.

CNSs should be actively engaged in product and device identification, selection, and evaluation. Product and device possibilities should be considered methodically with a clear idea to the intent and need underlying the review process (Table 10-7). Deliberate review processes may be enhanced by using a product evaluation tool that

Table 10-7	PRODUCT AND DEVICE EVALUATION CHECKPOINTS WITH EXEMPLARS
Product/Device Consideration	**Suggestions**
1. Carefully review the manufacturer claims (Carroll, 1992)	CNSs should make certain that manufacturer claims are accurate. Products may not perform as promised during clinical use. CNSs should thoroughly review the "fine print" of claims and make certain that these attestations are accurate when products are actually put to the test in clinical situations.
2. Product comparison (Carroll, 1992)	CNSs should compare products during clinical use. Select a few competing products or devices and compare them.
3. Ease of use (Carroll, 1992)	Consider how easy the product or device is to use. This consideration includes ease of cleaning and storing.
4. Ergonomics	CNSs should pay attention to the influence the product has on body mechanics. If a product requires repetitive movements, muscle straining, or periods of prolonged standing, CNSs should solicit input from staff and other healthcare professionals as to the potential for injury, particularly given the aging nursing workforce.
5. Manufacturer instructions (Carroll, 1992)	Review the written instructions for clarity and accuracy. CNSs should explore whether troubleshooting information is available in print and/or Web forms. It may be reasonable to ascertain whether a 24-hour contact is accessible for troubleshooting, particularly if a product or device is new to the setting.
6. Safety features (Carroll, 1992)	CNSs should encourage staff to think about what could go wrong and ways in which the device might be misused. It's important to make certain that critical safety features cannot be turned off.

(continues)

Table 10-7   (continued)

Product/Device Consideration	Suggestions
	Some devices may have delay switches that reset after a period of time to avoid the need to deliberately reset safety features once discontinued.
7. Education expenses	CNSs should calculate the training costs associated with assuring competent use of new devices and equipment. Some products are quite sophisticated and may require hours of training. Others may warrant competency assessments.
8. Ease of repair	Many devices and products are sophisticated by design and require experts for repairs or maintenance activities. If the institution cannot afford the cost of backup equipment or cannot justify the expense of developing in-house repair expertise, it may be difficult for staff to work without equipment when it malfunctions. Consider the expenses associated with repair, replacement, and/or warranties.
9. Security	Consider the "theft factor" (Lyons, 1992). Is this a product or device that is likely to be appealing to would-be thieves? Can the product be used outside of the healthcare facility? If thievery is a concern, consider strategies for securing the product, restricting its access, or monitoring its use.
10. Environmental impact	CNSs should investigate the costs associated with cleaning or disposing of the product. Environmental impacts are important not only in terms of the chemicals or processes necessary for cleaning but also the biodegradability and bulk of items when no longer useful.
11. Device safety reports	Review MAUDE and MDR databases for information about reported safety concerns that may be relevant to the devices that are under consideration.

can be used to solicit feedback from nurses and other involved healthcare professionals (Table 10-8).

Healthcare resources are limited, and CNSs are obliged to participate in activities that promote the highest quality of care using the dollars that are available. Understanding the budget process, engaging in conversations and data collection activities

Table 10-8   PRODUCT EVALUATION TOOL

Characteristic	Evaluation 1 = unacceptable 2 = poor 3 = adequate 4 = good 5 = highly beneficial	Rank importance of this characteristic to the purchase decision 1–20	Comments: details, suggestions, and recommendations
1. Simplicity of use			
a. Size of print on buttons			
b. Manipulability of equipment			
c. Weight			
d. Height (Does it fit in the patient room?)			
e. Portability			
f. Amount of space required for storage			
2. Instructions			
a. Readability of written instructions			
b. Availability of additional instructional materials (e.g., DVD, laminated information cards, signs, computer-based instruction)			
c. Vendor-provided education programs			
d. Step-by-step guidelines for competency development			
3. Safety features			
a. Alarm features			

(continues)

Table 10-8 (continued)

Characteristic	Evaluation 1 = unacceptable 2 = poor 3 = adequate 4 = good 5 = highly beneficial	Rank importance of this characteristic to the purchase decision 1–20	Comments: details, suggestions, and recommendations
b. Battery life and indicators			
c. Default settings			
d. Most common errors and failures with related safeguards			
e. Reset buttons			
f. Expiration dates (on products)			
g. Allergens			
h. Risk to staff			
4. Amount of time needed to initially learn how to use the equipment			
a. Preliminary in-service time			
b. Predicted frequency of use and impact on nurse competence			
c. List of users and associated education needs			
5. Repair services			
a. In-house repair versus contracted repair			
b. Guaranteed turnaround time for repairs			

Table 10-8 (continued)

Characteristic	Evaluation 1 = unacceptable 2 = poor 3 = adequate 4 = good 5 = highly beneficial	Rank importance of this characteristic to the purchase decision 1–20	Comments: details, suggestions, and recommendations
c. Replacement policy			
d. Weekend/after business hours/holiday support			
e. Repair expense			
f. Availability of replacement parts			
6. Shared dependency on other departments			
a. Components stored and managed off nursing unit?			
b. Materials management training			
c. Consistent coding and identification of parts between nursing and other departments			
d. Distribution and clear designation of "who-does-what and when"			
e. Off hours responsibilities for each department			
7. Ergonomics			
a. Repetitive motions			
b. Impact on standing/sitting			
c. Potential for staff injury			
d. Required dexterity for safe use			

(continues)

Table 10-8 (continued)

Characteristic	Evaluation 1 = unacceptable 2 = poor 3 = adequate 4 = good 5 = highly beneficial	Rank importance of this characteristic to the purchase decision 1–20	Comments: details, suggestions, and recommendations
8. Environmental impact			
a. Discard versus clean, sterilize			
b. Recyclable, if discard			
c. Product ingredients			
d. Efficiency of product packaging and impact on trash volume			
9. Expense			
a. Purchase cost			
b. Maintenance cost			
c. Miscellaneous costs			
10. Security			
a. Theft prevention			
b. Tracking location			
c. Physical security options (e.g., locks, mounting)			
11. Impact on patient care outcomes			
a. Potential impact on outcomes of concern			

Table 10-8 (continued)

Characteristic	Evaluation 1 = unacceptable 2 = poor 3 = adequate 4 = good 5 = highly beneficial	Rank importance of this characteristic to the purchase decision 1–20	Comments: details, suggestions, and recommendations
12. Patient perspective			
a. Alarm noise			
b. Transportability for mobile patients			
c. Patient safety			
13. Impact of misuse			
a. Worst-case scenario when equipment fails			
b. Opportunities for incorrect use			
14. What patient care problems does this product fix?			
15. Product capabilities that are useful in this clinical setting as compared to capabilities not useful/required			
16. Gaps in processes, within and/or between departments, that this product may create			
17. Gaps in processes, within and/or between departments, that this product may solve			
18. Clinical and nonclinical stakeholders			
a. Who is potentially affected by this purchase decision?			

(continues)

Table 10-8 (continued)

Characteristic	Evaluation 1 = unacceptable 2 = poor 3 = adequate 4 = good 5 = highly beneficial	Rank importance of this characteristic to the purchase decision 1–20	Comments: details, suggestions, and recommendations
19. Time required from securing the product (start) to finishing with the product (end). (Nursing time utilized by this product per usage)			
20. References or commentary from nonbiased users			

that inform the budget, teaching and coaching staff to develop a better sense of the fiscal realities of care, and contributing to capital budgets through product and device evaluations are CNS responsibilities. Many teaching moments related to healthcare administration processes are experienced by CNSs as they work closely with nurses at the point of care. Having a good understanding of the business basics of nursing is an excellent way to contribute to the managerial functions of the institution, functions that are critical to the overall success of the organization.

References

Aiken, L. H., Clarke, S. P., Sloane, D. M., Sochalski, J., & Silber, J. H. (2002). Hospital nurse staffing and patient mortality, nurse burnout, and job dissatisfaction. *Journal of the American Medical Association, 288*, 1987–1993.

American Association of Preferred Provider Organization. (2004). *Learn more about PPOs: PPO overview.* Retrieved February 12, 2006, from http://aappo. org/ppo_about.html

American Nurses Association. (1999). *Principles for nurse staffing.* Retrieved May 6, 2006, from http://www.NursingWorld.org/readroom/stffprnc.htm

AORN Recommended Practices Committee. (1998). Recommended practices for the evaluation and selection of products and medical devices used in the perioperative practice settings. *Association of periOperative Nurses, 67*(1), 270–272.

Bureau of Labor Statistics (BLS). (2002). *National Compensation Survey. Definitions of health insurance terms.* Retrieved February 12, 2006, from http://www.bls.gov/ncs/ebs/sp/healthterms.pdf

Carroll, P. (1992). Nursing input into the purchase decision reveals costs not included in the price tag. *Hospital Materiel Management Quarterly, 13*(4), 63–68.

Center for Devices and Radiological Health (CDRH). (2008a). *MAUDE.* Retrieved August 31, 2008, from http://www.accessdata.fda.gov/scripts/cdrh/cfdocs/cfMAUDE/search.CFM

Center for Devices and Radiological Health (CDRH). (2008b). *Adverse reporting data files.* Retrieved August 31, 2008, from http://www.fda.gov/cdrh/mdr/mdr-file-general.html

Center for Devices and Radiological Health (CDRH). (2008c). Home page. Retrieved August 31, 2008, from http://www.fda.gov/cdrh

Centers for Medicare & Medicaid Services (CMS). (2005). *Medicare program. General information. Overview.* Retrieved December 6, 2008, from http://www.cms.hhs.gov/MedicareGenInfo/

Centers for Medicare & Medicaid Services (CMS). (2006). *National health expenditure data.* Retrieved April 7, 2006, from http://www.cms.hhs.gov/NationalHealthExpendData/downloads/highlights.pdf

Centers for Medicare & Medicaid Services (CMS). (2008). National health expenditure projections 2007–2017. Retrieved July 13, 2008, from http://www.cms.hhs.gov/NationalHealthExpendData/Downloads/proj2007.pdf

Centers for Medicare & Medicaid Services (CMS). (n.d.). *Mission vision goals.* Retrieved December 6, 2008, from http://www.cms.hhs.gov/MissionVisionGoals/Downloads/CMSStrategicActionPlanExecSummary06-09_061016.pdf

Cho, S. H., Ketefian, S., Barkauskas, V. H., & Smith, D. G. (2003). The effects of nurse staffing on adverse events, morbidity, mortality, and medical costs. *Nursing Research, 52*(2), 71–79.

Contino, D. (2001). Proposing the "capital" in capital budgets. *Nursing Management, 32,* 10, 13.

Halvorson, C., & Chinnes, L. (2007). Collaborative leadership in product evaluation. *AORN Journal, 85*(2), 334–352.

Hankin, C., Schein, J., Clark, J., & Panchal, S. (2007). Adverse events involving intravenous patient-controlled analgesia. *American Journal of Health-System Pharmacists, 64,* 1492–1499.

Kaiser Family Foundation. (2006). *Employer health benefits 2006 annual survey.* Retrieved July 13, 2008, from http://www.kff.org/insurance/7527/

Lyons, D. (1992). Making the purchase decision: Factors other than price. *Hospital Materiel Management Quarterly, 13*(4), 55–62.

Malloch, K. (2000). Purchasing pointers. Wise buys. *Nursing Management, 31*(5), 30.

Pelter, M., & Stephens, K. (2008). Evaluation of a device to facilitate female urethral catheterization. *Medical-Surgical Nursing, 17*(1), 19–25.

Shi, L., & Singh, D. (2005). *Essentials of the U.S. health care system.* Sudbury, MA: Jones and Bartlett.

Sovie, M. (2001). Hospital restructuring and its impact on outcomes: Nursing staff regulations are premature. *Journal of Nursing Administration, 31*(12), 588–600.

Zuzelo, P., Fallon, R., Lang, A., Lang, C., McGovern, K., Mount, L., et al. (2004). Clinical nurse specialists' knowledge specific to Medicare structures and processes. *Clinical Nurse Specialist, 18,* 207–217.

Index

Page numbers followed by *t* or *f* denote tables and figures respectively.